Register Now for Online Access to Your Book!

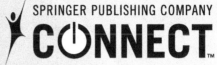

SPRINGER PUBLISHING COMPANY

CONNECT™

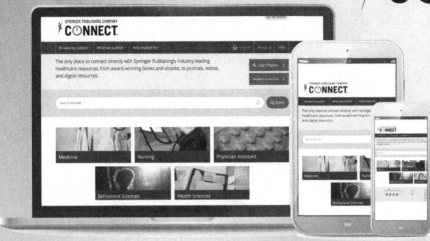

Your print purchase of *Nurses Improving Care for Healthsystem Elders* **includes online access to the contents of your book**—increasing accessibility, portability, and searchability!

Access today at:

http://connect.springerpub.com/content/book/978-0-8261-7082-8 or scan the QR code at the right with your smartphone and enter the access code below.

LHMR6NHB

Scan here for quick access.

If you are experiencing problems accessing the digital component of this product, please contact our customer service department at cs@springerpub.com

The online access with your print purchase is available at the publisher's discretion and may be removed at any time without notice.

Publisher's Note: New and used products purchased from third-party sellers are not guaranteed for quality, authenticity, or access to any included digital components.

Nurses Improving Care for Healthsystem Elders

NICHE™

Terry Fulmer, PhD, RN, FAAN

Kimberly Glassman, PhD, RN, NEA-BC, FAAN

Sherry Greenberg, PhD, RN, GNP-BC, FGSA

Peri Rosenfeld, PhD

Mattia Gilmartin, PhD, RN, FAAN

Mathy Mezey, EdD, PhD, FAAN

EDITORS

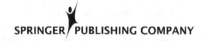

SPRINGER PUBLISHING COMPANY

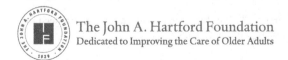

The John A. Hartford Foundation
Dedicated to Improving the Care of Older Adults

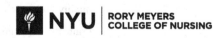

NYU | RORY MEYERS COLLEGE OF NURSING

Springer Publishing Company, LLC
11 West 42nd Street
New York, NY 10036
www.springerpub.com
http://connect.springerpub.com

Acquisitions Editor: Elizabeth Nieginski
Compositor: S4Carlisle Publishing Services

ISBN: 978-0-8261-7081-1
ebook ISBN: 978-0-8261-7082-8
DOI: 10.1891/9780826170828

19 20 21 22/5 4 3 2 1

The author and the publisher of this Work have made every effort to use sources believed to be reliable to provide information that is accurate and compatible with the standards generally accepted at the time of publication. Because medical science is continually advancing, our knowledge base continues to expand. Therefore, as new information becomes available, changes in procedures become necessary. We recommend that the reader always consult current research and specific institutional policies before performing any clinical procedure. The author and publisher shall not be liable for any special, consequential, or exemplary damages resulting, in whole or in part, from the readers' use of, or reliance on, the information contained in this book. The publisher has no responsibility for the persistence or accuracy of URLs for external or third-party Internet websites referred to in this publication and does not guarantee that any content on such websites is, or will remain, accurate or appropriate.

Library of Congress Cataloging-in-Publication Data

Names: Fulmer, Terry T., author.
Title: Nurses Improving Care for Healthsystem Elders : NICHE / Terry Fulmer,
    Kimberly Glassman, Sherry Greenberg, Peri Rosenfeld, Mattia
    Gilmartin, Mathy Mezey.
Other titles: Nurses Improving Care for Healthsystem Elders
Description: New York : Springer Publishing, [2019] | Includes
    bibliographical references and index.
Identifiers: LCCN 2019009601 | ISBN 9780826170811
Subjects: | MESH: Nurses Improving Care for Healthsystem Elders. | Geriatric
    Nursing–methods | Geriatric Assessment | Nursing Assessment | Health
    Services for the Aged | Models, Nursing | Aged
Classification: LCC RC954 | NLM WY 152 | DDC 618.97/0231–dc23 LC record available at https://
lccn.loc.gov/2019009601

Publisher's Note: New and used products purchased from third-party sellers are not guaranteed for quality, authenticity, or access to any included digital components.

Printed in the United States of America.

This book is dedicated to NICHE nurses around the world.
Thank you for your courage and leadership!
Your commitment to excellence in the care of older adults is both
humbling and inspiring.
—Terry Fulmer, PhD, RN, FAAN
New York City 2019

Contents

About the Editors

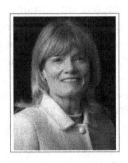

Terry Fulmer, PhD, RN, FAAN, is the President of The John A. Hartford Foundation in New York City, an organization dedicated to improving the care of older adults. Established in 1929, the Foundation has a current endowment of over $560 million and is world renowned for philanthropy devoted exclusively to the health of older adults. She serves as the chief strategist for Foundation giving and is also the chief spokesperson for advancing the Foundation's mission. She is the lead voice for the Age-Friendly Health System initiative now underway.

Dr. Fulmer previously served as distinguished professor and dean of the Bouve College of Health Sciences at Northeastern University, and prior as the Erline Perkins McGriff Professor of Nursing and founding dean of the New York University (NYU) College of Nursing. She received her bachelor's degree from Skidmore College, her master's and doctoral degrees from Boston College, and her Geriatric Nurse Practitioner Post-Master's Certificate from New York University. She is an elected member of the National Academy of Medicine (formerly the Institute of Medicine).

Dr. Fulmer is nationally and internationally recognized as a leading expert in geriatrics and is best known for conceptualization and development of the national *Nurses Improving Care for Healthsystem Elders (NICHE)* program and research on the topic of elder abuse and neglect, work that has been funded by the National Institute on Aging and the National Institute of Nursing Research. Her recent effort with the *Age-Friendly Health Systems* initiative in partnership with the Institute for Healthcare Improvement (IHI) is a potential game changer for how we think about care for older adults.

She has received many prestigious awards and invitations for named lectureships from noted universities. She has previously held faculty appointments at Columbia University, where she held the Anna Maxwell Chair in Nursing and has also held appointments at Boston College, Yale University, and the Harvard Division on Aging. She has served as a visiting professor of nursing at the University of Pennsylvania and Case Western University. She received an honorary doctorate from the University of South Florida in 2018. She is a trustee for the Josiah Macy Jr. Foundation, The Clark Foundation, Springer Publishing Company, and chair of the Bassett Medical Center Board of Trustees. She is co-chair of the National Academy of Medicine's Forum on Aging, Disability, and Independence.

Dr. Fulmer is dedicated to the advancement of interprofessional science, education, and practice that advances the health of older adults. Her clinical appointments have included the Beth Israel Hospital in Boston, the Massachusetts General Hospital, and the NYU-Langone Medical Center. She is an attending nurse at the Mount Sinai Medical Center in New York, NY. She is a Distinguished Practitioner of the National Academies of Practice. She has served as the first nurse on the board of the American Geriatrics Society and as the first nurse to serve as president of the Gerontological Society of America.

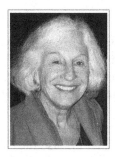 **Mathy Mezey, EdD, RN, FAAN,** Dr. Mezey's interest and scholarship have centered on nursing ethics and care of older adults, focusing on assuring that nurses have the necessary skills and knowledge to provide quality care to this potentially vulnerable population. She directed two major national initiatives focused on care of older adults, the Robert Wood Johnson Foundation Teaching Nursing Home Program (1981–1987) and the Hartford Institute for Geriatric Nursing, NYU College of Nursing (founding director 1996–2009). She has written or edited 16 books and written over 70 articles on topics related to geriatric nursing, the education and practice of geriatric nurse practitioners, care in nursing homes, and ethical decision making. Dr. Mezey holds honorary degrees from Case Western Reserve and Fairfield University, is a fellow of the American Academy of Nursing, the Gerontological Society of America, and the New York Academy of Medicine, is an Emerita member of the Board of the Visiting Nurse Service of New York, and is Trustee Emerita, Columbia University.

Dr. Mezey has been involved in numerous national initiatives that focused on undergraduate and graduate nursing education. In collaboration with the American Association of Colleges of Nursing (AACN), she was codirector in the development of the national standards for Gerontological Nurse Practitioner education. Again, with AACN, she directed the Geriatric Nursing Education Consortium (GNEC) which involved over half the bachelor's in science in nursing (BSN) programs nationally in a 3-year project to strengthen their geriatric curriculums. At the Hartford Institute, she directed Nurse Competence in Aging, a national initiative to assure that specialty nurses are prepared in geriatrics. She was a Woodrow Wilson Fellow at Lindfield College in McMinnville, OR, and a visiting fellow of Greene College, Neufield College, Oxford, England. At Monmouth College, she has been invited to the Nursing Program twice, most recently last year when she was the speaker at the Nursing Program's Inaugural White Coat Ceremony.

Dr. Mezey received a BSN from Columbia University Nursing (1960), an MEd, Teachers College, Columbia University (1973), and an EdD, (1977). She spent 50 years in nursing, first working in home care (Visiting Nurse Service of New York) and at a city hospital in New York (Jacobi Hospital, New York Health and Hospitals Corporation), and then having a career as a nurse educator: at Lehman College, City University of New York (assistant professor, 1973–1980), at the University of Pennsylvania (clinical associate professor, 1980–1991), and New York

University (professor, Independence Professor, 1991–2013). She is currently professor emerita, New York University. Mathy Mezey joined the Nurses Educational Funds, Inc. Board of Directors in April 2017 and will be chairing the Thelma Schorr Society.

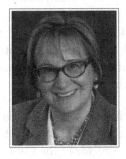

Kimberly Glassman, PhD, RN, NEA-BC, FAAN, is the senior vice president of patient care services and chief nursing officer at NYU Langone Health. She holds an endowed position as the Lerner Director of Health Promotion at NYU Langone, where she oversees the integrative health programs, including stress reduction, tobacco cessation, and mind–body programs for staff, patients, and families. Dr. Glassman serves as the associate dean for Partnership Innovation at the NYU Rory Meyers College of Nursing, where she also holds a faculty position. Dr. Glassman joined the Medical Center as a clinical nurse in critical care and has held many leadership positions in nursing over her 40-year career at Langone. Dr. Glassman is a graduate of the Johnson & Johnson Wharton Fellows Program in Management for Nurse Executives at the University of Pennsylvania, a Robert Wood Johnson Nurse Executive Fellow Alumna, a fellow in the New York Academy of Medicine, and a fellow in the American Academy of Nursing. She serves as an advisory board member for EBSCO Health, chairs the NYU Meyers Board of Advisors, and serves on the board of the NYU-Hartford Institute for Geriatric Nursing, and the Visiting Nurse Service of New York Quality Committee. She is the past president of the New York Organization of Nurse Executives and Leaders and is the Nursing Alliance for Quality Care representative to the National Quality Forum Measures Application Partnership (MAP) Hospital Workgroup that advises performance metrics to the Center for Medicare and Medicaid Services (CMS).

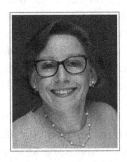

Sherry Greenberg, PhD, RN, GNP-BC, FGSA, is a courtesy-appointed associate professor at New York University Rory Meyers College of Nursing. Dr. Greenberg is editor-in-chief of the Hartford Institute for Geriatric Nursing's *Try This:*® series that promotes evidence-based assessment practices and approaches to care of older adults. She recently helped expand Nurses Improving Care for Healthsystems Elders (NICHE) into long-term care. Dr. Greenberg is a nurse practitioner faculty consultant on the IHI's Age-Friendly Health Systems Action Community initiative. Dr. Greenberg currently serves on the Board of Directors of the Gerontological Advanced Practice Nurses Association as director-at-large and on the Jonas Scholars Alumni Council. Dr. Greenberg is a fellow in the Gerontological Society of America and New York Academy of Medicine, as well as Distinguished Educator in Gerontological Nursing through the National Hartford Center of

Gerontological Nursing Excellence. She is the recipient of the Gerontological Advanced Practice Nurses Association Foundation Education Poster Award (2016), Outstanding Podium Presentation Award (2013), and Research Project Award (2012). Dr. Greenberg earned her academic nursing degrees—bachelor's, master's, and PhD—from the University of Pennsylvania School of Nursing and was a Jonas Nurse Leaders Scholar. Her research has focused on fear of falling among older adults and the relationship with the neighborhood-built environment. Dr. Greenberg has worked as a certified gerontological nurse practitioner in acute, long-term care, and outpatient primary care practices and has taught at undergraduate and graduate nursing levels.

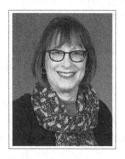

Peri Rosenfeld, PhD, a sociologist and health services researcher, is the director of Outcomes Research & Program Evaluation and the director of the Center for Innovations in the Advancement of Care at the Departments of Nursing at NYU Langone Health. She is also a professor (adjunct) at the NYU Meyers College of Nursing. Her 30-year career has been devoted to health services research, with specific content expertise in health professions workforce (particularly nursing); quality of care across hospital and home care settings, and access to care among underserved populations. Prior to joining NYU Langone Health, she served as senior evaluation scientist at the Center for Home Care Policy and Research at the Visiting Nurse Service of New York; senior research associate at the New York Academy of Medicine; executive director of the New York State Council on Graduate Medical Education and vice president for research at National League for Nursing (NLN). While at NLN, Dr. Rosenfeld compiled a range of data books on nursing workforce and, more recently, she was coauthor with Kim Glassman, PhD, RN, FAAN, of *Data Makes the Difference: The Smart Nurse's Handbook for Using Data to Improve Care* (2015). In addition, she has published more than 70 peer-reviewed articles and book chapters, presented over 100 conference podium and poster presentations, and serves as review editor for several journals including *Policy, Politics & Nursing Practice, Medical Care,* and *American Journal of Hospice & Palliative Medicine*. She is a fellow of the New York Academy of Medicine and an inaugural fellow of the Center for Healthcare Innovation and Delivery Science (CHIDS) at NYU School of Medicine.

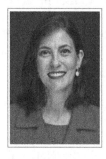

Mattia Gilmartin, PhD, RN, FAAN, is the executive director of Nurses Improving Care for Healthsystems Elders (NICHE) at the New York University Rory Meyers College of Nursing, where she is responsible for leading efforts to spread the NICHE model in the United States and abroad. Dr. Gilmartin's research focuses on strategic management, chronic disease management, organizational change, performance improvement, and leadership development. Dr. Gilmartin has published widely for both academic and practitioner audiences.

Prior to joining the NYU Meyers College of Nursing in 2011, Dr. Gilmartin managed an interdisciplinary research group at INSEAD (European Institute of Business Administration), a leading international business school in France and designed and implemented a three-semester specialty track for the Clinical Nurse Leader master's degree program at the Hunter-Bellevue School of Nursing, City University of New York (CUNY). Dr. Gilmartin holds a bachelor's and master's degree in nursing, a Master of Business Administration from the University of San Francisco, and a PhD degree from the University of Virginia. She completed a postdoctoral fellowship at Cambridge University, Judge School of Management. Dr. Gilmartin is a fellow of the American Academy of Nursing, the National Academies of Practice, and the New York Academy of Medicine. She received the Raven Award in 2000 for her outstanding achievements and service to the University of Virginia (UVA), and in 2018, she received the Distinguished Alumna award from the UVA School of Nursing.

Contributors

Ivo Abraham, PhD, RN, FAAN   Professor of Pharmacy and Medicine, University of Arizona, Tucson, Arizona

Amy Berman, RN, LHD, FAAN   Senior Program Officer, The John A. Hartford Foundation, New York, New York

Marie Boltz, PhD, RNP-BC, FAAN   Professor, Penn State University College of Nursing, State College, Pennsylvania

Melissa M. Bottrell, PhD, MPH   Executive Director, Ethics Quality Consulting, Berkeley, California

Barbara Bricoli, MPA   B2 Advisory Group, LLC, Cedar Grove, New Jersey

Elizabeth Capezuti, PhD, RN, FAAN   W. R. Hearst Foundation Chair in Gerontology, Hunter College School of Nursing, New York, New York

Deirdre M. Carolan Doerflinger, PhD, ANP, GNP, BC, FAANP   NICHE Coordinator, Nurse Practitioner, Geriatrics, Inova Fairfax Hospital; Assistant Professor, The Catholic University of America, Falls Church, Virginia

Tara A. Cortes, PhD, RN, FAAN   Executive Director, Hartford Institute for Geriatric Nursing, New York University Rory Meyers College of Nursing, New York, New York

Catherine O'Neill D'Amico, PhD, RN, NEA-BC   Director, Programs and Operations, NICHE, New York, New York

Susan Fairchild, PhD, MPH   Senior Program Officer, Bill and Melinda Gates Foundation, Seattle, Washington

Donna Marie Fick, PhD, RN, FGSA, FAAN   Professor of Nursing and Medicine; Director, Center of Geriatric Nursing Excellence, The Pennsylvania State University College of Nursing, University Park, Pennsylvania

Kathleen Fletcher, RN, DNP, GNP-BC, FAAN   Clinical Assistant, Professor of Nursing, University of Virginia, Charlottesville, Virginia

Marquis D. Foreman, PhD, RN, FAAN   John L. and Hellen Kellogg Dean of Nursing, Rush University College of Nursing, Chicago, Illinois

Flora B. Haus, MSN, RN-BC, NEA-BC   Education Coordinator, Cedars Sinai Medical Center, Los Angeles, California

Hongsoo Kim, PhD, MPH, MSN, RN   Professor, Graduate School of Public Health, Seoul National University, Seoul, South Korea

Denise Kresevic, PhD, APN-BC, RN, FGSA, FAAN   Certified Nurse Specialist/ Nurse Practitioner, University Hospitals of Cleveland, Cleveland, Ohio

Dennise R. Lavrenz, MBA, BSN, RN, CENP   Chief Clinical Officer, Milwaukee Center for Independence, Milwaukee, Wisconsin

Carrie Lehman, MA   Coordinator, Osher Lifelong Learning Institute, College of William and Mary, Williamsburg, Virginia

Marilyn Lopez, MA, RN, GNP-BC, IIWCC-NYU   Administrative Nurse Practitioner Coordinator, NICHE Program, NYU Langone Health, New York, New York

Denise L. Lyons, DNP, APRN, AGCNS-BC   NICHE Program Manager, Christiana Care Health System, Newark, Delaware

Karen Mack, MS, MBA, APRN, RN-BC, CCNS, ACPNC, ACNP-BC   Clinical Practice Program Specialist, MedStar Health, Columbia, Maryland

Kedar S. Mate, MD   Chief Innovation Officer, Institute for Healthcare Improvement, Boston, Massachusetts

Maureen P. McCausland, DNSc, RN, FAAN   Senior Vice President and Chief Nursing Officer, MedStar Health, Columbia, Maryland

Carrie Hays McElroy, MSN, RN-BCACM   VP Clinical Operations, Chief Nursing Compliance Officer, Trinity Health PACE (Program of All-Inclusive Care for the Elderly), Livonia, Michigan

Leslie J. Pelton, MPA   Senior Director, Institute for Healthcare Improvement, Boston, Massachusetts

Inna Popil, DNP, RN, ACNS-BC, CCM   Director, System Care Coordination Education, Northwell Health, Manhasset, New York

Susan C. Reinhard, PhD, RN, FAAN   Senior Vice President, American Association of Retired Persons Public Policy Institute, Washington, District of Columbia

Mildred Z. Solomon, EdD   President, The Hastings Center and Professor of Anaesthesia, part-time, at Harvard Medical School, Boston, Massachusetts

Judy Santamaria, MSPH   Elder Care Advocate, Judy Santamaria LLC, Mamaroneck, New York

Foreword

I miss Joyce Clifford. I met her first when I was a medical student, and, happily for me, our paths crossed frequently thereafter as my career matured. Joyce died in 2011, but I think of her often as a model of the leader-scholar-activist upon whose shoulders the possibility of truly systemic, disruptive change rests.

Joyce headed nursing at Boston's Beth Israel (BI) Hospital. Every classmate of mine knew Joyce's force of character and the intensity of her devotion to nursing as a calling. But not nursing as some static, closely defended professional guild; rather, nursing as a dynamic, ever-changing, searching citizen in an enterprise much bigger than itself. Like all great leaders, Joyce asked not only, "What do we do?" but also, "What are we part of?" I knew that this search had led Joyce to be a founder of "primary nursing," placing the nurse at the very center of the coordinative and authentically respectful activity that we now call "patient-centered care" (or, more recently and ambitiously, "person-centered care"). It was for that reason more than any other that medical students who wanted to train in an environment that deeply and above all valued the humanity of the patient, family, and staff competed to land rotations at the BI.

Until reading this book—*NICHE: Nurses Improving Care for Healthsystem Elders*—I was less aware of Joyce's pivotal role in what I daresay is the majestic modern story of the evolution of theory and practice for proper care of older people. She was not alone in that expedition. The editors and other scholars whose work is so well catalogued here had DNA like Joyce's—genes for clarity, extreme patient focus, impatience with what is wrong, and courage to birth change.

I am not surprised to find Joyce's name prominently among them, nor to see the profession of nursing at the vanguard of disruptive improvement. On practically my first day of medical training on a hospital ward, a wise supervising resident, a year or two ahead of me, pulled me aside gently and gave me advice I never forgot: "If you want to be successful here, Don, just remember one thing: You are a guest of the nurse." I took that advice then to be tactical—a way to stay out of trouble. Now, decades later, I see it as a much deeper comment on the culture and sociology of the healthcare we have built—the facts on the ground. In the words of an explanation herein of the three key principles underlying the Geriatric Resource Nurse model at Yale New Haven Hospital: "(a) the nurse at the bedside has the best knowledge of how the older patient is responding to treatment and care, (b) the bedside nurse is the one most likely to be engaged with the family, and (c) she can apply key principles of geriatric nursing with the support of a master's-prepared geriatric nurse specialist."

More simply put, the nurse at the bedside is in the best position to "know" and to "do." A slight update would draw on the insights of Susan Edgman-Levitan, Michael Barry, and Maureen Bisognano: "Who better than the nurse can know, not just 'what is the matter' with the patient, but, maybe more important, 'what matters' to the patient?"

As a pediatrician, I am delighted that the needs of children—what matters to them—were recognized in a certified branch of the healthcare world, my branch, many decades ago. But, as a student of the performance and improvement of healthcare, I am embarrassed that it took so much longer for the needs and circumstances of people in older age to get such specialized recognition. NICHE represents a potential turning point, at scale, for redressing that lapse. This book offers a sweeping historical perspective on the evolution of NICHE and its ancestors, and of the scholars and activists who made that happen. Many were nurses, because nurses were in a position most clearly to see what was wrong.

The story unfolds in waves, each connected to its forerunners. The Hospital Outcomes Project for the Elderly (HOPE) sets the stage—an empirically based action project to find formulae for better care in participating hospitals. In the early 1990s, HOPE had built enough confidence in the feasibility of breakthroughs that philanthropists, researchers, and healthcare delivery leaders converged to found NICHE, with the express intent to bring scientifically sound changes in care of elders (initially mostly in hospitals) to very broad scale. On a parallel path, creating needed tools for NICHE and related efforts, these pioneers were learning how to assess the progress of hospitals in acquiring and implementing the needed skills, importantly with the Geriatric Institutional Assessment Profile (GIAP), which is now already in its eighth iteration. Many helped in all of this, but any honest historian has to give a shout-out to the John A. Hartford Foundation, whose constancy of purpose and repeated investments were (and remain) a *sine qua non* for this evolution.

That is one impressive characteristic of the story of NICHE, as told in this book: continuity, not just in the Hartford Foundation's level-headed support, but also in the apparent connectivity among the researchers and change agents on this expedition. The same names, like Joyce Clifford's, arise again and again, decade upon decade, of people whose dedication to better geriatric care was not just sincere but perpetual. They were, and are, tenacious, to say the least.

Another characteristic is cooperation among these scholar-activists. Academic politics can be tightly self-interested, and even frankly vicious. Maybe there were such tough rivalries over the three or four decades under scrutiny in this book, but the main feeling the observer has is of a community of connected effort—researchers and practitioners generally trying to build on each other's insights, not to shoot them down.

I had personal experience with this in my involvement as a coach to a current descendant of NICHE—the Age-Friendly Health Systems (AFHS) initiative of the John A. Hartford Foundation and the Institute for Healthcare Improvement.

The first steps in that project were to convene the varsity of researchers on the design of age-friendly care (many of who had had support from the Hartford Foundation) to sit together and explore their learnings, agreements, and disagreements.

This was a model of respectful, collaborative inquiry that many other disciplines in healthcare (not to mention Congress) can only envy. The resulting "4M" model (what Matters, Mentation, Mobility, and Medication) that emerged from those conversations is an easily explained distillation of the hard-won insights of world-class researchers over many years. Astonishingly, those researchers have assented to rallying around that model in an effort to help the dozens of organizations now trying to become more "Age Friendly." What the researchers did not do is defend their turf and skulk back home. Bravo!

If you want to get a vivid sense of the scale of this learning enterprise overall, spend some extra time with Chapter 10 in this volume. It is a wide, embracing catalogue of real-world trials (of archival value in itself), revealing the richness of experience upon which the change agents of now, and the future, can draw, thanks to the intentionality of so many champions of better care.

A third property that infuses NICHE and its forerunners is combining pragmatism with intellectual discipline. The researchers on geriatric care whose work converges so well on these pages successfully walked a tightrope that many do not: between obsessive and constipating insistence on evaluation methods that, in the end, stall progress, discourage risk-taking, and fail to take appropriate account of contexts and localities, on the one hand, and, on the other hand, unsupported mere storytelling claims that reflect more enthusiasm than knowledge. The NICHE story, to me, is a story of the right way to learn in complex systems. The researchers overall used the right assessment methods in the right way.

A fourth impressive property is related to the third: the intimate, continual juxtaposition of theory and action (à la Joyce Clifford, actually). The knowledge-growing enterprise that climaxed at present in NICHE and AFHS at every step of the way seems to have involved collaborations among active sites of care and academic theoreticians. This was learning in the "real world," not just in laboratories, and, in my view, the advances in NICHE and the benefits to elders would not be anywhere nearly as large if the researchers had avoided the messiness of practice.

The journey, of course, is not over. The authors in the volume chart a course that aims at obdurate problems, such as the design and performance of long-term care, and promising innovations, like telemedicine and artificial intelligence, which may offer entirely new levels of responsiveness to the needs of Healthsystem Elders. NICHE's track record so far bodes well.

Joyce Clifford, my heroine, scholar, change agent, champion of healing, destroyer of walls, builder of bridges, would be smiling broadly to read this ambitious book. She would be waving—thumbs up—at the authors and those whose work these authors summarize, people of similar ilk and welcome, intense impatience. As an aging person, myself, I can only offer thanks for what this promises for the chances of my thriving in the years ahead.

Donald M. Berwick, MD, MPP
President Emeritus and Senior Fellow
Institute for Healthcare Improvement
Boston, Massachusetts

Preface

This book is a gift back to all the staff nurses, nurse leaders, nurse educators, and system leaders who have helped us think deeply about what it means to provide excellent care to older adults. Our goal is to tell the story of how *Nurses Improving Care to the Hospitalized Elderly* evolved into the national and international program it is today and what some of the essential elements are to ensure program success. We are deeply grateful to the John A. Hartford Foundation and Donna Regenstreif for their support and ongoing commitment to the NICHE program. Thank you, as well, to all the students who worked with us throughout this journey!

As we began our work over 30 years ago, we were building the evidence as we went along and few funding sources had the confidence to make a calculated risk and invest in us. Over time, the maturation of the program along with the engagement of pivotal organizations and leaders in the field have solidified the work and we are proud that today, we do have the evidence to show that NICHE really works. In the first section of the book (Chapters 1–5), we provide the historical underpinnings of the program and the nurse leaders who helped conceptualize and shape the program.

We follow with chapters that describe the approach to NICHE and how the geriatric institutional assessment profile along with a readiness assessment for the geriatric resource nurses and assurance of leadership support are crucial to have in place at the outset of the program (Chapters 6–10). Over time, we have moved from paper to computerized formats and from charts to electronic health records but the basics remain the same. Careful assessment, person-centered care, planning, and reliable follow-through with the geriatric syndromes most likely to create difficulties for older people are at the heart of the program. The soul of the program is the leadership commitment of geriatric resource nurses who take it upon themselves to self-identify as champions for best practice for older adults. This is no small task and over time we have learned that the geriatric resource nurse model really serves as a nurse empowerment strategy. Nurses gain great agency and practice far more independently when they understand their roles and responsibilities and NICHE provided strong guidance to that end.

We believe the experience shared by the nurse authors who have breathed life into NICHE in their hospitals is instrumental in enticing a whole new cohort of nurses to embrace the NICHE journey. The chapters serve as a road map to plan and implement improved care of older adults in hospitals nationwide. They direct nurse administrators on how to make a case for NICHE to other hospital administrators. They advise nurses as to how to gauge commitment of clinicians to best practices in geriatric care. Further, they help nurses to reach out to the extensive reservoir of information and experience that lies in existing NICHE hospitals.

The final section of our book relates to the business proposition for NICHE and how external regulations and consumers are central to refinement of the program on an ongoing basis. The international context is exceptionally important as our world becomes more and more integrated in our practice approaches and concepts (Chapters 11–20). As global demography shifts toward older adults, every older person in a family should expect and demand age-friendly healthcare. NICHE is the backbone of an age-friendly health system and the very special vignettes provided by nurses who have traveled the geriatric resource nurse journey are inspiring. From the beginning, Trish Gibbons inspired so many of us to lead with the authority and responsibility that goes with expertise. Thank you, Trish.

Best wishes to all of you in your NICHE journey.

Terry Fulmer
Kimberly Glassman
Sherry Greenberg
Peri Rosenfeld
Mattia Gilmartin
Mathy Mezey

NICHE Timeline

GRN and HOPE Development Phase

1981–1988

Terry Fulmer, PhD, RN
Geriatric Resource Nurse (GRN) model initiated in 1981 at
Boston's Beth Israel Hospital

1989–1991

Geriatric Resource Nurse model adapted within a geriatrician-led
care team at Yale New Haven Hospital as part of The John A. Hartford
Foundation's Hospital Outcomes Program for the Elderly (HOPE) initiative

NICHE Phase 1

1992 HOPE Becomes NICHE

**1992–1998 Mathy Mezey and Terry Fulmer (Terry Fulmer moved from
Columbia University to New York University in 1994)**

HOPE models served as the basis for what becomes known as Nurses Improving Care
for Hospitalized Elderly (NICHE);
First John A. Hartford Foundation grant to Terry Fulmer at Columbia University School
of Nursing, 1992–1993: *Building on HOPE Projects to Improve Geriatric Nursing Care*;
with Mathy Mezey at NYU and Cheryl Vince at EDC;
Four NICHE workshops, 23 hospitals participate; four sites selected to test NICHE;
Geriatric Institutional Assessment Profile (GIAP) in development

**1993 NICHE Tools and
Processes Field Tested**

More organizations join the
original four sites

**The John A. Hartford Foundation
Grant 1995–1998**

Grant to New York University: *Nurses
Improving Care to the Hospitalized Elderly*
- Annual NICHE conference begins with
  2-day preworkshops for new sites

NICHE at NYU and HIGN Phase 2

1996–2002

**1996 NICHE Is Integrated
Into The Hartford Institute
for Geriatric Nursing**

Many accomplishments; NICHE
has grown to include a national
network of hospitals

1999 NICHE Toolkit Launched

Findings from field tests result in the NICHE Toolkit: *The NICHE Planning and
Implementation Guide*
- Effective nursing care models, including
  – Geriatric Resource Nurse (GRN) model
  – Acute Care for Elders (ACE) model
- Revised Geriatric Institutional Assessment Profile (GIAP) at Epsilon Group
- *Try This* Series
- Listserv for NICHE hospitals
- NICHE portal on HIGN website
- Expanded clinical practice protocols that reflect the standards of nursing
  practice on 13 important geriatric syndromes, published by Springer
  Publishing Company, 1999, now in its 5th edition

2003–2006

**Elizabeth Capezuti comes to NYU
as Faculty and Director of NICHE &
Marie Boltz joins NICHE as Director
of Practice**

Expanded with two new initiatives:
- GIAP Benchmarking Service moved from
  Epsilon Group to NYU
- GIAP Research Group was organized to
  develop research initiatives

Expansion—Building the Business Phase 3

2007 NICHE Received Major Expansion Grant

Atlantic Philanthropies fund the 5-year business plan
2008—revised NICHE website
2009—Online Knowledge Center

2007–2012 Expansion Plan or Building the Business Model

Elizabeth Capezuti, Director and PI

2007 Barbara Bricoli joins NICHE as Managing Director

**2012 NICHE Celebrates
500 Members**
NICHE continues to build
capacity and grow

Postexpansion Grant—Continued Growth Across Settings and Globally Phase 4

2013—Eileen Sullivan Marx at NYU, Dean

2014—Barbara Bricoli, Executive Director

2014—Expands Internationally

2014—NICHE Mexico

2014—NICHE Singapore

2015—NICHE Australia

Other international expansion includes Bermuda and testing the GIAP in Portugal and Brazil

NICHE Expands Across the Continuum of Care

2016–2018 NICHE receives grant from The John A. Hartford Foundation
to expand to LTC, *Nurses Improving Care for Healthsystem Elders in Long-
Term Care (NICHE-LTC)*
NICHE in over 700 hospitals and other healthcare settings in the United
States, Canada, Singapore, Australia, Bermuda

2016—Next Phase

**Mattia Gilmartin joins NICHE as Executive
Director**

Overview of NICHE

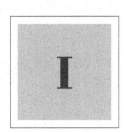

The Compelling Context for NICHE

Terry Fulmer and Mathy Mezey

It's hard to realize that NICHE was started more than 30 years ago. It was a spectacular innovation then and still feels fresh and new. Its contribution to the care of elders has been significant and equally important has been its contribution to the caring professions.
—Claire Mintzer Fagin, PhD, RN, FAAN, Professor and Dean Emerita, University of Pennsylvania School of Nursing

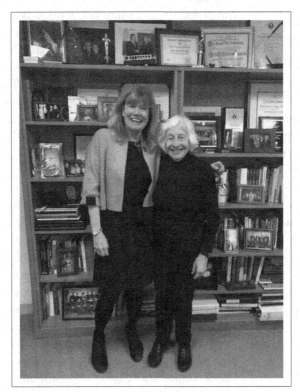

From left: Terry Fulmer, Mathy Mezey (2019).

> ### CHAPTER OBJECTIVES
>
> 1. Provide an overview of the genesis of the NICHE program
> 2. Discuss how the context of contemporary health systems has influenced NICHE
> 3. Review the evolution of the NICHE program

INTRODUCTION

What would a hospital visit or healthcare encounter that truly met the needs of older adults with complex care needs, functional limitations, multiple medications, and a set of geriatric syndromes look like? Nurses Improving Care for Healthsystem Elders (NICHE) set out to answer that question over 30 years ago. NICHE, originally conceived of in the mid-1980s at Boston's Beth Israel Hospital (today the Beth Israel–Deaconess Medical Center), is an extraordinary program that is dedicated to improving care for older adults. Originally focused on hospital care, today NICHE spans care settings. In large part, NICHE has adapted to the cataclysmic changes in healthcare and been able to innovate and adapt to the changing needs of older patients. Critical to NICHE's success had been support from the John A. Hartford Foundation (JAHF) and The Atlantic Philanthropies (TAP). These foundations recognized early the value of capturing the attention and talent of the nursing community, over 3.2 million strong, as leaders in the architecture of care for the elderly (Fulmer, 2015; Fulmer & Mezey, 1994; Mezey & Fulmer, 2002).

NICHE has adapted to the cataclysmic changes in healthcare and been able to innovate and adapt to the changing needs of older patients.

Not a new concept, the alignment of nursing practice with the maintenance and improvement of function for older people during the recovery process from illness (Fulmer & Mezey, 1994) was initially introduced by Florence Nightingale and followed by many others, including Lavinia Dock, Virginia Henderson, and an array of other nurse leaders and theorists (Henderson, 1964; Henderson & Nite, 1978). Terry Fulmer, PhD, RN, FAAN, who founded NICHE, was able to apply and disseminate the principles put forth by these leaders as a structured program that is nationally and internationally recognized as a proven model for improving hospital care for older adults. NICHE has been successfully executed around the country and around the world. Today, Dr. Mattia Gilmartin, PhD, RN leads the program, based at the Rory Meyers College of Nursing at New York University. Over 700 healthcare organizations are NICHE members and they convene annually at the NICHE Conference to discuss best practices and approaches to care improvement for older adults (www.nicheprogram.org).

Over 700 healthcare organizations are NICHE members and they convene annually at the NICHE Conference to discuss best practices and approaches to care improvement for older adults

A BRIEF OVERVIEW OF HOSPITALS AND NURSING CARE

The hospitals of the late 1800s bear little resemblance to the hospital experience of today. Early almshouses preceded hospitals as charitable housing for those who could no longer work to pay rent. They also served as homes to "contain" those with mental illness, developmental disabilities, the crippled, blind, deaf, and dumb, and vagrants (Spencer-Wood, 2001). Hospitals gained in number with both religious and secular support in the late 1800s and early 1900s. As medical and surgical breakthroughs began to emerge and more patients needed care, it was clear that hospital facilities with well-trained nursing staff were of the utmost importance for the healing and recovery processes. Bellevue Hospital in New York City, cited as America's first hospital, was founded in 1852 and soon after came the founding of the Bellevue Hospital School of Nursing (1873), which was an absolute necessity in order to prepare nurses to care for those hospitalized (Oshinsky, 2017). It was widely understood that hospitals came into being for the purpose of nursing care and to this day, this largely holds true (Figure 1.1). The Social Security Act of 1935 permanently established a national old-age pension system that was extended to many who had previously required almshouses (Social Security Administration, n.d.). Many have written about the history of nursing and the amazing progress in the discipline since the 1900s (Dock & Stewart, 1920;

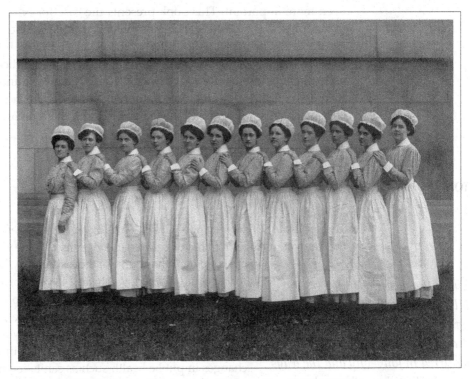

FIGURE 1.1 *Nurses at the Bellevue Hospital School of Nursing.*

TABLE 1.1 Number of U.S. Hospitals by Type (Total = 5,534, Fiscal Year 2016)

HOSPITAL TYPE	NUMBER OF HOSPITALS	PERCENTAGE
Community (nonfederal acute care)	4,840	88
Nonfederal Psychiatric	397	7
Federal Government	209	4
Nonfederal Long-term Care	78	1
Hospital Units of Institutions	10	<1

Source: Data from American Hospital Association. (2018). Fast facts on U.S. hospitals—2018 pie charts. Retrieved from https://www.aha.org/statistics/2018-01-09-fast-facts-us-hospitals-2018-pie-charts

Kalisch & Kalisch, 2004). Our disciplinary work builds on the extraordinary progress that evolved under our world-class leaders in nursing. Here, we focus on the genesis and trajectory of a special program, NICHE, that had its origins in hospital-based nursing and came of age during an era of primary nursing and the emergence of nurse-led models of care (Fulmer, 2015; Fulmer & Gibbons, 2015). Today, the American Hospital Association (AHA) reports that there are 5,534 registered hospitals in the country (Table 1.1) with 894,574 registered beds.

The demand for nurses and reliable, evidence-based nursing care has never been more important. This book presents the case for NICHE as a model of care that addresses those needs. The most recent count for nurses as of October 2018 by the Bureau of Labor Statistics (BLS) and the Kaiser Family Foundation is 3,378,669 registered nurses and 821,000 licensed practical nurses, indicating there are almost 4.2 million professionally active nurses (Kaiser Family Foundation, 2018). Imagine the power of those 4 million nurses if they were well versed in the NICHE protocols available today and had the leeway to implement them autonomously within the team context.

TODAY'S HEALTHCARE ENVIRONMENT FOR AN AGING POPULATION

The enthusiastic adoption of NICHE by healthcare systems reflects their awareness of the dramatic changes that have occurred in longevity and the ways that our lives have changed over the course of the last century. In 1900, life expectancy for men and women was 46 and 48 years of age, respectively, while now it is in the mid 80s. The idea that people would live to be 80 or 90 years old was thought of as exceptional, while today we see it with regularity, as a person turns 65 every 8 seconds (U.S. Census Bureau, 2000). How do we account for this progress? Certainly, changes in public health such as sanitation and clean water along with vaccinations and preventive care have brought an enormous reduction of mortality at childbirth and during youth. Further, the

The enthusiastic adoption of NICHE by healthcare systems reflects their awareness of the dramatic changes that have occurred in longevity and the ways that our lives have changed over the course of the last century.

advent of antibiotics, pacemakers, organ transplants, and more recently our under-standing of genomics and "designer medicine" is creating what some have called the "longevity dividend" (Fried, 2016). With all these extra years, however, we have also seen, as would be expected, an increase in chronic disease and functional decline. Today the number one reason for death is cardiac disease followed by cancer. Both of these diseases can now span decades in a person's life, where previously they would have been death sentences. Thus, today, we grapple with the question of how we are dealing with quality of life in these additional years. Some data would suggest not very well (Foley, Ancoli-Israel, Britz, & Walsh, 2004; Wilson et al., 2006).

We know that there is a dramatic cohort effect taking place related to how peo-ple approach aging and healthcare access and utilization. In previous generations, for example, people in "the greatest generation" (Brokaw, 2000) thought that an appointment with the doctor meant that you would go to your visit, listen carefully, and do as you were instructed. There was very little discussion or questioning on the part of the patient and, in most cases, doctors had an authoritarian approach to their practice. One need only look at old movies and television shows like *Marcus Welby, M.D.* to get a sense of how things have changed. Today, as Baby Boomers move into their later years, they are unwilling to be silent partners in their plan of care. The advent of the Internet with information readily available along with a differ-ent mind-set regarding the role in the doctor–patient relationship has dramatically changed the patient–provider relationship (Forkner-Dunn, 2003). People expect to be educated about choices and ultimately make choices that suit their goals and preferences (Reuben & Tinetti, 2012). Those of us who are trying to improve care for older adults need to examine our own values and beliefs related to the healthcare experience and determine how we can improve care and assure quality and value for those receiving care. NICHE has been successful, in part, because it gives nurses the knowledge and resources required to assess, listen to, and work with older adults to improve both their care and their quality of life.

NICHE has been successful, in part, because it gives nurses the knowledge and resources required to assess, listen to, and work with older adults to improve both their care and their quality of life.

In many ways, the early NICHE leaders were flying the plane while building it, especially when it came to developing the evidence base for geriatric nursing practice. The National Institute on Aging was not established until 1974 and its founding director, Robert Neil Butler, MD, understood very well the limitations of care for the elderly. His groundbreaking Pulitzer Prize–winning book, *Why Survive? Being Old in America*, laid out the unimaginable challenges that people face as they grow old and try to receive the care they need in a context of dignity and respect (Butler, 1975). More recently, Gawande (2014) has documented how far we still have to go in delivering exemplary care. We are only beginning to see some of the sorely needed changes that address the concerns of these leaders, including beginning to draw on the talent from the entire healthcare team. The National Institute for Nursing Research (NINR) began life as the National Center for Nursing Research (NCNR) in 1986. Within only 30-plus years, nursing has made remarkable progress in the development of the evidence base that is essential to defining best practice for all patients and, in this case, older adults.

The development of the field of geriatric nursing and medicine along with the growth and development of interdisciplinary healthcare teams has also been a 30-year endeavor (Fulmer, Flaherty, & Hyer, 2004; Hyer, Fairchild, Abraham, Mezey, & Fulmer, 2000).

Today it is widely recognized that we will never have an adequate number of geriatrically prepared healthcare workforce personnel. *Retooling for an Aging America: Building the Health Care Workforce*, a report from the Institute of Medicine (IOM; now the National Academy of Medicine), clearly documented the dearth of those so trained, and the need for new strategies (IOM, 2008). To address the issue, several specialties in medical and surgical physician practice and in nursing practice have recognized the need to integrate geriatrics into the specialties of internal medicine and adult nurse practitioner preparation as well as encourage comanaged care (Friedman, Mendelson, Kates, & McCann, 2008; Hazzard, Woolard, & Regenstreif, 1997). Nurses have long understood the essential nature of interdisciplinary teams for optimal patient care outcomes, especially for older adults, and serve as the essential linchpin for coordination across disciplines. As the only discipline with 24-hour presence in acute care critical access hospitals and the dominant clinical practice professionals in all care settings, nurses have a responsibility to lead the care plan for older adults (McClure & Nelson, 1982). The NICHE program is the embodiment of this philosophy.

This book represents the collective efforts of many who have helped establish NICHE and who have gotten us to this point in history. Our goal in writing this book is to make evident how NICHE is now a mainstream program and the backbone of an age-friendly health system (Fulmer & Berman, 2016). In 2016, the JAHF of New York City in partnership with the Institute for Healthcare Improvement (IHI) in Cambridge, Massachusetts formally announced a new program entitled "Age Friendly Health Systems," which will capitalize on lessons learned from NICHE and focus on creating seamless care across settings and disciplines that improve care outcomes for older adults. This book provides a comprehensive reference for the NICHE program, including the background and history of the program along with the strategies that have been employed over the past 30 years to build on nursing leadership in order to accelerate the progress in momentum of care improvement for older adults.

CHAPTER SUMMARY

NICHE can help health organizations meet the increasing demand for care of older adults and their complex healthcare needs resulting from the dramatic increase in longevity over the past century.

NICHE was founded by Terry Fulmer, PhD, RN, FAAN, over 30 years ago with the goal of improving healthcare for older adults. In developing NICHE, Fulmer built on nursing principles established by Florence Nightingale, Lavinia Dock, Virginia Henderson, and others. Today, based at the Rory Meyers College of Nursing at New York University, NICHE has over 700 healthcare organization members internationally.

NICHE provides a model of care to address the current need for evidence-based nursing care. In particular, NICHE can help health organizations meet the increasing demand for care of older adults and their complex healthcare needs resulting from the dramatic increase in longevity over the past century. Furthermore, in an era in which patients have easy access to healthcare information and increasingly expect to participate actively in their own care, NICHE is effective in equipping nurses to listen well to their patients and collaborate with them in their care. This program also prepares nurses to work well as members of interdisciplinary teams in caring for older adults.

REFERENCES

American Hospital Association. (2018). Fast facts on U.S. hospitals—2018 pie charts. Retrieved from https://www.aha.org/statistics/2018-01-09-fast-facts-us-hospitals -2018-pie-charts

Brokaw, T. (2000). *The greatest generation*. New York, NY: Random House.

Butler, R. N. (1975). *Why survive? Being old in America*. Baltimore, MD: Johns Hopkins University Press.

Dock, L. L., & Stewart, I. M. (1920). *A short history of nursing from the earliest times to the present day*. New York, NY: G. P. Putnam's Sons.

Foley, D., Ancoli-Israel, S., Britz, P., & Walsh, J. (2004). Sleep disturbances and chronic disease in older adults: Results of the 2003 National Sleep Foundation Sleep in America Survey. *Journal of Psychosomatic Research, 56*(5), 497–502. doi:10.1016/ j.jpsychores.2004.02.010

Forkner-Dunn, J. (2003). Internet-based patient self-care: The next generation of health care delivery. *Journal of Medical Internet Research, 5*(2), e8. doi:10.2196/jmir.5.2.e8

Fried, L. P. (2016). Investing in health to create a third demographic dividend. *The Gerontologist, 56*(Suppl. 2), S167–S177. doi:10.1093/geront/gnw035

Friedman, S. M., Mendelson, D. A., Kates, S. L., & McCann, R. M. (2008). Geriatric co-management of proximal femur fractures: Total quality management and protocol-driven care result in better outcomes for a frail patient population. *Journal of the American Geriatrics Society, 56*(7), 1349–1356. doi:10.1111/j.1532-5415.2008.01770.x

Fulmer, T. (2015) Geriatric nursing 2.0! *Journal of the American Geriatrics Society, 63*(7), 1453–1458. doi:10.1111/jgs.13492

Fulmer, T., & Berman, A. (2016) Age-friendly health systems: How do we get there? Retrieved from http://healthaffairs.org/blog/2016/11/03/age-friendly-health-systems-how-do-we-get-there

Fulmer, T., Flaherty, E., & Hyer, K. (2004). The geriatric interdisciplinary team training (GITT) program. *Gerontology & Geriatrics Education, 24*(2), 3–12. doi:10.1300/J021v24n02_02

Fulmer, T., & Gibbons, M. P. (2015). Joyce Clifford the scholar: In her own words. *Advances in Nursing Science, 38*(4), 347–354. doi:10.1097/ANS.0000000000000093

Fulmer, T. T., & Mezey, M. (1994). Nurses improving care to the hospitalized elderly. *Geriatric Nursing, 15*(3), 126. doi:10.1016/S0197-4572(09)90035-0

Gawande, A. (2014). *Being mortal: Medicine and what matters in the end*. New York, NY: Metropolitan Books.

Hazzard, W. R., Woolard, N., & Regenstreif, D. I. (1997). Integrating geriatrics into the subspecialties of internal medicine: The Hartford Foundation/American Geriatrics Society/Wake Forest University Bowman Gray School of Medicine Initiative. *Journal of the American Geriatrics Society*, 45(5), 638–640. doi:10.1111/j.1532-5415.1997.tb03102.x

Henderson, V. (1964). The nature of nursing. *The American Journal of Nursing*, 64(8), 62–68. doi:10.2307/3419278

Henderson, V., & Nite, G. (1978). *Principles and practice of nursing*. London, England: Macmillan.

Hyer, K., Fairchild, S., Abraham, I., Mezey, M., & Fulmer, T. (2000). Measuring attitudes related to interdisciplinary training: Revisiting the Heinemann, Schmitt and Farrell "attitudes toward health care" teams scale. *Journal of Interprofessional Care*, 14(3), 249–258. doi:10.1080/jic.14.3.249.258

Institute of Medicine. (2008). *Retooling for an aging America: Building the health care workforce*. Washington, DC: The National Academies Press.

Kaiser Family Foundation. (2018). Total number of professionally active nurses, October 2018. Retrieved from https://www.kff.org/other/state-indicator/total-registered-nurses/?currentTimeframe=0&sortModel=%7B%22colId%22:%22Location%22, %22sort%22:%22asc%22%7D

Kalisch, P. A., & Kalisch, B. J. (2004). *American nursing: A history*. Philadelphia, PA: Lippincott Williams & Wilkins.

McClure, M., & Nelson, J. (1982). Trends in hospital nursing. In L. Aiken (Ed.), *Nursing in the 1980s: Crises, opportunities, challenges* (pp. 59–73). Philadelphia, PA: Lippincott.

Mezey, M., & Fulmer, T. (2002). The future history of gerontological nursing. *The Journals of Gerontology Series A: Biological Sciences and Medical Sciences*, 57(7), M438–M441. doi:10.1093/gerona/57.7.M438

Oshinsky, D. (2017). *Bellevue: Three centuries of medicine and mayhem at America's most storied hospital*. New York, NY: Doubleday.

Reuben, D. B., & Tinetti, M. E. (2012). Goal-oriented patient care—An alternative health outcomes paradigm. *New England Journal of Medicine*, 366(9), 777–779. doi:10.1056/NEJMp1113631

Social Security Administration. (n.d.). Historical background and development of Social Security. Retrieved from https://www.ssa.gov/history/briefhistory3.html

Spencer-Wood, S. M. (2001). Introduction and historical context to the archaeology of seventeenth and eighteenth century almshouses. *International Journal of Historical Archaeology*, 5(2), 115–122. doi:10.1023/A:1011317109050

U.S. Census Bureau. (2000). Population projections of the United States by age, sex, race, Hispanic origin, and nativity: 1999 to 2100. Retrieved from https://www.census.gov/prod/1/pop/p25-1130/p251130.pdf

Wilson, R. S., Arnold, S. E., Schneider, J. A., Kelly, J. F., Tang, Y., & Bennett, D. A. (2006). Chronic psychological distress and risk of Alzheimer's disease in old age. *Neuroepidemiology*, 27(3), 143–153. doi:10.1159/000095761

NICHE: The Formative Years

2

Terry Fulmer, Mathy Mezey, and Mildred Z. Solomon

Implementation of the NICHE model in health systems throughout the United States has motivated and positioned frontline nurses and other health team members to deliver the highest quality of care to older adults. The NICHE model is an outstanding example of the positive outcomes that can be achieved by committed healthcare teams who are positioned to maintain an unwavering focus on what older adults need, want, and deserve. Kudos to the NICHE leadership and teams past and present!
—Mary D. Naylor, PhD, RN, FAAN, Marian S. Ware, Professor in Gerontology
Director of the NewCourtland Center for Transitions and Health

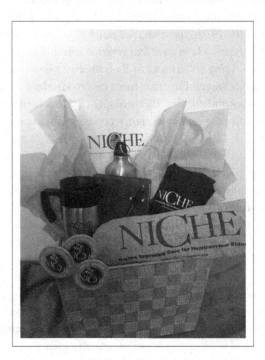

CHAPTER OBJECTIVES

1. Discuss the climate for the early phases and maturation of the NICHE program
2. Describe the impact of foundation funding
3. Relate the influence of Education Development Center's Decisions Near the End of Life model to the progression of NICHE
4. Describe the early developments in the implementation of NICHE

INTRODUCTION

The genesis of Nurses Improving Care for Healthsystem Elders (NICHE) is largely attributable to the willingness, in 1974, of the leadership of the then Beth Israel Hospital in Boston (Joyce Clifford, RN, Trish Gibbons, RN, and Mitchell Rabkin, MD) to support the primary nursing model, a model of practice that recognizes and empowers nurses to act with autonomy, authority, and responsibility over their practice. Much of the care that nurses provided at Beth Israel was to older adults. The supported model of practice encouraged, in fact required, that nurses exercise autonomy and responsibility to manage the nursing care of older patients, for example their skin care, decubitus ulcer prevention, ambulation, sleep, and continence needs. Thus, this model of practice had a profound impact on how nurses thought about and cared for older patients.

Until the 1970s, there was not much of an evidence base for geriatric nursing or geriatric medical care. There were few geriatricians and geriatric-trained nurses. The National Institute on Aging (NIA) was in its formative phase and the science of geriatric care was in its neophyte stages. Care was based on "received wisdom" passed down through generations of nurses and doctors. Poor nursing care was correctly recognized as a source of complications and poor outcomes, but recommended management strategies were very much anecdotal. For example, Minnie Goodnow correctly wrote in her textbook, The Technic of Nursing (Goodnow, 1927) that "a pressure sore, except in the rarest of instances, proclaims poor nursing." Her best prevention techniques were clean linen, bathing with soap and water, and rubbing the skin with alcohol and dusting powder, since rubbing stirred circulation, a contraindicated practice that persisted into the 1970s. For treatment of decubiti, without any proven efficacy, she advocated the use of zinc oxide, castor oil, camphorated oil, or a mixture of mutton tallow and olive oil with 1% carbolic acid. A thick layer of Castile soap was also deemed effective (p. 109). By the 1970s, it was still accepted that pressure ulcers were the result of poor nursing care, but, again with no scientific support, the commonly recommended treatment was Maalox and heat lamps, sugar applications, or simply wet to dry dressing. Further compounding the inability to prevent and treat pressure ulcers, there were no mobility programs and the use of physical restraints was the order of the day.

It would be several years before scientists like Rowe and Besdine (1982), Resnick and Yalla (1985), Lipsitz, Wei, and Rowe (1985), Strumpf and Evans (1988), and others would successfully compete for National Institutes of Health (NIH) funding to develop the definitive evidence base for the practice of geriatrics. Many investigators engaged in bench science that would lead to breakthroughs in understanding the hemodynamics and immune function in older adults as distinct from younger people. Scientists such as Leonard Hayflick described cellular aging in 1975, which ushered in a new era for the science in support of geriatric care (Hayflick, 1975). The Baltimore Longitudinal Study of Aging (Shock, 1984) was extraordinarily important to the prodromal years leading up to the founding of the NIA in 1974.

Slowly, evidence-based geriatric knowledge was incorporated into nursing and medical care for older patients. Skillman's (1975) book described the parameters necessary for surgical care of the elderly and documented the widely accepted practice that age was an exclusionary factor to admission to intensive care. Early pioneers in nursing including Mezey, Wells, Ebersole, and Wykle began defining the science that would underpin best practices in geriatric nursing care (Ebersole & Hess, 1985; Wells, Brink, & Diokno, 1987). The Journal of Gerontological Nursing issued its first volume in 1978, signaling a new era of geriatric nursing practice. Documented elsewhere (Fulmer, 2015) are the other extraordinary markers of progress in a relatively short period of time that would bring about changes in the care of older adults. The pilot work at Beth Israel and early enthusiasm for a NICHE-type initiative were occurring during this period of enhanced geriatric activity in nursing and medical education. The NIA-funded geriatric centers of excellence for physicians and the Veterans Administration (VA) did a remarkable job accelerating the pace of practice change for older veterans (Schneider, Ory, & Aung, 1987). American nursing gained strength through the acceleration of baccalaureate education and the emergence of advanced practice nurses. The Health Resources and Services Administration (HRSA) increased geriatric funding in baccalaureate and masters nursing programs. The Robert Wood Johnson Foundation funded the Teaching Nursing Home Program, soon followed by NIA funding of Academic Teaching Nursing Homes (Mezey & Lynaugh, 1989). The National Gerontological Nursing Association (NGNA) was founded along with a special geriatric nursing interest group at the Gerontological Society of America (GSA) in 1982. Funding for this first GSA interest group was provided by the Harvard Division on Aging under the leadership of Jack Rowe.

Early pioneers in nursing including Mezey, Wells, Ebersole, and Wykle began defining the science that would underpin best practices in geriatric nursing care.

In this ripe climate, NICHE began to take shape at Beth Israel. Clifford and Gibbons funded the development of geriatric nursing care protocols to be used in the hospital. Understanding that it would take champions to get the care protocols embedded into nursing practice, Fulmer worked with nurse managers to identify "geriatric resource nurses" (GRNs), floor nurses who had an interest in older adults and were willing to complete a specified in-hospital education program.

GERIATRIC RESOURCE NURSE MODEL DEVELOPMENT

The GRN model became fully developed when Gibbons and Fulmer were recruited to Yale New Haven Hospital (YNHH) in 1989, with Gibbons as chief nursing officer. Holding a joint appointment at the Yale School of Nursing and the YNHH, Fulmer led geriatric nursing both in the academic and practice settings. An early training grant from the Department of Health and Human Services was essential to implementing a geriatric curriculum at the School of Nursing. With the strength of the Yale School of Medicine geriatric faculty (led by Dr. Leo Cooney, with Drs. Tinetti, Inouye, Maritoli, Miller, and others), an influential critical mass of geriatric healthcare professionals garnered the attention of the John A. Hartford Foundation (JAHF) in New York City.

THE HOSPITAL OUTCOMES PROJECT FOR THE ELDERLY

The JAHF was conceptualizing a new project, the Hospital Outcomes Project for the Elderly (HOPE), under the leadership of Dr. Donna Regenstreif, JAHF senior program officer in 1988. Yale was selected as one of the six HOPE sites. Each of the HOPE sites used a different model of care as the intervention in this case–control study. Yale used the GRN model. Marquis Foreman, PhD, RN, at the University of Chicago used the clinical nurse specialist model (Fulmer, 1991a, b). In Cleveland, Case Western Reserve University faculty used an acute care of the elderly (ACE) unit approach with Denise Kresevic, PhD, RN, as the nurse leader (Kresevic & Naylor, 1995; Palmer, Landefeld, Kresevic, & Kowal, 1994).

At the completion of the HOPE grant, the three HOPE models, in which nursing care was key in achieving positive outcomes, captured the attention of the JAHF. Again under Dr. Regenstreif's leadership, in 1992 the JAHF Board approved the first nurse-led grant to Dr. Fulmer at the Columbia University School of Nursing for a pilot program to further test these hospital-based nursing models in four hospitals nationwide (Fulmer et al., 2002; Mezey, Fulmer, & Fletcher, 2002; NICHE Project Faculty, 1994). Appendix 2.1 shows a personal letter Dr. Fulmer received during this time describing the launch of NICHE at the University of Virginia Health System. A subsequent 3-year grant from the JAHF, awarded in 1995 to Mezey and Fulmer at the New York University (NYU) Division of Nursing (now known as the NYU Rory Meyers College of Nursing), became the basis for the full implementation of the NICHE program.

JAHF funding was the critical accelerant for development of the NICHE program.

JAHF funding was the critical accelerant for development of the NICHE program. It was a remarkable accomplishment for geriatric nursing to have the support and funding of one of the nation's most prestigious foundations. At that time the JAHF was one of the only national foundations that focused solely on geriatrics and care of older adults. JAHF Board chairs, initially James Farley and then Norman Volk, cemented the Foundation's commitment to geriatrics and care of older adults, and specifically to geriatric nursing, now continuing over 35 years.

NICHE, EDUCATION DEVELOPMENT CENTER, AND THE ADVISORY BOARD

In 1992, the first critical step in developing NICHE was to convene an Advisory Board and to enter into a collaboration with Education Development Center (EDC; Table 2.1). EDC, a freestanding educational research institution based in

TABLE 2.1 NICHE Advisory Board (1992)

NAME	DEGREE	LOCATION
Priscilla Ebersole	PhD, RN, FAAN	University of San Francisco
Marquis Foreman	PhD, RN	University of Chicago
Denise Kresevic	MSN, RN	University Hospitals of Cleveland
Mary Naylor	PhD, RN, FAAN	University of Pennsylvania
Neville Strumpf	PhD, RN, FAAN	University of Pennsylvania
Mary Walker	PhD, RN, FAAN	University of Kentucky
May Wykle	PhD, RN, FAAN	Case Western Reserve University

Massachusetts, is world renowned for designing highly participatory educational materials and strategies that can effectively empower learners. In the 1980s, their researchers and curriculum designers were actively applying innovative educational approaches to the design of health behavior change interventions to enable individuals to make healthy choices. Then, with a major grant from the Kellogg Foundation, the EDC researchers began an ambitious program in collaboration with The Hastings Center in Garrison, New York to enhance the care of people near the end of life. The goal of this project, *Decisions Near the End of Life*, was not behavioral change on the part of individuals to enhance their own health, but rather organizational change that would result in better care for populations of patients near the end of life. The need for this program was clear: too many older adults were dying in pain, because of common myths and misunderstandings about the use of pain medications; when patients could no longer speak for themselves, there was great uncertainty about the authority of their loved ones to make treatment decisions for them; and physicians were reluctant to ever withdraw or forgo life-sustaining treatments without court orders—a process that disenfranchised patients and their families.

The EDC researchers saw the power in developing an educational program, akin to quality improvement programs today, in which attending physicians, medical residents, nurses, social workers, and other healthcare professionals involved in the care of the critically ill would learn together in interdisciplinary teams, and often in workplace units such as an intensive care unit (ICU) or other medical units (Solomon, Jennings, Guilfoy et al., 1991). *Decisions Near the End of Life* began with a national survey of healthcare professionals' knowledge, attitudes, and beliefs about the current quality of care of patients at their institutions and their views on critical national policies. Publication of the results (Solomon et al., 1993) stirred broad national debate, including coverage by *The New York Times* and the Associated Press. But a national survey did not answer a key stumbling block to local learning and improvement: many health systems could just say "Those problems may exist elsewhere, but what do they have to do with us? The care we are giving is optimal and our clinicians are all on the same page."

To spur self-reflection and openness to organizational improvement at the local level, it became clear to the EDC researchers that each institution should begin by completing its own institutional assessment. The EDC researchers made the national survey available to health systems willing to undertake this process. Systems were encouraged to survey critical care physicians, critical care nurses, and any specialists like cardiologists and oncologists likely to care for patients near the end of life. These local results nearly always made explicit the irrefutable: many nurses and physicians in their system are unaware of best practices and national policies, and there was troubling disagreement on key issues, particularly between physicians and nurses. With this reality in hand, ultimately more than 200 health systems became motivated to participate in the *Decisions Near the End of Life* leadership training program and to use its case-based curriculum (Solomon, Guilfoy, O'Donnell et al., 1991, revised 1997), designed for interdisciplinary learning in small groups at the workplace (see also O'Donnell & Solomon, 1994; Solomon, 1995). This approach was later adopted and translated into German for use in Germany and Switzerland, and the EDC team developed a similar program, *The Initiative for Pediatric Palliative Care (IPPC)*, which engaged many U.S. children's hospitals across the nation during the early 2000s (Browning & Solomon, 2005, 2006; curriculum available at www.ippcweb.org).

Early in 1991, Fulmer and Mezey saw the power of beginning with data about one's own institution as an important spur to organizational learning. Using the Decisions Institutional Assessment Profile as a guide, they developed the Geriatric Institutional Assessment Profile (GIAP), modeled after the IAP from the EDC Decisions Project, with the input of the expert NICHE Advisory Board and EDC senior staff. The GIAP was constructed to elicit nurses' knowledge, attitudes, and beliefs about the current quality of care of geriatric patients at their institutions. This assessment provided a means for potential NICHE hospitals to assess the baseline knowledge and attitudes of their staffs to care for older adults, and then to reassess staff knowledge and attitudes once NICHE had been implemented to discern improvement. Data from the GIAP were analyzed by NICHE staff at NYU and sent back to each hospital, benchmarking the hospital against other NICHE hospitals of similar size and configuration. The early phases of GIAP construction are discussed in detail in Chapter 5.

Fulmer and Mezey saw the power of beginning with data about one's own institution as an important spur to organizational learning.

SCALING NICHE

It was crucial to develop a strategy for scaling NICHE and much had been learned from EDC. NICHE began to solicit applications from hospitals in 1993. The competitive application process required a description of the current care for older adults, evidence of administrative support, and expertise in nursing and other disciplines in order to implement NICHE. Upon review by the Advisory Board, the first four hospitals were enrolled. In year 2, four additional sites were added and with each successive year, the number of applications has grown. In 2002, there were 105 hospitals, and today there are over 700. The original NICHE Toolkit (tools developed specifically for NICHE) included the GIAP, three nursing care models developed in the HOPE sites, clinical practice protocols (initially 14 and now 39), and self-reported clinical outcome indicators along with a consumer survey to understand the impact of NICHE. Hospitals received consultation from the NICHE office at NYU to assist with interpretation of GIAP data and to implement a practice model and protocols. An annual NICHE conference, first held in 1993, brought together a team from each NICHE hospital and allowed for sharing of strategies, tactics, and outcomes. New NICHE sites were required to attend a 2-day, face-to-face Pre-Conference Workshop that introduced them to NICHE.

The NICHE Advisory Board (Priscilla Ebersole, PhD, RN, Denise Kresevic, MSN, RN, Mary Naylor, PhD, RN, May Wykle, PhD, RN, Neville Strumpf, PhD, RN, Marquis Foreman, PhD, RN, and Mary Walker, PhD, RN) adopted the name Nurses Improving Care to Hospitalized Elders (NICHE), subsequently changed, in 1997, to Nurses Improving Care for Healthsystem Elders.

GERIATRIC PROGRAMS AT NYU NURSING

Initially, the NICHE program at the then NYU Division of Nursing was a standalone program supported by JAHF from 1995 to 1998. Subsequently, in 1998, administratively NICHE was incorporated into the newly funded Hartford Institute for Geriatric Nursing (HIGN), a national initiative of the JAHF also housed at the NYU Division of Nursing (now the Rory Meyer College of Nursing). In 2015, the NICHE program began a new administrative structure in which the NICHE director reported directly to the dean of the Rory Meyer School of Nursing, with a collaborative arrangement with the HIGN. The mission of the HIGN is to develop materials to assist practicing nurses better assess and manage the nursing care of older adults. NICHE became the flagship program of the HIGN. Materials created by the HIGN are user friendly and disseminated on the HIGN clinical website, www.ConsultGer.org. This website is the "go to" authoritative resource on geriatric nursing for practicing nurses, educators, and students. The *Try This* Assessment Series is one HIGN product developed as an open-source resource but extensively used by NICHE hospitals. *Try This* is a series of assessment strategies commonly accepted as representing best practice in care of older adults. NICHE hospitals extensively use the SPICES (see Table 2.4) assessment, assessment of activities of daily living (ADLs), and assessment of cognitive status (Beecroft, 2000; Fulmer, 2007). The Geriatric Practice Protocols, described in this chapter, were developed by NICHE and the HIGN and again, were originally open source and now are a major resource of NICHE (Boltz, Capezuti, Fulmer, & Zwicker, 2016).

In 1995, the JAHF funded the Geriatric Interdisciplinary Team Training (GITT) program also at the NYU Division of Nursing. GITT developed alongside the HIGN and was also a major resource for NICHE. The Foundation's GITT

> *In 1998, administratively NICHE was incorporated into the newly funded Hartford Institute for Geriatric Nursing (HIGN), a national initiative of the JAHF.*

TABLE 2.2 New York University Grants

GRANT NAME	GRANT NO.	DATE AWARDED	AMOUNT
GITT Program: Resource Center	95228	9/22/1995	$1,549,981
GITT Program: Resource Center Renewal	990003	3/19/1999	$1,326,202
GITT Dissemination	2002-0030	3/15/2002	$373,967
Restoration to The John A. Hartford Foundation Institute for Geriatric Nursing	2004-0152	6/11/2004	$250,000
The John A. Hartford Foundation Institute for the Advancement of Geriatric Nursing Practice	95325	6/10/1996	$5,000,000
The John A. Hartford Foundation Institute for Geriatric Nursing: Phase II	2000-0546	3/16/2001	$4,600,000
How to Try This: Geriatric Assessment Nursing Resources	2006-0410	3/16/2007	$2,622,560

GITT, Geriatric Interdisciplinary Team Training.

national initiative addressed the need to train multiple health professionals to work as a team in providing comprehensive healthcare for elders (https://consultgeri.org/tools/gitt-2.0-toolkit). The GITT Resource Center (originally funded in 1995) greatly enhanced the success of the initiative by facilitating and supporting activities of the nine GITT training sites. Table 2.2 lists grants received by NYU related to geriatric nursing. The Resource Center activities were intended to maximize the impact of the GITT initiative by pursuing three interrelated tasks: first, gleaning the lessons of GITT through the evaluation of student outcomes; second, use of those lessons and the educational materials developed by GITT sites to produce refined models and materials adapted to the needs of a variety of potential educational institutions; and third, dissemination of the lessons and tools to institutions wishing to implement GITT models (Fulmer, Flaherty, & Hyer, 2004; Fulmer et al., 2005; Siegler, 1998).

GERIATRIC PRACTICE PROTOCOLS

In the first edition of *Geriatric Nursing Protocols for Best Practice* (Abraham, Bottrell, Fulmer, & Mezey, 1999, now in its fifth edition), Mezey and Fulmer wrote about a "crisis in caring for *older* (sick) patients who require a hospital stay" (p. XVII). We described the movement toward outpatient care for older patients with multiple, chronic conditions who leave the hospital "sicker and quicker." This had two

Geriatric Nursing Protocols for Best Practice, jointly developed by the HIGN and NICHE, was envisioned as a textbook that would be readily available to nurses who needed state-of-the-art clinical protocols in order to lead NICHE programs with the requisite practice expertise.

negative consequences. It meant that older people in the hospital were now the sickest of the sick. And it left very sick older patients and their families to manage their care at home. *Geriatric Nursing Protocols for Best Practice,* jointly developed by the HIGN and NICHE, was envisioned as a textbook that would be readily available to nurses who needed state-of-the-art clinical protocols in order to lead NICHE programs with the requisite practice expertise (Figure 2.1). Protocol development built on work begun in Boston and New Haven, as a compilation of evidence-based geriatric nursing care protocols, was needed. Protocols were created specifically for staff nurses with a keen interest in improving geriatric care. The authors in the first protocol book represent a compendium of extraordinary geriatric nursing pioneers (Table 2.3; Abraham, 1999). The practice protocols provided care objectives along with assessment parameters, care strategies, and a sense of the context of the person. Fulmer had previously used the acronym "SPICES" to delineate needed care protocols

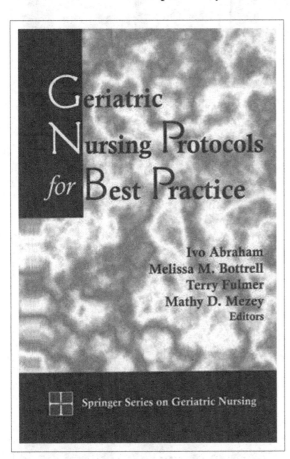
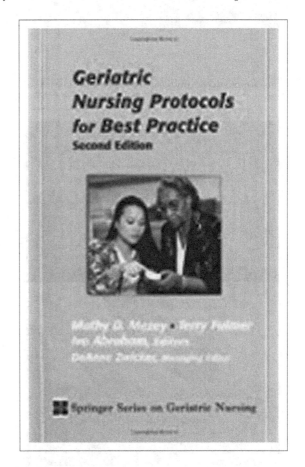

FIGURE 2.1 *Collection of Protocols covers. (continued)*

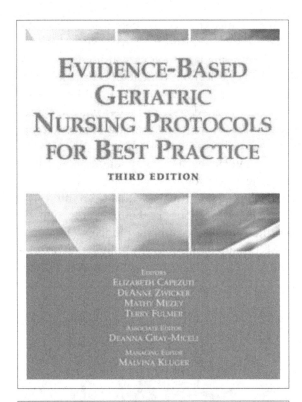

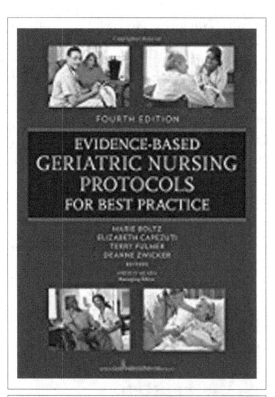

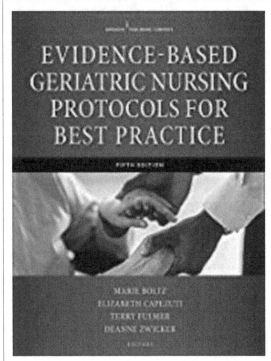

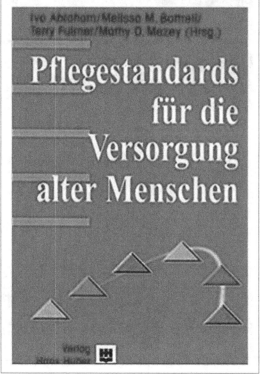

FIGURE 2.1 *(continued)*

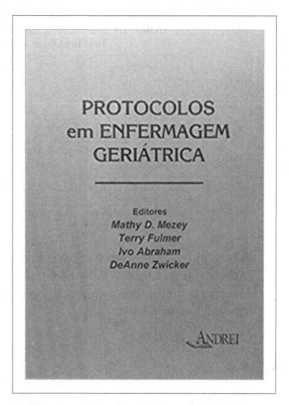

FIGURE 2.1 (*continued*)

TABLE 2.3 Geriatric Nursing Protocols for Best Practice Contributors (1999)	
Karen Allen MS, RN (as of 1999)	Lorraine C. Mion, PhD, RN, FAAN
Elaine Jensen Amella, PhD, RN, FGSA, FAAN	Janet Moore, PhD, RN, GCNS
Christine Bradway, PhD, RN, CRNP, FAAN	Mary D. Naylor, PhD, RN, FAAN
Roberta Campbell, MSN, RN (as of 1999)	Gloria Ramsey, JD, RN, FAAN
Barbara Corrigan, MS, RN, CS	Patricia Samra, MS, RN
Kathleen Fletcher, DNP, RN, NP-BC, FAAN	Cheryl Stetler, PhD, RN, FAAN
Marquis D. Foreman, PhD, RN, FAAN	Neville Strumpf, PhD, RN, FAAN
Deborah Francis, MSN, APRN, BC	Joyce Thielen, PhD, RN
Sharon Hernley, MS, GNP (as of 1999)	Lark J Trygstad, APRN
Denise M. Kresevic, PhD, RN, APN_BC, FGSA, FAAN	Mary K. Walker, PhD, RN, FAAN
Lenore H. Kurlowicz, PhD, RN, CS, FAAN	May L. Wykle, PhD, RN, FAAN, FGSA

(see Table 2.4 and Chapter 15 in Boltz et al., 2016). Skin problems, problems with eating and feeding, incontinence, confusion, evidence of falling, and sleep disorders readily helped frame common geriatric syndromes for staff nurses and served as a gateway into additional syndromes such as depression, mobility issues, and elder abuse. Little did Fulmer know that SPICES would soon be labeled "never events" by regulatory authorities (Fulmer, 2007). Protocols were available on the

TABLE 2.4 Fulmer SPICES: An Overall Assessment Tool for Older Adults		
Patient Name:	Date:	
	EVIDENCE	
SPICES	Yes	No
Sleep Disorders		
Problems with Eating or Feeding		
Incontinence		
Confusion		
Evidence of Falls		
Skin Breakdown		

website of the JAHF HIGN at NYU under a NICHE portal (see Table 2.3). Each protocol was arranged in three parts: need to know, which covered the very basic information on the topic; want to know more, which provided in-depth information; and a reference list.

CHAPTER SUMMARY

In this book, we highlight the extraordinary journey of NICHE from its inception, drawing on descriptions of the program's expansion, data as to outcomes, and vignettes from participating NICHE hospitals. Clearly, progress would not have been possible without funding from the JAHF and the visionary leadership of the program officers who understood the interrelationships among and across the project grants that were under way. From HOPE to NICHE to GITT to the HIGN, the interrelationships and synergy are clear, created the momentum for change, and will be underscored throughout this book.

REFERENCES

Abraham, I. L., Bottrell, M. M., Fulmer, T., & Mezey, M. D. (Eds.). (1999). *Geriatric nursing protocols for best practice*. New York, NY: Springer Publishing.

Beecroft, P. C. (2000). Try this: Best practices in nursing care to older adults. *Clinical Nurse Specialist, 14*(3), 138–140. doi:10.1097/00002800-200005000-00010

Boltz, M., Capezuti, E., Fulmer, T. T., & Zwicker, D. (Eds.). (2016). *Evidence-based geriatric nursing protocols for best practice* (5th ed.). New York, NY: Springer Publishing.

Browning, D. M., & Solomon, M. Z. (2005). The initiative for pediatric palliative care: An interdisciplinary educational approach for healthcare professionals. *Journal of Pediatric Nursing, 20*(5), 326–334. doi:10.1016/j.pedn.2005.03.004

Browning, D. M., & Solomon, M. Z. (2006). Relational learning in pediatric palliative care: Transformative education and the culture of medicine. *Child and Adolescent Psychiatric Clinics of North America, 15*(3), 795–815. doi:10.1016/j.chc.2006.03.002

Ebersole, P., & Hess, P. (1985). *Toward healthy aging.* St. Louis, MO: Mosby.

Fulmer, T. (1991a). The geriatric nurse specialist role: A new model. *Nursing Management, 22*(3), 91–93. doi:10.1097/00006247-199103000-00025

Fulmer, T. (1991b). Grow your own experts in hospital elder care: Geriatric clinical specialists can't be everywhere, but they can transform willing medical-surgical nurses into on-site geriatric resources. *Geriatric Nursing, 12*(2), 64–66. doi:10.1016/S0197-4572(09)90116-1

Fulmer, T. (2007). How to try this: Fulmer SPICES. *American Journal of Nursing, 107*, 40–48; quiz 48–49. doi:10.1097/01.naj.0000292197.76076.e1

Fulmer, T. (2015). Geriatric nursing 2.0! *Journal of the American Geriatrics Society, 63*(7), 1453–1458. doi:10.1111/jgs.13492

Fulmer, T., Flaherty, E., & Hyer, K. (2004). The Geriatric Interdisciplinary Team Training (GITT) program. *Gerontology & Geriatrics Education, 24*(2), 3–12. doi:10.1300/j021v24n02_02

Fulmer, T., Hyer, K., Flaherty, E., Mezey, M., Whitelaw, N., Jacobs, M. O., . . . Pfeiffer, E. (2005). Geriatric Interdisciplinary Team Training program: Evaluation results. *Journal of Aging and Health, 17*(4), 443–470. doi:10.1177/0898264305277962

Fulmer, T., Mezey, M., Bottrell, M., Abraham, I., Sazant, J., Grossman, S., & Grisham, E. (2002). Nurses Improving Care for Healthsystem Elders (NICHE): Using outcomes and benchmarks for evidenced-based practice. *Geriatric Nursing, 23*(3), 121–127. doi:10.1067/mgn.2002.125423

Goodnow, M. (1927). *The technic of nursing.* Philadelphia, PA: W. B. Saunders.

Hayflick, L. (1975). Current theories of biological aging. In G. J. Thorbecke (ed.), *Biology of aging and development* (pp. 11–19). New York, NY: Plenum Press.

Kresevic, D., & Naylor, M. (1995). Preventing pressure ulcers through use of protocols in a mentored nursing model. *Geriatric Nursing, 16*(5), 225–229. doi:10.1016/s0197-4572(05)80169-7

Lipsitz, L. A., Wei, J. Y., & Rowe, J. W. (1985). Syncope in an elderly, institutionalised population: Prevalence, incidence, and associated risk. *QJM: An International Journal of Medicine, 55*(1), 45–54. doi:10.1093/oxfordjournals.qjmed.a067852

Mezey, M., Fulmer, T., & Fletcher, K. (2002). A perfect NICHE for gerontology nurses [Editorial]. *Geriatric Nursing, 23*(3), 118. doi:10.1067/mgn.2002.126417

Mezey, M. D., & Lynaugh, J. E. (1989). The teaching nursing home program: Outcomes of care. *The Nursing Clinics of North America, 24*(3), 769–780.

NICHE Project Faculty. (1994). Geriatric models of care: Which one's right for your institution? *American Journal of Nursing, 94*, 21–23. doi:10.2307/3464687

O'Donnell, L., & Solomon, M. Z. (1994). The role of the physician in decisions to use or forgo life-sustaining technologies. In F. Homburger (Ed.), *The rational use of advanced medical technology with the elderly*. New York, NY: Springer Publishing.

Palmer, R. M., Landefeld, C. S., Kresevic, D. M., & Kowal, J. (1994). A medical unit for the acute care of the elderly. *Journal of the American Geriatrics Society, 42*(5), 545–552. doi:10.1111/j.1532-5415.1994.tb04978.x

Resnick, N. M., & Yalla, S. V. (1985). Management of urinary incontinence in the elderly. *New England Journal of Medicine, 313*(13), 800–805. doi:10.1056/nejm198509263131307

Rowe, J. W., & Besdine, R. W. (Eds.). (1982). *Health and disease in old age*. Boston, MA: Little, Brown and Company.

Schneider, E. L., Ory, M., & Aung, M. L. (1987). Teaching nursing homes revisited: Survey of affiliations between American medical schools and long-term–care facilities. *Journal of the American Medical Association, 257*(20), 2771–2775. doi:10.1001/jama.1987.03390200111024

Shock, N. W. (1984). Normal human aging: The Baltimore longitudinal study of aging (NIH Publication #84-2450). Washington, DC: U. S. Government Printing Office.

Siegler, E. L. (1998). *Geriatric interdisciplinary team training*. New York, NY: Springer Publishing.

Skillman, J. (Ed.). (1975). *Surgical intensive care*. Boston, MA: Little, Brown and Company.

Solomon, M. Z. (1995). Seizing the moment: How academic health centers can improve end of-life care. In D. Korn, C. McLaughlin, & M. Osterweis (Eds.), *Academic health centers in the managed care environment*. Washington, DC: Association of Academic Health Centers. Retrieved from https://www.worldcat.org/title/academic-health -centers-in-the-managed-care-environment/oclc/31815017

Solomon M. Z., Guilfoy, V., O'Donnell, L, Jackson, R., Jennings, B., Wolf, S., . . . Koch-Weser, D. (1997). *Faculty guide: Decisions near the end of life*. Newton, MA: Education Development Center. (2nd edition 1997, with Fins, J. J., Crigger, B., & Heller, K. S.).

Solomon, M. Z., Jennings, B., Guilfoy, V., Jackson, R., O'Donnell, L., Wolf, S. M., . . . Donnelley, S. (1991). Toward an expanded vision of clinical ethics education: From the individual to the institution. *Kennedy Institute of Ethics Journal, 1*(3), 225–245. doi:10.1353/ken.0.0051

Solomon, M. Z., O'Donnell, L., Jennings, B., Guilfoy, V., Wolf, S. M., Nolan, K., . . . Donnelley, S. (1993). Decisions near the end of life: Professional views on life-sustaining treatments. *American Journal of Public Health, 83*(1), 14–23. doi:10.2105/ajph.83.1.14

Strumpf, N. E., & Evans, L. K. (1988). Physical restraint of the hospitalized elderly: Perceptions of patients and nurses. *Nursing Research, 37*(3), 132–137. doi:10.1097/00006199-198805000-00002

Wells, T. J., Brink, C. A., & Diokno, A. C. (1987). Urinary incontinence in elderly women: Clinical findings. *Journal of the American Geriatrics Society, 35*(10), 933–939. doi:10.1111/j.1532-5415.1987.tb02295.x

Appendix 2.1

Tracie Nolan Kientz
3544 Dutchman Rd.
Charlottesville, VA 22901

Terry Fulmer
Columbia University School of Nursing
630 West 168th St.
New York, NY 10032

June 30, 1994

Dear Terry,

It's been in my mind to write you for a while. I think now is a good time because it is truly NICHE EVE here for me at UVA. Kathy Fletcher and I will begin rounds in the CCU early in July. Two of my co-workers had the opportunity to meet Kathy at a physical assessment class given at the School of Nursing this past week. They both said they now see why I've been so excited to work with Kathy. They found her a wonderful teacher and could tell how much she cares about the elderly. I'm excited that they feel this way and think it can only help the whole process we are about to begin.

I had a difficult spring but have bounced back nicely. I had a cervical laminectomy April 5. Talk about a threat to one's functional capacity! But what good lessons I learned as a nurse—especially one that wants to help our elderly patients. I'm doing very well, with complete relief of my symptoms.

When I got back to work after my surgery I felt a little overwhelmed by all of the geriatric issues I saw in our patients. There really are many issues once your assessment skills expand beyond the immediate concerns of blood pressure and oxygenation. It seems I see the issues more clearly than before and I'm learning all the time.

I am feeling more and more support towards improving the care of our geriatric patients. One of our nursing attendants told me she was glad someone was bringing this information into the unit. This same person figured out how to clear up a skin problem in one of our long-term patients. She received written praise for this.

We had an elderly patient from a nursing home this week. The RN caring for her was concerned about the patient's mental status and anxiety level. This RN called the nursing home from which the elderly woman came and discovered she was on Ativan TID. The RN obtained an order for the Ativan and the patient was able to relax and have a good visit with her family. This same woman died the next night.

Another RN I work with did a wonderful pre-op assessment of an elderly woman going for coronary bypass.

This RN found out information about the patient's history of urinary incontinence, difficulty ambulating, and history of a fecal impaction on a previous hospitalization. As you know, any one of these issues could have a huge impact on the woman's post-op course. We wrote the information in the chart for her post-op nurses. I told my coworkers what a great job they did and how much they helped these two elderly patients.

It was such a wonderful experience to be able to spend time with you back in March. There are times and people in one's career that turn out to be real pointers for the future. I will never forget how you bent down to speak to that elderly patient we visited, or how you spoke to and praised the nurse that was caring for that patient. That's the essence of all this for me, right there, in that moment.

It's the magic part of leadership in nursing that we both get to share. Thanks for bringing me in and I hope our paths cross again.

Sincerely,

Tracie Nolan Kientz

Tracie Nolan Kientz

Initial NICHE Momentum: The Hospital Outcomes Program for the Elderly (HOPE) Project

3

Terry Fulmer, Marquis D. Foreman, and Denise Kresevic

Having the NICHE program as part of Ascension Health has been a foundational element for strengthening our holistic care models, that are team-based, with an emphasis on highly reliable care. The learning and journey of NICHE will surely inform today's healthcare systems as they build integrated systems of care across the continuum with a special focus on needs and individual desires of each older adult. This will be a crucial part of health and healthcare delivery for the foreseeable future that will decrease unnecessary cost from preventable harm and promote wellness and healthy aging across the care continuum.

—Ann Hendrich, PhD, RN, FAAN, Senior Vice President and Chief Quality/Safety and Nursing Officer

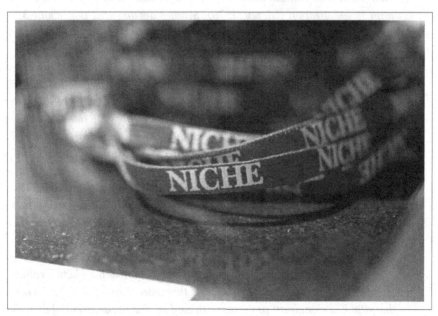

CHAPTER OBJECTIVES

1. Describe the components and evaluation of the HOPE project
2. Describe the three nursing models tested in the HOPE project
3. Discuss the foundational impact of HOPE on NICHE
4. Review the selection and implementation of the four hospitals that served as pilot sites for full-scale NICHE implementation

INTRODUCTION

The John A. Hartford Foundation (JAHF) was one of the first foundations to take on the thorny work of improving hospital care for older adults. The Hospital Outcomes Project for the Elderly (HOPE) was conceptualized under the leadership of the then senior program officer Donna I. Regenstreif, PhD, who worked with the trustees to conceive a program that would focus on the reduction of functional decline during hospitalization. The reasons for this work were many. There was mounting evidence that functional status decline was prevalent in hospitalized older adults (Margitić et al., 1993). It was recognized that while nurses were in a pivotal position to prevent this decline, few had sufficient training to do so.

Patients aged 65 years and older in the early 1990s constituted more than 40% of patients hospitalized on medical and surgical units of acute hospitals (Fulmer et al., 2002). U.S. hospital beds were increasingly becoming filled with adults over 65 and each year the acuteness of elder patients in hospital expanded. Many older individuals were discharged in poorer health than when they were admitted and found it took longer to recover after hospitalization (Mezey, 1979). Studies documented that about 33% of individuals were not able to perform daily living activities any better than they could before admission (Landefeld, Palmer, Kresevic, Fortinsky, & Kowal, 1995). In fact, many were less functional at discharge than prior to admission. This phenomenon appeared to be multifactorial and included the influences of acute illness superimposed on chronic illness as well as iatrogenic factors including bedrest and nothing by mouth (NPO) status.

Older adults, then and now, have preexisting functional dependencies that make them more vulnerable to further decline and functional loss. Up to 50% of older hospitalized patients experience functional decline, that is, a reduction in physical or cognitive function. Functional decline occurs when a person is unable to engage in daily living activities and typically begins a day after hospital admission. The loss of function is correlated with prolonged hospital stays, mortality rate increase, institutionalization, rehabilitation, and healthcare expenditure increase (Inouye et al., 1990). An acute hospitalization can be a life-changing event for an older person because the independence that has been supported for years is suddenly gone. Loss of independence can be explained through enforced bedrest, use of sedating drugs, indwelling bladder catheters, and physical restraints. Warshaw et al. (1982) found that more than 50% of elderly patients in a general hospital had significant problems with confusion and the essential daily functions of walking, bathing, dressing, and eating. Acute confusion is also a common disorder among hospitalized patients. When a patient with dementia or other mental illness becomes delirious, the acute confusion is often overlooked by healthcare professionals because of the dementia label on their medical record.

Care of older adults in all clinical settings needed to shift to prevent the problematic geriatric syndromes.

It was in this context that the JAHF initiated the HOPE project. Care of older adults in all clinical settings needed to shift to prevent the problematic geriatric syndromes. In the acute care setting, the most common approach was to treat the illness rather than employ preventive techniques to ensure the safety and comfort of the older patient. The purpose of this chapter is to describe the HOPE project and explain its foundational relationship to Nurses Improving Care for Healthsystem Elders (NICHE).

THE HOPE PROJECT (1989–1992)

HOPE consisted of a series of six interdisciplinary clinical studies aimed at reducing functional decline in the acutely ill hospitalized elderly. It was a prospective, multicenter pooled analysis project involving collection of a common set of data from a group of related but distinct intervention trials with similar objectives. The enrollment settings were five university-affiliated hospitals and one community hospital that formed the settings for enrollment of older patients (age minimums from 65 to 75 years) admitted for a range of acute illnesses. Site-specific interventions included exercise and physical therapy; developing and implementing methods to improve detection and evaluation of delirious patients; a multidisciplinary geriatric care unit; a multidisciplinary intervention implemented in-hospital that included some post discharge care; and a nursing-centered geriatric care program (GCP; Landefeld et al., 1995; Table 3.1). The prospective, multicenter design of HOPE provided an innovative approach for analysis of hospital outcomes in the elderly. The differences in study populations and interventions were examined through qualitative comparisons across sites, which enhanced generalizability. The pooled analysis of HOPE was extremely rigorous and conceptualized to detect the primary and secondary outcomes at the six sites. The stated primary meta-analytic outcomes were functional status measures and there were eight secondary domains: neurocognitive function, mobility, healthcare utilization, hospital costs, quality of life, all-cause mortality, number of hospital readmissions, and nursing home placements.

THE HOPE NURSING MODELS

What is most germane to NICHE (Margitić, Morgan, Sager, & Furberg, 1995) from the HOPE program were the three nurse-led geriatric care models that were imbedded and de facto funded as a part of the study. This was an enormous boon to these three nursing models in that HOPE provided rigorous evidence for the success of the models. These models would not have been funded by the National

TABLE 3.1 Original HOPE Sites

SITE	PURPOSE
Cedars-Sinai Medical Center (Los Angeles, CA)	For the development of an in-hospital "conditioning" program to maximize physical fitness, and the testing of this program in a randomized trial of acute hospital patients over the age of 70.
St. Mary's Hospital Medical Center (Madison, WI)	For a clinical test of a multidisciplinary intervention program, both preventive and therapeutic in nature, for elderly patients admitted for problems typically associated with a high degree of functional dependency at discharge (e.g., stroke, pneumonia, hip and other joint procedures). The Medical Center will compare the functional status of three groups of patients after discharge—a control group of those who have received usual care, a group which has received an intervention via a multidisciplinary team, and a group which has received not only the inpatient team intervention but also follow-up care after discharge.
Stanford University (Stanford, CA)	For a program specifically geared to address loss of mobility among elderly patients. This project will not only compare the functional outcomes of patients in a control group with those who have undergone a specially designed regimen of physical therapy but will also focus on evaluating the impact of personal attention and optimism on the part of caregivers in the patient's improvement.
University Hospitals of Cleveland (Cleveland, OH)	For a two-phased program aimed at a better understanding of the causes, and the potential prevention, of what University researchers have identified as "Hospital Dysfunctional Syndrome" among elderly patients. To curtail the tendency toward this syndrome, University Hospitals will test the effectiveness of a special unit for the acute care of the elderly (ACE), a unit characterized by an atmosphere of special treatment, caring, and concern for functional preservation and independence.
University of Chicago (Chicago, IL)	For a two-pronged approach to identifying and treating delirium among hospitalized elderly, since patients who develop delirium during their hospital stay are among those at high risk for the personal, social, and financial trauma of subsequent nursing home placement. The specific goal of this project is to test whether the use of a standardized assessment protocol, administered by geriatric and nursing consultants, can reduce the morbidity associated with delirium, and thus improve the short- and long-term functioning of elderly patients.

Institutes of Health (NIH) or other major foundations at that time, largely because nursing was emerging as a scientific discipline and few nurses had PhDs or a track record of research that would merit such funding. Fulmer (NICHE), Foreman (delirium nurse specialist), and Kresevic (acute care of the elderly [ACE] unit) all had the unique opportunity to engage in a prospective meta-analysis study in an interdisciplinary context. Dr. Curt Furberg, one of the nation's leading scientists in meta-analysis at Bowman Gray Medical Center, was the principal investigator of the data-coordinating center, lending enormous intellect and credibility to the study and to the nursing model outcomes. As noted earlier, six medical centers received grants totaling over $2.5 million to develop, implement, and evaluate interventions designed to reduce functional deterioration of "hospitalized elders," the term then used (Landefeld et al., 1995). The inception of HOPE was linked to a recognition that hospitals, oriented to high technology and life-threatening acute illnesses, do not attach as high a priority to the preservation of patients' function. These awards began in July 1989 and were completed by 1992. Three of the projects (University of Chicago, University Hospitals of Cleveland, and Yale New Haven Hospital) underlined the role of nursing in achieving better patient outcomes and had embedded nursing models.

> *The inception of HOPE was linked to a recognition that hospitals, oriented to high technology and life-threatening acute illnesses, do not attach as high a priority to the preservation of patients' function.*

The Chicago Nursing Model

The Chicago Nursing Model, developed at the University of Chicago Hospitals, provided for consultation and education by a doctorally prepared gerontological nurse specialist (GNS) to improve nurses' accuracy and speed in detecting and managing delirium in hospitalized elderly patients. Specifically, nurses were taught (a) the use and interpretation of simple bedside tests for assessing cognition; (b) the clinical features that distinguish delirium, dementia, and depression; (c) when and how to communicate symptoms to physicians; (d) common causes of delirium in this patient population; (e) independent, interdependent, and dependent strategies for preventing and managing delirium; and (f) how to document findings in the hospital record. Nurses received direct instruction on all study units and on every shift. The instruction was repeated once for reinforcement. Nurses were given preprinted assessment forms and a large poster summarizing all essential aspects of instruction was placed in a prominent location in each nursing station. In addition, the model provided for consultation from the GNS. While the GNS model had been used in a few other hospitals to provide geriatric support to nurses in hospitals, no prior program had measured the effect of the GNS model in alleviating one discrete clinical problem.

The Cleveland Nursing Model

The Cleveland Nursing Model, developed at University Hospitals of Cleveland in conjunction with the Frances Payne Bolton School of Nursing at Case Western Reserve University, tested the efficacy of a specialty unit in preventing functional decline in acutely ill medical patients. A 29-bed medical–surgical nursing unit was renovated in preparation for the study. This ACE unit was designed with special attention to the physical environment, interdisciplinary rounds, collaborative team building, and development of nurse-initiated clinical protocols of care. Clinicians worked with designers to adapt the environment in ways that enhance function. Soft colors, which have a calming effect, were used for patients' rooms. Geometrical hallway carpeting helped patients pace their activity. An activity room for congregate meals, visiting, and art and music therapy was decorated in vivid colors. Levers replaced doorknobs for easy access. Patients' rooms contained recliners and low beds with automatic night lights. Collaborative team building began with interdisciplinary in-service education and workshops. Nurses working closely with an interdisciplinary team developed preventive and restorative clinical protocols as appropriate. And, unlike previous models using geriatric experts as consultants, in this model the geriatric medical director and clinical nurse specialist held complementary roles that included direct care, mentoring, and education.

Sustaining the ACE units has continued to be a challenge. However, the original Cleveland ACE unit has been expanded to two units: one surgical with an emphasis on orthopedic surgery patients and a medical ACE unit. The protocols and geriatric resource nurse (GRN) training has been disseminated throughout the healthcare system. Currently, there are over 200 ACE units internationally.

The Yale GRN Model

The objective of the Yale New Haven Hospital model was to develop and implement an integrated, unit-based, nurse-centered GCP involving an integrated model of GRNs, gerontological nurse specialists (GNSs), primary nurses, and a geriatrician on the geriatric care team (GCT). From the outset, the overall project was divided into two parallel programs: the GCP, concerned with the clinical intervention, and the GCP Evaluation Project, concerned with evaluating the efficacy of the intervention. Four target conditions, referred to as "geriatric vital signs," were selected to serve as markers of general functional decline in the hospitalized elderly: delirium, decline in physical functioning, incontinence, and decubiti. The overall hypothesis of the study was that, through improved recognition, prevention, and effective remedial therapy, the target conditions would be reduced in the intervention group as compared with the nonintervention group. High-level, mid-level, and control interventions were implemented on both medical and surgical services. The high-level units received the full intervention model (GRNs, GNSs, and a physician-based GCT). The so-called mid-level units received only the nursing component (GRNs and GNSs) but not the physician-based GCT. Standard care was provided on the control units.

The program was based on the following beliefs:

1. Primary nurses know the most about the day-to-day patterns and problems of the elderly who come to their units.

2. Primary nurses, by serving as GRNs, are more likely to integrate new behaviors into practice because of the unit-based visibility and regular feedback available.

3. A GRN program can provide recognition of expertise and later might be reflected in a clinical ladder program for primary nurses. To support the learning needs of the GRNs, a monthly geriatric nursing interest group conference was established for teaching purposes and the exchange of ideas (Fulmer, 1991b).

Today, there are well over 1,000 GRNs functioning in a variety of settings and capacities across the country and around the world. The model has been disseminated broadly through the NICHE program at New York University (NYU) and the body of literature in Medline shows the evidence and impact of GRNs.

These three models from the HOPE project were and are exciting for several reasons. They underscore that there is a variety of ways to improve nursing care for geriatric patients. While commonalities of the models are translatable irrespective of setting, the models also need to be "customized" to allow for differences in nursing systems and hospital environments. For those systems that do not have dedicated geriatric evaluation units, the geriatric nurse resource model provides an excellent alternative. The geriatric nursing models also suggest that improvements in nurses' attitudes toward the elderly and higher work satisfaction can go hand in hand with improvements in care.

HOPE NURSING MODEL OUTCOMES

The project at the University Hospitals of Cleveland demonstrated that ACE unit patients had better function at discharge when compared with controls. ACE unit nursing appeared to be a key component in this achievement. It consisted of an individualized patient-centered care program that varies in accordance with nurses' diagnoses of patients' needs. ACE unit nurses were empowered to initiate patient management interventions developed in consultation with a geriatric nurse clinician. They also presented information on each of their patients (i.e., admission status, progress, discharge plans) at daily multidisciplinary meetings held on the unit.

Yale's HOPE intervention used a GRN (trained and supported by a geriatric clinical nurse specialist) as the primary care nurse of elders at greatest risk of functional deterioration (Fulmer, 1991a, 1991b). This GRN also served as a unit-based consultant to other primary care nurses for patients under their care. Yale's high-risk experimental patients experienced 30% to 40% less functional loss than controls.

The Chicago HOPE project involved education and consultation for staff nurses relative to assessment, prevention, and management of delirium. While it failed to show any statistically significant changes in the detection of delirium in hospitalized elders, it did demonstrate the utility of enhancing nurses' capacity for such a role (Foreman, 1984, 1986).

Because of the high level of nursing interest at the meeting of HOPE sites held in San Francisco in June 1991, provision was made in the 1992 JAHF

Aging and Health Program budget to convene a meeting of leading hospital nurse executives to review the HOPE projects' nursing components and suggest ways in which they might be used to improve hospital care of the elderly. At an April 1992 meeting of JAHF staff and HOPE faculty, a strategy was developed involving (a) workshops on geriatric inpatient care for diverse hospital nursing audiences and (b) assistance to hospital administrators in assessing and improving their institutions' geriatric nursing. Both components of the strategy would draw primarily on new knowledge gained through HOPE projects.

STARTING NICHE (1992–1994)

Columbia University's School of Nursing with the NYU Division of Nursing (Terry Fulmer, Mathy Mezey) sought Foundation support for a project to improve inpatient geriatric nursing through the workshops and assessments proposed in the April 1992 meeting.

Four workshops would take place under the proposed project in conjunction with annual meetings of the following: American Association of Colleges of Nursing, which represents educators and administrators from 424 undergraduate and graduate programs in nursing; the Association of Nurse Executives, which then had over 5,000 members made up of nurse executives and managers in acute care hospitals; the Gerontological Society of America, which included about 1,000 nurses in its Clinical Medicine Section; and Sigma Theta Tau International, the 160,000-member nursing honor society. A portion of the cost of the conferences was supported by the Foundation, but a registration fee was charged to defray some expenses and ensure commitment from attendees and their sponsoring hospitals.

Under the proposed project, hospitals sponsoring nurses' attendance at the above conferences would be eligible to compete for assistance in assessing and improving their geriatric nursing care. The organizational assessment component would have several phases. "Best Nursing Practice" protocols reflecting consensus of an expert panel would be developed in key areas. These would build on HOPE project protocols for such syndromes as confusion, incontinence, skin breakdown, and so on. The protocols, which would be published, would become the basis of an organizational Geriatric Institutional Assessment Questionnaire (GIAP). Four hospitals chosen competitively from a pool of applicants would receive technical assistance in the form of both a site visit and subsequent consultation to make changes identified through their organizational assessments. The approach could be easily replicated if well received by the four "pilot" hospitals.

The project, led by Fulmer, at Columbia would be accomplished in partnership with the New York University School of Nursing and Education Development Center (EDC), Inc. of Newton, MA. Mathy Mezey, EdD, RN, then director of the Geriatric Nurse Clinician Program at NYU, would be responsible for the national nursing conference workshops and publications. EDC, under the direction of its Vice President Cheryl Vince-Whitman, MEd, would provide administrative support for the workshops and aid in development of the organizational assessment tool and the design of on-site technical assistance. This work provided an opportunity for the Foundation to build on the nursing advances of its HOPE project to improve inpatient care consistent with the goals of that program. The project implemented a strategy conceived by hospital nursing leaders regarding effective ways to use HOPE findings for the much needed goal of care improvement for older persons in hospitals.

In September 1992, the first nurse-led project was successfully taken to and approved by the Board of Trustees of the JAHF, entitled "Building on HOPE Projects to Improve Geriatric Nursing Care."

In September 1992, the first nurse-led project was successfully taken to and approved by the Board of Trustees of the JAHF, entitled "Building on HOPE Projects to Improve Geriatric Nursing Care." The Columbia University School of Nursing (TF), with the NYU Division of Nursing (MM) and EDC (CVW), had as its goals:

- To convene four conferences linked to national professional meetings

- To publish articles in nursing journals

- To develop an assessment tool that hospitals can use to evaluate the quality of their geriatric care

- To provide on-site technical assistance to the four hospitals as they implement the assessment tool to increase the skill of their nursing staff and improve the hospital environment in care of elderly patients

With this approval, NICHE was underway. The NICHE Advisory Board was convened to construct the GIAP and a call for applications was announced to interested clinical sites. Twenty-three applications resulted in the selection of four hospitals. Each hospital was required to complete the GIAP prior to the first site visit. This strategy served to engage hospitals early on in thinking about their own care and practices and set the stage for the establishment of an ambitious time table for project completion. Monthly phone calls (not originally planned for) provided the much needed additional support at each site. Information was then shared across all hospitals to maximize the learning experience of each.

Key factors for institutional success as cited by the investigators were leadership skills of the on-site project leader, including depth of geriatric expertise and organizational savvy in implementing change, administrative support for the project leader as well as the project goals, and, finally, mentoring by advance practice nurses with experience in interdisciplinary work.

Key factors for institutional success as cited by the investigators were leadership skills of the on-site project leader, including depth of geriatric expertise and organizational savvy in implementing change, administrative support for the project leader as well as the project goals, and, finally, mentoring by advance practice nurses with experience in interdisciplinary work. The mandate for interdisciplinary work is patient driven. The care of elders often requires nurses, physicians, and other professionals to function as an integrated team capable of forming goals that incorporate the services of more than one discipline. Each of the four hospitals benefited by early dissemination of the knowledge gained in the HOPE projects and by the carefully constructed processes of technical assistance. This formed the basis of the project, that is, utilization of guidelines to support decision making, accessibility to experts in the field, and ongoing coaching as new skills are developed.

After review and deliberation, the University of Virginia Medical Center (Ivo Abraham), the University of California Davis Medical Center (Deborah Francis), Methodist Hospital of Indiana (Anne Hendrich), and Northern Iowa Mercy Health Centers (Lark Simon) were selected as the inaugural NICHE sites. Over 18 months, five conferences served as the vehicle to educate nurse leaders about geriatric care models offered at well-attended national professional meetings. The project team also developed two generic tools to help hospital nursing staffs improve their care. The first was the GIAP, created and used to evaluate the quality of care. The other tool was the clinical protocol set (sleep disorders, incontinence, restraint management, and decubitus ulcers) for nurses to use in treating hospitalized elders, which was completed and published.

The four hospitals received help in adapting a geriatric nursing model on pilot units. Each was provided technical assistance in the form of site visits, conference calls, and written materials to assess and improve practice. Project implementation costs (estimated to be about $5,000 per site) were assumed by the hospitals, each of which involved its senior executives. The hospitals soon after began to export the models to units beyond those used as pilots to initiate the spread and scale, which was important to embedding the new models. The clinical protocols, now a book in its fifth edition, have been published or accepted for publication in prominent nursing journals and are raising awareness about effective hospital geriatric nursing care (Boltz, Capezuti, Fulmer, & Zwicker, 2016). The Foundation saw promise in the work and at the March 1995 Trustee Board meeting another grant was made to the NYU Division of Nursing to ensure the spread and scale of NICHE as we know it today.

CHAPTER SUMMARY

The JAHF initiated the HOPE project in 1989 to reduce functional decline and harm in older adults during hospitalization. This project was intended to address the prevalence of a loss of physical or cognitive function in older adults during hospitalization, which results in longer hospital stays, increased mortality rates, and greater expense. HOPE consisted of six interdisciplinary clinical studies conducted at six different sites that compared the outcomes of various interventions—such as exercise, physical therapy, detection and evaluation of delirium, and several forms of multidisciplinary geriatric care—in older hospitalized patients who were acutely ill.

HOPE incorporated three different nurse-led geriatric care models: the Chicago, Cleveland, and Yale GRN nursing models. The Chicago model involved a GNS training nurses on how to improve their accuracy and speed in detecting and managing delirium in older hospitalized patients. The Cleveland model involved creating and implementing a special unit focused on providing acute care for older adults. The Yale GRN model involved developing and implementing an integrated, unit-based, nurse-centered program providing geriatric care via a team consisting of GRNs, GNSs, primary nurses, and a geriatrician. The Cleveland and Yale models resulted in significant reduction in functional loss among older hospitalized patients compared with controls, whereas the Chicago model did not. Today there are several evidence-based geriatric care models that improve care for older adults (Malone, Capezuti, & Palmer, 2015).

The HOPE project spawned a proposed strategy developed by attendees of a meeting of JAHF staff and HOPE faculty in April 1992 to implement workshops on geriatric inpatient care and to provide assistance to hospital administrators to assess and improve geriatric nursing. Dr. Fulmer at Columbia University's School of Nursing and Dr. Mezey at the New York University School of Nursing then sought and received funding from the JAHF to develop a project to implement these proposed interventions. After successful implementation of this project at four initial sites, additional funding was provided to establish NICHE as a permanent organization.

REFERENCES

Boltz, M., Capezuti, E., Fulmer, T. T., & Zwicker, D. (Eds.). (2016). *Evidence-based geriatric nursing protocols for best practice* (5th ed.). New York, NY: Springer Publishing.

Foreman, M. D. (1984). Acute confusional states in the elderly: An algorithm. *Dimensions of Critical Care Nursing, 3*, 207–215. doi:10.1097/00003465-198407000-00003

Foreman, M. D. (1986). Acute confusional states in hospitalized elderly: A research dilemma. *Nursing Research, 35*(1), 34–38. doi:10.1097/00006199-198601000-00008

Fulmer, T. (1991a). The geriatric nurse specialist role: A new model. *Nursing Management, 22*(3), 91–93. doi:10.1097/00006247-199103000-00025

Fulmer, T. (1991b). Grow your own experts in hospital elder care. *Geriatric Nursing, 12*(2), 64–66. doi:10.1016/s0197-4572(09)90116-1

Fulmer, T., Mezey, M., Bottrell, M., Abraham, I., Sazant, J., Grossman, S., & Grisham, E. (2002). Nurses Improving Care for Healthsystem Elders (NICHE): Using outcomes and benchmarks for evidenced-based practice. *Geriatric Nursing, 23*(3), 121–127. doi:10.1067/mgn.2002.125423

Inouye, S. K., van Dyck, C. H., Alessi, C. A., Balkin, S., Siegal, A. P., & Horwitz, R. I. (1990). Clarifying confusion: The confusion assessment method: A new method for detection of delirium. *Annals of Internal Medicine, 113*(12), 941–948. doi:10.7326/0003-4819-113-12-941

Landefeld, C. S., Palmer, R. M., Kresevic, D. M., Fortinsky, R. H., & Kowal, J. (1995). A randomized trial of care in a hospital medical unit especially designed to improve the functional outcomes of acutely ill older patients. *New England Journal of Medicine, 332*(20), 1338–1344. doi:10.1056/nejm199505183322006

Malone, M. L., Capezuti, E., & Palmer, R. M. (Eds.). (2015). *Geriatric models of care.* New. York, NY: Springer.

Margitić, S. E., Inouye, S. K., Thomas, J. L., Cassel, C. K., Regenstreif, D. I., & Kowal, J. (1993). Hospital Outcomes Project for the Elderly (HOPE): Rationale and design for a prospective pooled analysis. *Journal of the American Geriatrics Society*, *41*(3), 258–267. doi:10.1111/j.1532-5415.1993.tb06703.x

Margitić, S. E., Morgan, T. M., Sager, M. A., & Furberg, C. D. (1995). Lessons learned from a prospective meta-analysis. *Journal of the American Geriatrics Society*, *43*(4), 435–439. doi:10.1111/j.1532-5415.1995.tb05820.x

Mezey, M. (1979). *Stress, hospitalization and aging*. In American Nurses Association (Ed.), Clinical and Scientific Sessions [NP-59] (pp. 123–132). Kansas City, MO: American Nurses Association Publication Unit.

Warshaw, G. A., Moore, J. T., Friedman, S. W., Currie, C. T., Kennie, D. C., Kane, W. J., & Mears, P. A. (1982). Functional disability in the hospitalized elderly. *Journal of the American Medical Association*, *248*(7), 847–850. doi:10.1001/jama.1982.03330070035026

The NICHE Theory of Change: The Power of Convening and Evidence

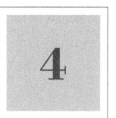

Terry Fulmer and Mathy Mezey

Our NICHE program has assisted us in transforming the care of our older patients and energizing a staff that is very proud of that care. The geriatric resource nurse training has led our teams to modify practices to promote the evidence-based best care to our patients. We now identify with every patient and family what matters to them so that we can personalize care. As we recognize the specialty care that our older patients require, I strongly recommend the NICHE program to assist staff in developing the education and skills to help patients maintain the highest quality of life.
—Barbara Jacobs, PhD, RN, FAAN, Senior Vice President and Chief Quality / Safety and Nursing Officer of Ascension Healthcare

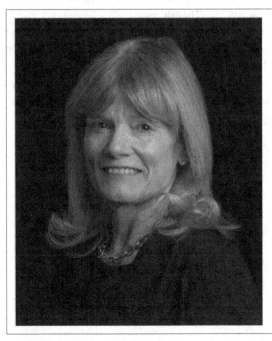 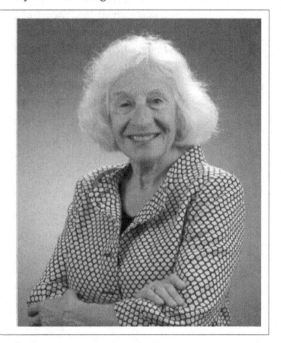

From left: Terry Fulmer, Mathy Mezey.

CHAPTER OBJECTIVES

1. Understand the theory of change for NICHE
2. Reflect on using evidence as a lever for change
3. Discuss the power of convening for accelerating change

INTRODUCTION

The original Nurses Improving Care for Healthsystem Elders (NICHE) grant, awarded by The John A. Hartford Foundation in 1992, used the principles described in Chapter 2 with the Education Development Center (EDC) framework for change. Today, this is often referred to as a "theory of change." Solomon noted that in order to spur self-reflection and change, institutions need data that reflect their reality. The theory of change, first conceptualized by Thomas Kuhn in 1963, was developed specifically to discuss change in the world of science and to debunk the notion that scientific change is linear in process (Kuhn, 1963). Kuhn discussed the "concept of development by accumulation." Kurt Lewin was a major figure in bringing the theory of change to the forefront, describing a three-stage model that has been extremely influential in helping organizations consider the approach and steps included in the change process (Figure 4.1; Lewin, 1947). Decades later, we use the theory of change to articulate how an organization is going to achieve its objectives. Berman has written about the "theory of the foundation" (2016) and how once a foundation expresses its core purpose and mission for social change, it will use active partnerships, collaborations, advocacy, and communication to make change. The foundation will draw talent from a much broader array of sectors and try to develop a social compact to drive change around a particular issue. In retrospect, it seems clear that The John A. Hartford Foundation was doing just that. The change envisioned was better care for older adults and NICHE was one strategy that fit their theory of change.

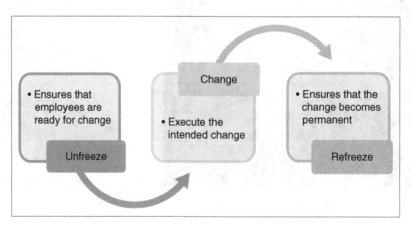

FIGURE 4.1 *Lewin's three-stage model of change.*

THE NICHE THEORY OF CHANGE

NICHE itself, as a program for improving nursing care of older adults, had a theory of change, although it was not articulated in these words at that time. The NICHE theory of change included the belief that in order to improve the care of older adults in the practice of nursing, it was essential to have baseline evidence related to nurses' perceptions of the practice environment, their own knowledge, and their attitudes about care of older adults in order to create goals for improvement. Another key component of the change theory was the requisite use of evidence-based practice protocols that could be used uniformly across NICHE settings. A further component of the NICHE theory of change was the requirement for the hospital to identify NICHE leaders and geriatric resource nurse (GRN) champions who could implement the evidence-based practice protocols on a day-to-day basis. Finally, the theory of change incorporated what we refer to as the "power of convening." The first NICHE conference took place in 1993 with the goal of gaining support and influencing key stakeholders, such as chief nursing officers and academic leaders, to accelerate the spread and scale of the ideas embedded in the NICHE model. The NICHE program had three key constructs in the theory: evidence, communication, and influence.

The NICHE program had three key constructs in the theory: evidence, communication, and influence.

Building upon the knowledge gained from the Hospital Outcomes Project for the Elderly (HOPE; Chapter 3), the objectives of this ambitious project as originally defined and slightly expanded after 6 months included:

- Development of practice protocols for frequently encountered problems of hospitalized elderly (EVIDENCE)

- Development of a Geriatric Institutional Assessment Protocol (GIAP) for assessing the perceived quality of geriatric care (EVIDENCE)

- On-site technical assistance to four competitively selected hospitals as they implemented the GIAP (INFLUENCE)

- Implementation of a HOPE practice model, and use of evidence-based geriatric practice protocols (EVIDENCE)

- Convening in the form of four conferences to disseminate outcomes of the HOPE projects (INFLUENCE/COMMUNICATION)

- Dissemination strategies including publication of the work in professional journals and national presentations (EVIDENCE/COMMUNICATION/INFLUENCE)

The NICHE approach encompassed a philosophy of parsimony, for example, the use of existing talent and resources to efficiently maximize outcomes. The NICHE program leaders appointed an Advisory Board of national geriatric nurse experts for protocol development, development, and review of the GIAP and development and review of the application packet (including a Request for Proposals). Finally, the NICHE Advisory Board served as the review body for the competitive selection process. Four protocols (physical restraints, sleep disorders, urinary incontinence, and pressure ulcers) were developed, reviewed, and finalized. These syndromes were selected for their representativeness of common geriatric problems that make care of older adults complex and lead to harm.

The GIAP was modeled after the "Decisions Near the End of Life Institutional Profile." It was designed to test attitudes regarding elder care, knowledge of institutional guidelines, care involving practice areas covered by the protocols, and perceived impediments to care and demographic data. This instrument was appropriately piloted and tested in phase 1 of the NICHE program for reliability and validity before use with the selected hospitals (see Chapter 3). The NICHE staff quickly provided GIAP data to hospitals regarding current care and therefore offered each institution the ability to selectively intervene to improve care.

Joining the original NICHE cohort of hospitals was a competitive process. In the first round, 23 applications resulted in the selection of four hospitals. Getting selected was perceived by hospitals as an extremely beneficial and prideful moment (INFLUENCE). Each selected hospital was then required to complete the GIAP prior to the first site visit by NICHE faculty consultants (EVIDENCE). This strategy served to engage hospitals early on in thinking about their own care practices and to set the stage for the establishment of an ambitious time table for project completion (EVIDENCE/COMMUNICATION). Monthly phone calls between the NICHE directors (Terry Fulmer, Mathy Mezey, and Cheryl Vince-Whitman) and the four sites, not originally planned for in the work (COMMUNICATION), provided additional support at each and across sites. New learnings were shared across all hospitals to maximize the experience of each site (COMMUNICATION/ INFLUENCE/EVIDENCE).

Key factors for institutional success as noted by the four sites included the leadership skills of the on-site project leader, including depth of geriatric expertise and organizational savvy in implementing change; administrative support for the project leader; clarity of the project goals; and finally, evidence of experience with and to some degree success with interdisciplinary work. The need for interdisciplinary work was patient driven. The care of older adults requires nurses, physicians, and other professionals to function as an integrated team capable of forming goals that incorporate the services of more than one discipline. This was a shared experience across the sites (Fulmer, Flaherty, & Hyer, 2004; Hyer, Fairchild, Abraham, Mezey, & Fulmer, 2000).

Each of the four hospitals benefited by early dissemination of the knowledge gained in the HOPE projects and by the carefully constructed processes of technical assistance that formed the basis of this project, that is, utilization of guidelines to support decision making, accessibility to experts in the field, and ongoing coaching as new skills were developed (COMMUNICATION/INFLUENCE).

A limitation of the early model was that the evaluation component required more time and resources than originally anticipated. This issue was identified early on by the sites; they requested a 6-month extension without funding to complete their GIAP and protocol work. This extension enabled better review of GIAP results on-site, but did not address the further goal of systematic review and data sharing across settings.

The importance of evaluation data linked to outcomes of patient care is more critical now than ever given the complexity of care and multiple chronic conditions that coexist in older adults. Competing demands for resources highlight the need for data-based decisions that are readily available and understood at the point of care. As successful strategies in the care of older adults are achieved, quantified results are essential factors for institutional decision making (EVIDENCE/INFLUENCE/COMMUNICATION).

As successful strategies in the care of older adults are achieved, quantified results are essential factors for institutional decision making.

POWER OF CONVENING

The power of convening cannot be overestimated. In the first 18 months of NICHE, five conferences were held that were linked to national meetings across the country. Attendance was estimated at approximately 150 to 160 individuals per conference. One measure of the effectiveness of this approach was the request of NICHE faculty to speak at meetings, such as the Annual American Journal of Nursing Medical-Surgical/Gerontological Nursing Conference and a preconference workshop of the Gerontological Society. This program objective for national presentations was fully met and exceeded.

By 1995, six articles were published or accepted for publication in nursing journals (COMMUNICATION/EVIDENCE). These two forms of dissemination allowed thousands of nurses to benefit from the knowledge gained in both the HOPE and NICHE projects. In summary, the breadth and depth of the early phase of NICHE were impressive.

IMPACT/DISSEMINATION

Professionals strive to provide the best care possible. One way to do this is to make new knowledge available for utilization in practice. NICHE successfully fast-tracked knowledge utilization by skillfully combining multiple strategies that have been refined over time. The application process in the early days engaged hospitals in thinking through their own issues in the care of the elderly; it was not simple and required commitment from not only those completing the application but also senior executives, who had to sign a letter of commitment to the process (Appendix 4.1). This was extremely important to gain complete buy-in across the organization. From data gathering to model selection and implementation, each hospital "owned" their project. Thus, the NICHE project leaders were able to facilitate institution-specific work by bringing resources to the staff based on their identified needs. In addition, through conferences and the literature, thousands of nurses have been informed about this work with the ability to positively improve the care and lives of hospitalized elders across the country. Today, the membership model is another method of showing commitment to practice change for older adults.

EARLY NICHE EVALUATION

Experts were brought in by The John A. Hartford Foundation to evaluate NICHE progress and Mary Patricia (Trish) Gibbons, PhD, RN was the 1995 evaluator who commented at that time:

> Suggestions have already been made concerning the need to further evaluate the outcomes of the NICHE program. A next step would be to support a more extensive evaluation and subsequent dissemination to facilitate NICHE application nationwide. Nurses are an appropriate professional group to discover and advance the knowledge necessary to provide care to the nation's elders.

Her wise words have been guideposts for our work.

Today, the NICHE program can boast of 26 successful years of conferencing—an opportunity that provides staff nurses and nurse leaders from around the country to convene and compare best practices related to care of older adults.

Today, the NICHE program can boast of 26 successful years of conferencing—an opportunity that provides staff nurses and nurse leaders from around the country to convene and compare best practices related to care of older adults. The opportunity to network should be particularly highlighted. It is an honor and a privilege for nurses to be supported from their institutions to join the NICHE conference as there is a required registration fee that is significant in both travel and hotel. This means that institutions are aware of and making a very substantial and visible commitment to assuring that their staff are getting the state-of-the-art knowledge and skills that improve care for older adults. This type of visibility in a national meeting is also a very strong and positive indicator for the progression of staff nurses on the clinical ladder. NICHE is recognized by The Joint Commission (www.jointcommission.org) and the clinical work conducted by the NICHE staff at any given institution goes beyond simple local recognition. This is an influential element of the process of being a NICHE team at any given site and is important to note.

The ability and capacity to readily access best practice protocols is another dominant feature of the NICHE model success.

The ability and capacity to readily access best practice protocols is another dominant feature of the NICHE model success. From the inception of the program, evidence-based practice protocols were a defining feature of NICHE. The initial four protocols (physical restraints, sleep disorders, urinary incontinence, and pressure ulcers) were the base for a textbook, *Evidence-Based Geriatric Nursing Protocols for Best Practice*, which is now in its fifth edition (Boltz, Capezuti, Fulmer, & Zwicker, 2016). Published by the Springer

Publishing Company in New York City since the first edition in 1999, today there are 39 practice protocols and over 75 authors of those protocols. The book is widely used and evidence based, which is another influential feature of the NICHE program. Another added value is that GRNs often become protocol authors and are able to participate in a textbook that was recognized with *the American Journal of Nursing Book of the Year Award* in 2016 in the category of gerontological nursing. This enhances program reputation and credibility and adds joy to the work of GRNs.

CHAPTER SUMMARY

The NICHE theory of change including evidence, convening, and influence has stood the test of time. Since 1993, the NICHE program has gained national and international momentum and is widely recognized as a powerful vehicle for improvement in the care of older adults.

REFERENCES

Berman, M. (2016, March 21). The theory of the foundation. *Stanford Social Innovation Review*. Retrieved from http://ssir.org/articles/entry/the_theory_of_the_foundation

Boltz, M., Capezuti, E., Fulmer, T. T., & Zwicker, D. (Eds.). (2016). *Evidence-based geriatric nursing protocols for best practice* (5th ed.). New York, NY: Springer Publishing.

Fulmer, T., Flaherty, E., & Hyer, K. (2004). The Geriatric Interdisciplinary Team Training (GITT) Program. *Gerontology & Geriatrics Education, 24*(2), 3–12. doi:10.1300/j021v24n02_02

Hyer, K., Fairchild, S., Abraham, I., Mezey, M., & Fulmer, T. (2000). Measuring attitudes related to interdisciplinary training: Revisiting the Heinemann, Schmitt and Farrell attitudes toward health care teams scale. *Journal of Interprofessional Care, 14*(3), 249–258. doi:10.1080/jic.14.3.249.258

Kuhn, T. S. (1963). *The structure of scientific revolutions* (Vol. 2). Chicago, IL: University of Chicago Press.

Lewin, K. (1947). Frontiers in group dynamics: Concept, method and reality in social science; social equilibria and social change. *Human Relations, 1*(1), 5–41. doi:10.1177/001872674700100103

Appendix 4.1 Letter of Commitment

Draft Text for Memo to Nursing Staff
(for discussion at Friday meeting)

Finding our NICHE at "Institution Name"

TO: Nursing Staff

This is an exciting but critical time for nursing. The combination of rapid changes in healthcare with a graying population challenges us in ways we have not seen in the profession. Our knowledge and skills are put to test daily as we care for increasingly older, frailer, and sicker patients. Our patients and their families have become knowledgeable consumers as well. They expect quality nursing care, and they will hold us to this expectation.

The word may have become overused, but "empowerment" of nursing staff has become more critical than ever. We may feel at times that healthcare and demographics push us to work harder, when the key is to "work smarter, not harder." At "Institution Name," we want to know how we can assist you in this—how we can empower you to provide the best possible nursing care to older adults and their families.

Patients aged 65 and older make up about half of our admissions and about two-thirds of our hospital days. We strive to provide the best possible care to older adults, and to achieve the highest possible patient satisfaction. How prepared are we for this challenge? What are our strengths, and what are our weaknesses? How can we build on these strengths to improve where we need to? How can we empower our nursing staff in caring for older adults and their families?

In the next month or so, "Institution Name" will be conducting a survey on geriatric care among its nursing staff—part of NICHE (Nurses Improving Care to Hospitalized Elderly), a national initiative to assist healthcare organizations around the country in meeting the needs of acutely ill elderly. The survey, the Geriatric Institutional Assessment Profile (GIAP), assesses nurses'

- Attitudes toward caring for the elderly

- Knowledge of guidelines for care of the elderly

- Knowledge of common geriatric syndromes

- Perceptions of barriers to best nursing practice for elderly patients

The findings will be critical in our efforts to provide quality care to our older patients and their families. In addition, by linking our results to a national database, we will be able to assess how we compare to other healthcare providers.

NICHE hospitals have used the survey data in a variety of ways:

- Highlight staff strengths and weaknesses regarding care for the elderly, and use these data as a baseline against which to judge the effectiveness of CQI efforts
- Identify areas for staff development and recruitment
- Redesign services and care processes
- Identify areas of concern for accreditation
- Document strengths and expertise to negotiate contracts with insurers

Surveys will be distributed the week of Date???. Your responses will be anonymous and will be analyzed as a group data. It will be impossible to identify individual responses, nor do we want to do so. The data will be analyzed by an external group, which will present the results to us in the (Season???). We are planning several ways of sharing the results with you.

Please take the time to respond to the survey. We want to hear your voice! We will listen attentively.

To Be Named
Example: Vice President for Hospital Services

Contact Person: TBD

Dear NICHE Captain:

Thank you very much for agreeing to become involved in the NICHE project and administer the GIAP. This project is a wonderful kickoff to the Geriatric Program we are developing at (site name) _____ and your participation is very important.

We are hoping for at least a 75% return on each unit and encourage you to rally your staff members to complete a questionnaire. It will take them approximately 20 to 30 minutes to complete. The sooner they do it the less likely they are to forget or lose the questionnaires. Ideally they will complete the questionnaire and return it the same day you give it to them. The following are guidelines we wish you to follow.

Guidelines for Administering the Geriatric Assessment Profile (GIAP)

- Obtain a list of all RNs and LPNs who are either full- or part-time employees of your designated area (not per diems).
- Schedule times and places where you or someone whom you designate is available to hand out questionnaires.
- Delegate a central location for questionnaires to be returned in a closed envelope or box.
- Place name(s) of captains on flyers.
- Place flyers in various places on your unit that will be clearly visible (e.g., bathrooms, conference rooms, locker rooms).
- Hand out questionnaire and informed consent form.
- Have them sign the second page of informed consent and return them to you.
- Identify a 2-week time span during which you are able to administer the questionnaire and have them return them to you.
- If the participants are interested in participating in a raffle, obtain the numbers of the questionnaires and put them next to their names. Assure them that this is for the purpose of the raffle only.
- Check off returned questionnaires on numbered list.
- Call _____ when questionnaires are ready to be picked up.
- Have ready for him/her the completed questionnaire, the signed informed portion of the informed consent, and the list of those people who will be entered in the raffle.
  Notify _____ when:
  a. You do not have enough questionnaires.
  b. Questionnaires are lost.
  c. There are questions about the project that you cannot answer.

The Geriatric Institutional Assessment Profile and Measurement

The Original Geriatric Institutional Assessment Profile: Vision, Development, and Validation[1]

5

Ivo Abraham, Mathy Mezey, and Terry Fulmer

NICHE not only addresses the knowledge base of frontline staff but just as important their attitudes toward the care of older adults. The Geriatric Institutional Assessment Profile (GIAP) helps determine where the gaps are, including attitudes that may be interfering with improving care. Developing the empathy that complements the evidence-based approaches is key to successful outcomes.
—Eric Coleman, MD, MPH/MSPH, Professor of Medicine and Director of the Care Transitions Program, University of Colorado Anschutz Medical Campus

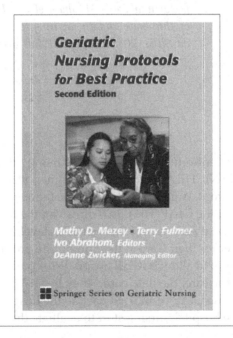

---

[1] This chapter is focused on the first version of the GIAP. For purposes of transparency, this chapter follows closely, and ties together, two publications describing this first version of the instrument (Abraham et al., 1999; Fulmer at al., 2002). Any similarities in text between these two prior publications and this chapter are with due acknowledgment of these two publications.

CHAPTER OBJECTIVES

1. Describe the vision for GIAP development
2. Describe the process for GIAP development and validation
3. Discuss data from piloting the GIAP

INTRODUCTION

The intent of the GIAP was to allow NICHE hospitals to conduct an initial survey of their staff as to geriatric care; the data could then be analyzed by the NICHE program centrally, with the GIAP results fed back to the hospital in a user-friendly format that allowed the hospital nursing staff to evaluate their strengths and weaknesses and establish priorities for interventions.

One of the four pillars supporting the Nurses Improving Care for Healthsystem Elders (NICHE) program when it was established in 1992 was the development of the Geriatric Institutional Assessment Profile (GIAP; Fulmer et al., 2002). The intent of the GIAP was to survey staff of NICHE health systems in terms of their attitudes, knowledge, and perceptions of care to older adults, and to use these data as measures for assessing geriatric care as these health systems implemented the NICHE program. In this chapter, we take a historical look at the vision for the GIAP, the key constructs and how these were operationalized into the items in the first version of the GIAP, and the validation of this version of the GIAP in a set of exploratory factor analyses (Abraham et al., 1999). As described in Chapter 7 of this book and in an integrative review (de Almeida Tavares & da Silva, 2013), the GIAP has evolved as the NICHE program has grown.[2]

VISION

A broad patient-centered as well as (nursing) staff-centered vision was put forward by the NICHE Advisory Board (Fulmer, Mezey, Ebersole, Foreman, Kresevic, Naylor, Strumpf, Walker, Wykle) to frame the conceptualization, development, and validation of the GIAP. The GIAP draws on the foundational work of the successful Institutional Assessment Profile (IAP) developed by the Educational Development Center for their Care at the End of Life project (see Chapter 2). The intent of the GIAP was to allow NICHE hospitals to conduct an initial survey of their staff as to geriatric care; the data could then be analyzed by the NICHE program centrally, with the GIAP results fed back to the hospital in a user-friendly format that allowed the hospital nursing staff to evaluate their strengths and weaknesses and

---

[2] Henceforth, unless otherwise specified, GIAP in this chapter refers to the original version of the instrument.

establish priorities for interventions. Built into the GIAP was the possibility that, at some later date, it could be administered a second time to assess the effectiveness of interventions put into place to improve care.

In its development, foremost, the GIAP should be based on the prevailing principles that geriatric care should maximize function and autonomy by ensuring the least restrictive environment, promoting awareness of the vulnerability of older persons, engaging the family, and ensuring continuity of care across settings (Abraham et al., 1999). The need for a rigorously validated, multidimensional, quantitative method for assessing the attitudes, knowledge, and perceptions of nursing and other health system staff along six dimensions was emphasized: (a) knowledge of institutional policies; (b) institutional obstacles to best practices; (c) conflict over appropriate care; (d) clinical knowledge; (e) liability for inadequate practice; and (f) supportiveness in the workplace (Abraham et al., 1999). Three key domains to be covered were identified: the perceived quality of geriatric practice, knowledge about geriatric practice, and the milieu or environment for geriatric practice. Further, it was recommended to focus on four disease-agnostic geriatric syndromes that, taken together, could be assumed to be quality proxies of geriatric care: (a) pressure ulcers; (b) incontinence; (c) confusion (including restraint use); and (d) sleep disturbances. The NICHE Advisory Board envisioned the GIAP to be a tool that could be used for cross-sectional assessments of a health system at one time point but would also be sufficiently sensitive to capture changes over time. Lastly, there was the desire for a methodology to benchmark individual health systems against other health systems in the aggregate.

The NICHE Advisory Board envisioned the GIAP to be a tool that could be used for cross-sectional assessments of a health system at one time point but would also be sufficiently sensitive to capture changes over time.

INSTRUMENT DEVELOPMENT

The vision for the GIAP was operationalized into 12 areas of assessment, for which questions and items were formulated. These were reviewed by the Advisory Board. The GIAP was amended based on the feedback received. As summarized in Table 5.1, the GIAP version that was retained for validation included a total of 67 questions and 152 items (Abraham et al., 1999). This version of the GIAP was distributed to staff in a 685-bed academic medical center. In total, 303 evaluable questionnaires were received with the majority coming from nurses (86.5%).

Internal Consistency Reliability

We used the data set to assess the internal consistency reliability (Cronbach's alpha) for several areas of assessment (treatments for geriatric patients; institutional commitment to geriatric care; institutional obstacles to geriatric care; vulnerability to

TABLE 5.1 Areas of Assessment, Description, Questions, and Items

AREA	DESCRIPTION	QUESTIONS	ITEMS
Professional demographics	Profession, years of experience and employment, clinical area of employment	4	4
Treatments for geriatric patients	Frequency of:		
	• Use of treatments	1	9
	• Disagreements among staff about treatments	1	10
	• Disagreements with patients and families about treatments	1	10
Institutional commitment to geriatric care	Satisfaction with the extent to which the institution facilitates, directly or indirectly, aging-sensitive and aging-relevant care to older patients and their families	1	10
Institutional obstacles to geriatric care	Perceived barriers to geriatric care from staff and unit to management levels	1	11
Staffing	Staffing resources across disciplines dedicated to geriatric care, including level of education and expertise	5	11
Vulnerability to legal liability	Perceived vulnerability to legal liability arising from falls, injuries, restraints, infections, and sedation	1	6
Demographics of patients	General and clinical demographics and referral/disposition status of geriatric patients	3	14
Frequency and burden of behavioral problems	Frequency of behavioral problems exhibited by patients and perceived burden (or reward) to work with patients	5	17
Institutional commitment to staff	Institutional commitment to support and empower staff to provide care to older adults	1	7
Knowledge about aging and geriatric care	General and applied knowledge related to aging and principles and practice of geriatric care	36	36
Personal demographics	Age, gender, religion, race/ethnicity, education	5	5
Free-text comments	Open-ended questions about most pressing issues and additional comments	2	5
	Total	67	152

TABLE 5.2 Internal Consistency Reliability

AREA	ALPHA
Treatments for geriatric patients (all items):	0.89
• Use of treatments	0.45
• Disagreements among staff about treatments	0.87
• Disagreements with patients and families about treatments	0.89
Institutional commitment to geriatric care	0.93
Institutional obstacles to geriatric care	0.89
Staffing	0.83
Vulnerability to legal liability	0.86
Frequency and burden of behavioral problems (all items):	0.77
• Frequency of behavioral problems	0.76
• Burden of behavioral problems	0.80
Institutional commitment to staff	0.84
Knowledge about aging and geriatric care	0.60

legal liability; frequency and burden of behavioral problems; institutional commitment to staff; and knowledge about aging and geriatric care [Abraham et al., 1999]). Internal consistency refers to the degree to which a set of items measure a common construct and is measured on a 0.00 to 1.00 scale.

Reported in greater detail elsewhere (Abraham et al., 1999), alpha coefficients ranged from 0.45 to 0.93, with 11 of the 13 coefficients being equal to or greater than 0.70, of which 9 were equal to or greater than 0.80 (Table 5.2). Thus, in general, this reliability assessment revealed that the initial GIAP had appropriate internal consistency in most of its areas of assessment. The two areas where the coefficient was less than 0.70 (frequency of use of treatments of geriatric patients; knowledge about aging and geriatric care) were flagged specifically for reevaluation later when larger data sets would be available (see Chapter 6).

Factor Analysis

We also used these data to conduct factor analyses to explore underlying dimensions of the GIAP that would enable additional differentiation in GIAP assessments. A successful factor analysis first yields a factor solution that shows which items in the analysis group together as "factors"—think of them as "dimensions" of geriatric care. In the next step, a panel of experts attempts to reach consensus on a name for each factor that represents the underlying concept. We conducted two factor analyses, the technical specifications of which are described elsewhere (Abraham et al., 1999). The first factor analysis included 35 knowledge items believed to be essential for best practice in geriatric nursing care (Best Practice—Knowledge), while the second comprised 28 items that addressed institutional barriers and facilitators (Best Practice—Institutional Environment).

The Best Practice—Knowledge factor analysis yielded a six-factor solution (Table 5.3). The first factor represented key indicators of best practices in geriatric nursing care, focusing mainly on the four geriatric syndromes that are core to the GIAP. Of note also is the inclusion of the item of staff members' opinions

TABLE 5.3 Best Practice Factors: Knowledge

Factor 1: Best practice principles

Time spent preventing sleep problems is valued at this institution.

Time spent managing urinary incontinence, without the use of diapers or catheters, is valued at this institution.

We do a good job identifying and preventing sleep disorders.

Time spent preventing pressure ulcers is valued at this institution.

At this institution, all reasonable alternatives are tried before restraining elderly patients.

I try to avoid indwelling catheters for elderly patients even if this means they are occasionally wet.

Clinicians need better guidelines to help determine what care is appropriate for the elderly.

My opinion about the proper care of geriatric patients is valued by my colleagues.

Factor 2: Knowledge—iatrogenic prevention

Nerve injuries can result from the use of restraints.

Using restraints often contributes to patient confusion.

Indwelling catheters are the single leading cause of septicemia in hospitalized elderly.

Sleep problems in hospitalized patients contribute to poor hospital outcomes.

Indwelling urinary catheters are appropriate in the management of incontinence as long as they are discontinued after 10 days.

We use diapers at night for most of our incontinent elderly patients.

When the use of mechanical restraints goes down, the use of sedating drugs goes up.

Factor 3: Inappropriate knowledge

Most sleeping problems in hospitalized elderly patients require the use of sedatives.

Confused elderly patients are safer when they are restrained in a bed or chair.

Sleep disturbances should always be aggressively treated.

Problems with urinary incontinence are a normal part of aging.

Reducing the use of indwelling catheters creates significant demands on staff time.

Sedatives prevent hallucinations and agitation in elderly patients with sleep disorders.

Regular massages over bony prominences reduces skin breakdown.

Factor 4: Knowledge—pressure ulcers

It is almost always possible to prevent skin breakdown.

Most pressure ulcers are preventable.

Pressure ulcers can lead to osteomyelitis.

(continued)

TABLE 5.3 Best Practice Factors: Knowledge (*continued*)
Heels are one of the most susceptible regions to break down in a bedridden patient.
Pressure ulcers occur in about half of the hospitalized elderly.
Factor 5: Clinical time management
I don't have time to perform daily skin assessments on my elderly patients.
I don't have time to help prevent sleep problems without relying on sedatives.
I check my restrained patients at least every hour.
Factor 6: Knowledge—health promotion
Kegel exercises are good for all types of incontinence problems.
Changes in sleep patterns are a normal part of aging.
Adequate nutrition is the most essential element in preventing skin breakdown.
Prevalence of incontinence in hospitalized elderly patients is about 20%.
Constipation can lead to urinary incontinence.

about the proper care of geriatric patients being valued by colleagues. The second knowledge factor focused on iatrogenic prevention. In particular, this factor incorporated items about staff's knowledge of the risks associated with the use of restraints and indwelling urinary catheters and the importance of assuring that patients have sufficient and adequate sleep. Inappropriate knowledge is measured by the third factor. It included items that represent poor geriatric care in the areas of sleep, the practice of chemical and mechanical restraints in confused patients, indwelling catheter use in patients with urinary incontinence, and the prevention of pressure ulcers. The latter was further explicated in the fourth factor, which targeted essential care aspects for preventing pressure ulcers. In addition, workflow-wise, providing best practice geriatric care may be time demanding and may also impose additional time-dependent actions. This was captured in the three items of the fifth factor, which queried staff whether they had time for daily skin assessments, for preventing sleep problems, and for checking restrained patients hourly. The final Best Practice—Knowledge factor shifted attention to integrating health promotion in geriatric nursing care. The emphasis of the items in this factor was on promoting continence, sleep, and skin integrity.

The Best Practice—Institutional Environment factor analysis revealed five factors (Table 5.4). The first and second factors were in counterbalance to each other. On the positive side, the first factor addressed the institutional facilitators of best practice in geriatric nursing care. In contrast, on the negative side, institutional obstacles to best practice were assessed by the second factor. The third factor, information transfer, emphasized communication to patients and families with regard to care; the availability of patient information to staff prior to admission; and continuity of care within and across care environments. The fourth factor appraises staff's perceptions of how the institution where they work values patients as well as staff. It provides critical information about the institutional context of care. The final factor in this analysis evaluates resource constraints within the institution.

TABLE 5.4 Best Practice Factors: Institutional Environment

Factor 1: Institutional facilitators of best practice

Staff are familiar with how aging effects response to treatment.

Issues about geriatric patient care are discussed by the staff.

Staff individualize care for the geriatric patients.

Geriatric patients get the care they need.

Aging is considered a factor in planning and evaluation.

Factor 2: Institutional obstacles to best practice

Lack of specialized equipment (e.g., raised toilet seats, special mattresses)

Lack of specialized services for the elderly (e.g., oral care, podiatry)

Lack of knowledge about care for the elderly

Exclusion of the elderly from care decisions

Differences in opinion among staff (disciplines) regarding common geriatric problems

Lack of or inadequate written geriatric policies and procedures

Confusion over who is the appropriate decision maker

Exclusion of nurses from geriatric care decisions

Factor 3: Information transfer

Patients received the information they need to make decisions about their care.

There is adequate continuity of care across settings.

Staff obtained information about elderly patients' prehospital baselines.

Families received information they need to help elderly patients.

There is adequate continuity of care between units.

Factor 4: Institutional values about patients and staff

Input from staff is sought in determining policies and guidelines about geriatric care.

Appropriate staff are involved with decisions about geriatric practice.

Personal growth is encouraged.

Clinicians and administrators work together to solve geriatric patient problems.

Geriatric patients are always treated with respect.

The rights of elderly patients are protected.

It is acceptable to disagree with your supervisor regarding geriatric patient care.

Factor 5: Time and resource constraints on best practice

Staff shortages/time constraints

Economic pressures to limit expensive treatment or length of stay

Communication difficulties with geriatric patients and their families

WHAT WE LEARNED FROM TESTING THE GIAP IN THREE PILOT SITES

Prevalence Rates of Common Clinical Syndromes in the Hospitalized Elderly

The GIAP was piloted at four hospitals, then called the University of Virginia Medical Center, Barnes Jewish Hospital in Missouri, University of California Davis Medical Center, and Methodist in Indiana. Methodist dropped out in the first year due to competing administrative demands. Generally, at that time, there was a lack of comparative national data on the prevalence of common clinical conditions in the hospitalized elderly. Today, this is not the case, but our work was early in understanding common geriatric clinical syndromes and their detection by practicing staff nurses. The use of the GIAP added to our knowledge as to the hospital prevalence of several of these syndromes (Table 5.5).

Changes in Capacity and Utilization Rates and Staffing Variability

After implementing the GIAP as a part of NICHE, hospital utilization rates for geriatric patients decreased within each hospital site, as evidenced by the decrease in hospital length of stay and in number of patient days for older adults (Table 5.6). However, as a proportion of hospital admissions, the percentage of geriatric patients had increased for each hospital during the study period. Thus, geriatric patients faced increasingly compressed lengths of stay and simultaneously constituted an increasing percentage of hospitalized patients. The higher turnover for geriatric patients results in increased demand for patient care at the time of admission and discharge. These findings

After implementing the GIAP as a part of NICHE, hospital utilization rates for geriatric patients decreased within each hospital site, as evidenced by the decrease in hospital length of stay and in number of patient days for older adults.

TABLE 5.5 Prevalence Rates of Common Clinical Conditions in the Hospitalized Elderly

CLINICAL CONDITION	PREVALENCE RATE
Urinary incontinence	2.7%–26.8%
Chronic urinary incontinence	0.0%–9.3%
Urinary incontinence on admission	0.0%–9.8%
Use of indwelling urinary catheter	3.9%–42.7%
Pressure ulcers on admission	0.0%–32.8%
Pressure ulcers during hospitalization	0.0%–13.9%
Falls	0.0%–2.8%
Use of restraints	1.7%–39.8%
Sleep disturbance	0.0%–58.3%

TABLE 5.6 Change in Hospital Length of Stay Subsequent to NICHE Program Implementation

HOSPITAL	CHANGE IN HOSPITAL LENGTH OF STAY
Hospital 1	−11.8%
Hospital 2	−14.8%
Hospital 3	−4.3%

TABLE 5.7 Staffing Variability Before and After NICHE Implementation

	STAFFING VARIABILITY	
STAFF ROLE	PRIOR TO IMPLEMENTATION	AFTER IMPLEMENTATION
Advanced practice nurse	0.0–0.4	0.0–0.9
Registered Nurse	4.6–6.9	4.8–6.9
Licensed practical nurse	0.4–0.6	0.3–0.7
Unlicensed assistive personnel	0.09–0.9	0.07–1.3
Total staff	6.0–12.6	6.5–11.5
Registered Nurse proportion	66.5%–89.2%	72.8%–80.4%

reinforce the necessity then and now to focus on the care of the hospitalized elderly as a particularly vulnerable patient segment.

Hospital readmission rates at 30 and 90 days, 13%, and 10% respectively, remained fairly constant across sites and subsequent to program implementation. Despite a lack of sufficient evidence regarding factors related to hospital readmission rates, the extent to which patients are readmitted may be viewed as an indirect measure of hospital care effectiveness and efficiency. Overall, the geriatric readmission rates for each hospital and year were greater than the respective readmission rates for the overall hospital population. The differences were generally higher for the 90-day rate.

Wide variability in staffing was seen for all hospitals, with little consistency across sites. The care of geriatric patients and the clinical performance measures are assumed to be related to the availability of nursing staff resources. Some changes were seen postimplementation, generally, an increase in advanced practice nurses and in unlicensed assistive personnel. The ranges for each variable, pre- and postimplementation, are shown in Table 5.7.

Changes and Change Patterns

Two distinct changes with respect to several prevalence rates for conditions, procedures, and outcome patterns emerged from this work. Change patterns were not consistent for specific variables across sites, but important information is derived from observing the trajectory of change. In some cases, as in urinary incontinence and sleep disturbance, the rates improved in the year following implementation, but then the improvements were not sustained. This pattern trajectory suggests that sustained change requires continued guidance and attention, subsequent to the initial improvements. In other cases, such as pressure ulcers and restraints, the rates deteriorated postimplementation, which likely is not the result of declining care quality, but rather is more suggestive of more accurate and consistent documentation.

Use of Data for Continuous Quality Improvement

As described by Donabedian (1979), there are administrative and research aspects to quality assessment and improvement. In research, new knowledge is sought about relationships between structures, processes, and outcomes. In administrative aspects of quality assessment and monitoring, knowledge of these relationships is used in the examination of organizational and system behaviors and outcomes.

Whereas rigorous design, methods, and statistical significance of data are essential elements of the research process, quality assessment and monitoring in the clinical setting rely on the operational significance of data and the meaning of the data within a specific applied context.

The significance of the findings related to the NICHE program relates primarily to the administrative aspect and the relevance and meaning of the data to the specific organizations under study. In addition, consistent with Donabedian's discussion of administrative and research aspects, data from this pilot can make a contribution to research by raising questions that can then be more rigorously pursued. The study findings suggest several promising areas for future research in clinical syndromes during a hospital stay. The positive relationship between urinary continence and the use of physical restraints has relevance to the seminal work of Strumpf and Evans (1988) in their examination of restraint use in hospitals. Our findings suggest promising areas for secondary data analysis of their study findings and for subsequent research. Further, the findings as to a high prevalence of sleep disturbance among hospitalized elderly underscore the need for further research in this area. Data on sleep patterns are clearly not collected in a reliable manner within and across hospitals. The fact that a substantial number of patients (13%) with no prior sleep disturbance left the hospital with impaired sleep patterns raises questions as to the role of sleep disturbance in recovery subsequent to hospital discharge.

Limitations in Studying the Prevalence Rates of Falls and Pressure Ulcers for the Elderly During Hospitalization

The low prevalence rates of falls and pressure ulcers in the NICHE hospitals raise methodological questions as to the value of outcome studies of these factors that look only at the hospital stay. Falls are consistently cited by hospital administrative staff as a priority area for geriatric research. Our data, however, suggest that the prevalence of falls during the hospital stay is very small. Given that major injury subsequent to a fall ranges between 1% and 5%, examining falls during a hospital stay is unlikely to yield fruitful findings. Rather, studying the consequences of falls for the hospitalized elderly is more fruitfully pursued by determining outcomes over a time period that encompasses discharge from hospital to home and a period (i.e., 6 months) following the hospital stay (Naylor et al., 1999). Similarly, research regarding pressure ulcers in the elderly is better pursued through methodologies that encompass the period prior to and subsequent to a hospital event.

Methodological Improvements for Studying Physical Restraint Use in the Hospitalized Elderly

Study of clinical syndromes in the hospitalized elderly is plagued by unreliable data sources (charts, incident reports), staff inaccuracy and lack of motivation for participating in data collection, and the expense of data collection. Our findings suggest that our methodology to determine the prevalence of physical restraints may provide a model for subsequent research. The methodology used yielded reliable data in studying patterns and trends of restraint use across hospitals and across years.

Relationship of Staffing to Quality of Care for the Hospitalized Elderly

Our data confirm the findings of others as to the large variation in nurse staffing patterns across hospitals and within hospitals over time. These findings suggest promising avenues for research in examining the relationship between nurse staffing and quality in hospital care of elderly patients, an area of research that is receiving increased attention (e.g., see Aiken, Clarke, Silber, & Sloane, 2003).

Case Mix Adjustment

The wide variation in the prevalence of clinical syndromes in the three pilot NICHE hospitals underscores what is already known about the need for careful case mix adjustment when comparing data about elderly patients across hospitals.

The wide variation in the prevalence of clinical syndromes in the three pilot NICHE hospitals underscores what is already known about the need for careful case mix adjustment when comparing data about elderly patients across hospitals. In longitudinal studies, such as ours, case mix needs to be adjusted at least annually, since our findings suggest that patient characteristics fluctuate from year to year. This is not surprising given changes in referral patterns and reimbursement that change where care is delivered (ambulatory/inpatient, hospital/nursing home) and sources of patient admissions (reduced admissions from nursing homes).

Our findings underscore the inaccuracies and inadequacy of data collection on clinical syndromes common to the elderly during a hospital stay. The wide variation in prevalence rates among hospitals for pressure ulcers and sleep disturbances is probably attributable in large part to inaccurate and/or absent assessment and inaccurate data reporting.

These issues of case mix adjustment have substantial ramifications for the cost of funding outcome research on hospitalization of the elderly.

Findings on NICHE Units

Our methodology yielded a sample of 357 patients, of whom 87 (24%) spent some time on NICHE units. In three areas—pressure ulcers, falls, and restraint use—the prevalence of these conditions was very low. Our sample size did not allow us to draw inferences as to the impact of the NICHE intervention on these patient outcomes. In urinary incontinence, NICHE patients did not have statistically significant differences in incontinence or catheter use as compared to other hospitalized elderly patients. The reasons for declines of 52% and 49% in restraint use in two hospitals are probably multifactorial: research findings supporting decreased restraint use; new Joint Commission recommendations and emphasis on decreasing the use of restraints; and the Nurses Improving Care to Hospitalized Elderly project.

CHAPTER SUMMARY

The first GIAP version, as reviewed in this chapter, provided a solid, though initial, foundation allowing the NICHE program to test at three pilot sites, facilitating evaluation of the reported care provided to older adults in health systems as viewed through the lens of their (nursing) staff. As such, it was used in the first phases of the NICHE program as both a tool to assess health systems and to benchmark these health systems against standards and against other health systems in the aggregate. Benchmark analysis would eventually allow hospitals to compare their results against all NICHE hospitals and NICHE hospitals similar as to size and sponsorship, for example, academic institutions, community hospitals, and so on. Importantly, the foresight of the Advisory Board in terms of vision and the diligence of many of the scientists involved in the development and initial validation of the GIAP translated into a clinical, conceptual, and methodological foundation. This has facilitated subsequent revisions of the GIAP as the NICHE program has aligned itself with changes in healthcare in general and geriatric care in particular and addressed other areas of geriatrics such as long-term care.

REFERENCES

Abraham, I. L., Bottrell, M. M., Dash, K. R., Fulmer, T. T., Mezey, M. D., O'Donnell, L., & Vince-Whitman, C. (1999). Profiling care and benchmarking best practice in care of hospitalized elderly: The Geriatric Institutional Assessment Profile. *The Nursing Clinics of North America, 34*(1), 237–255.

Aiken, L., Clarke, S., Silber, J., & Sloane, D. (2003). Hospital nurse staffing, education, and patient mortality. *Leonard Davis Institute Issue Brief, 9*(2), 1–4. Retrieved from https://ldi.upenn.edu/sites/default/files/pdf/issuebrief9_2.pdf

de Almeida Tavares, J. P., & da Silva, A. L. (2013). Use of the Geriatric Institutional Assessment Profile: An integrative review. *Research in Gerontological Nursing, 6*(3), 209–220. doi:10.3928/19404921-20130304-01

Donabedian, A. (1979). Needed research in the assessment and monitoring of the quality of medical care. Interim report. 1 May 1976–30 April 1979. DHEW/PUB/PHS-78/3219; NCHSR-78/145.

Fulmer, T., Mezey, M., Bottrell, M., Abraham, I., Sazant, J., Grossman, S., & Grisham, E. (2002). Nurses Improving Care for Healthsystem Elders (NICHE): Using outcomes and benchmarks for evidenced-based practice. *Geriatric Nursing, 23*(3), 121–127. doi:10.1067/mgn.2002.125423

Naylor, M. D., Brooten, D., Campbell, R., Jacobsen, B. S., Mezey, M. D., Pauly, M. V., & Schwartz, J. S. (1999). Comprehensive discharge planning and home follow-up of hospitalized elders: A randomized clinical trial. *Journal of the American Medical Association, 281*(7), 613–620. doi:10.1001/jama.281.7.613

Strumpf, N. E., & Evans, L. K. (1988). Physical restraint of the hospitalized elderly: Perceptions of patients and nurses. *Nursing Research, 37*(3), 132–137. doi:10.1097/00006199-198805000-00002

The Geriatric Institutional Assessment Profile: From Testing to Monitoring Change

6

Terry Fulmer, Marie Boltz, Kathleen Fletcher, Susan Fairchild, Melissa M. Bottrell, and Catherine O'Neill D'Amico

> *An essential element for a successful NICHE program is staff engagement. There are many daily competing demands and nurses need to understand and agree that NICHE will improve their practice and facilitate their nursing care.*
> —Marie Boltz, PhD, RN, Elouise Ross Eberly and Robert Eberly Professor of Nursing, Penn State College of Nursing

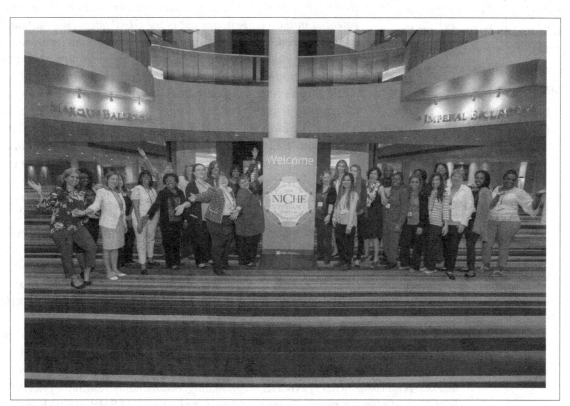

NICHE Conference Attendees. Atlanta, Georgia, April 2018.

CHAPTER OBJECTIVES

1. Appreciate the development of the Geriatric Institutional Assessment Profile (GIAP)
2. Understand the ways the GIAP assists practice improvement
3. Assimilate methods for advancing practice change through the experience of others
4. Recognize the need for continuous adaptation of the GIAP

INTRODUCTION

A paper entitled "Use of the Geriatric Institutional Assessment Profile: An Integrative Review" from 2013 provides an excellent summary of the ways in which the GIAP has enabled hospitals to characterize knowledge, attitudes, and perceptions of the staff as they provide care for older patients (de Almeida Tavares & da Silva, 2013).

By using the GIAP at the outset of an organizational change process to evaluate readiness to change, GIAP data can be used to set the direction of geriatric improvement interventions and prioritize among potential initiatives.

By using the GIAP at the outset of an organizational change process to evaluate readiness to change, GIAP data can be used to set the direction of geriatric improvement interventions and prioritize among potential initiatives. Repeated use of the GIAP offers data that can be used to evaluate the perceived practice response to interventions and over time it can identify areas in need of ongoing support in order to sustain excellence. It should be noted that the original GIAP was for the Nurses Improving Care for Hospitalized Elderly program. This meant that the assessment was conducted solely on older patients who were inpatients of the hospital. Since 2002, the title of the program has changed to Nurses Improving Care for Healthsystem Elders (NICHE) with a goal of cross-setting continuity of assessment and management of common geriatric syndromes. While there has been some progress in moving NICHE concepts across the care continuum, there is still much to do and this is in large part because of the difficulties clinicians have with sharing data across settings and systems, as well as the traditional siloed approach used in our care delivery models. A large literature has grown up around the problems of electronic health records (EHRs). With the advent of programs such as Epic and Cerner, one can hope that there will be better interoperability between various electronic medical record (EMR) systems that will facilitate communication between sites of care. Today, sharing material across settings is often done by transferring paperwork—an unreliable and incomplete yet practical solution at this time.

In this chapter, we discuss what we learned from using the GIAP over time to drive improvement in care of older adults and provide an exemplar from the University of Virginia Medical Center to underscore the application of GIAP data in helping institutions assess several components of NICHE programming: evaluation of readiness, prioritizing initiatives, evaluating practice response to data, and using GIAP data to sustain excellence (Note: the term "elderly," used in 1993, has largely been replaced today by the term "older adults").

CASE STUDY: UVAMC—IMPLEMENTATION PLAN FOR THE NICHE GERIATRIC RESOURCE NURSE MODEL

This case study is based on the 1993 progress report to The John A. Hartford Foundation (JAHF) and addresses evaluation of readiness, prioritizing initiatives, evaluating practice response to data, and using GIAP data to sustain excellence.

The Univeristy of Virginia Medical Center (UVAMC) is demonstrating strong commitment toward delivering quality healthcare services to older adults and their families. This commitment is illustrated in the plan created to establish a multidisciplinary geriatric initiative that will interface with the 10 vertically established service centers (Francis, Fletcher, & Simon, 1998). The Medical Center is one of four hospital sites chosen to implement the NICHE project. The goals of the project are to assist UVAMC to:

- Implement and analyze the geriatric institutional assessment of the needs of elderly patients

- Select and implement a nursing care model for care of elderly patients

- Implement one or more practice protocols on areas of nursing care for elderly patients with urinary incontinence, sleep disorders, pressure ulcers, and mechanical restraints

- Develop a database from which to monitor progress in achieving the hospital's goals for care of elderly patients (Figure 6.1)

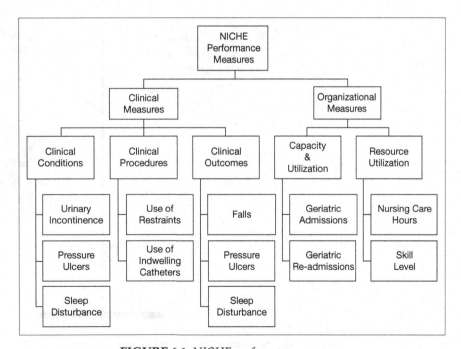

FIGURE 6.1 *NICHE performance measures.*

Although this new initiative was not officially announced at the time of inception due to organizational restructuring priorities, two major geriatric initiatives at UVAMC are already underway. A clinician with expertise in gerontology has been hired in Patient Care Services and the Medical Center was selected as a site for the grant from the JAHF ("Nurses Improving Care for Hospitalized Elderly" [NICHE] Project) to assist medical centers in improving care of older adults. An Advanced Practice Nurse in Geriatrics (Kathleen Fletcher) has been working primarily through the Center for Continuing Health Professions Education and the UVA School of Nursing for several months, developing and implementing geriatric educational programs to help prepare the current and future geriatric nursing workforce (Figure 6.2). Thirteen different geriatric educational programs have been developed for a broad audience consisting generally of hospital, nursing home, and home care nurses. Examples include falls, delirium, nutrition, pharmacology, and geriatric emergency programs, which are envisioned to become more portable, interdisciplinary, and packaged together as a Geriatric Enhancement Program. A core of approximately 15 UVAMC nurses from various care areas have attended

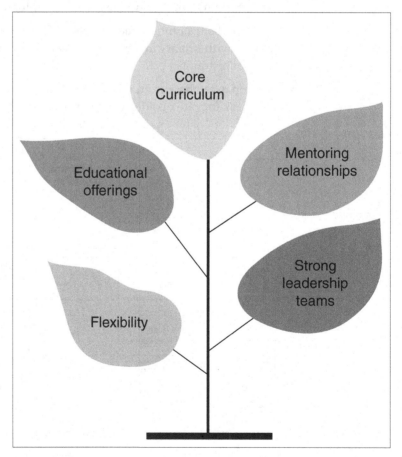

FIGURE 6.2 *Sustaining the Geriatric Resource Nurse Model at the University of Virginia. Source: Virginia K. Lee, APRN, BC, and Kathleen R. Fletcher, APRN, BC.*

these programs regularly; they would become the first geriatric resource nurses (GRNs) in the Medical Center. Recently, a geriatric nursing interest group (GNIG) was established at the Medical Center with the intent of sharing common concerns and for collaborative problem solving, developing basic and advanced competencies in geriatrics for acute care nurses, providing programs in geriatrics specifically addressing acute care issues, and creating quality improvement initiatives to address issues of concern. This group has monthly meetings and is open to other interested disciplines as well (Fletcher, Hawkes, Williams-Rosenthal, Mariscal, & Cox, 2007; Turner, Lee, Fletcher, Hudson, & Barton, 2001).

The Geriatric Institutional Assessment Profile (GIAP) has been completed and the results have been presented to the chief officer, Patient Care Service Division and the director, Center on Aging and Health. A decision was made to select the GRN model as this fits best the UVAMC nursing model (clinical ladder program) and with the previously established Geriatric Nurse Interest group.

In early March, UVAMC received 2 days of on-site consultation from project staff with expertise in this model, Terry Fulmer (Columbia University) and Lorraine Mion (Yale-New Haven Medical Center; now Cleveland Clinic Foundation). A brief overview of the GIAP data was presented and during Nursing Grand Rounds, Terry Fulmer described the GRN model. The project staff worked extensively with a defined UVAMC workgroup to detail how to implement the model at UVAMC. This workgroup consisted of Jean Sorrels-Jones, Chief Nursing Officer, Patient Care Services; Ivo Abraham, Director, Center on Aging and Health; Kathy Fletcher, Assistant Professor of Nursing and Geriatric Nurse Practitioner, Patient Care Services; Allene Brighton, Educational Coordinator, CCPNED; Vicki Hight, Project Director, Center on Aging and Health; and Tracy Kientz, Clinician 3 CCU. The plan for implementation of the GRN model emerged from these work sessions and can be found in Exhibit 6.1.

IMPLEMENTATION

The work described in the above case study provides an example of NICHE implementation in the first year at UVAMC. Data from the GIAP served as the basis for the implementation of the GRN model and also served as an essential element of the NICHE program and, with some exceptions, has been a requirement for institutions that wish to participate in the NICHE program. While driving change requires that an organization be open and ready, sustaining an interest in organizational change requires documentation of impact and also "early wins." To achieve those early wins, particularly when leaders or organizational managers might be less invested in an aging agenda, is challenging. This is especially true in the absence of compelling financial data that show NICHE care improvements reduce costs. The GIAP helps leaders look at a core set of clinical conditions that require evidence-based care for older adults. The GIAP data can help identify specific areas where change might be needed and help organizations target improvement initiatives and prioritize efforts.

The GIAP helps leaders look at a core set of clinical conditions that require evidence-based care for older adults.

Exhibit 6.1

UVAMC Implementation Plan for the NICHE Geriatric Resource Nurse Model

Objectives and Timetable for Year 1

MONTH 1

Objective: The Chief Nursing Officer, Patient Care Services announces geriatric nursing initiatives within a supportive interprofessional environment and the goal of improving the quality of care of older adults treated at the medical center.

Strategies

A general information meeting was conducted by Jean Sorrels-Jones and Ivo Abraham. A summary of the NICHE project and the Institutional Assessment Profile is presented, identifying both the strengths and opportunities for improvement in geriatric care. A brief overview of the geriatric resource nurse (GRN) model is presented and an announcement of the advanced practice nurse (APN) in Geriatrics, including the role and responsibilities of this position, is made. The two pilot units (CCU and Psychiatry) are identified and selected based on the geriatric interest and potential for GRNs on these units. The establishment and purpose of the institution-wide Geriatric Interest Group is announced. An advisory committee (AC) for the GRN model is established and the purpose of the group is announced.

MONTH 2

Objective: The GRN Model is initiated on the two identified pilot units.

Strategies

The APN meets with the nurse managers on both units to discuss implementation of the model and to select two GRNs from each unit to become the unit geriatric resource. The GRNs will meet with the APN and prepare self-learning strategies for developing/enhancing geriatric expertise. The APN will then orient the four selected GRNs to the SPICES card system to be used to guide the assessment of each person aged 70 or over admitted to the unit. The GRNs will role model the unit staff to the SPICES card system and SPICES assessment and management will become a unit competency. The APN will make rounds three times weekly with the GRNs to verify and discuss geriatric concerns, role model geriatric-focused assessment, and review the SPICES data. The APN will additionally be available for phone consultation to the GRNs. Two basic geriatric texts will be purchased for each pilot unit to be used as supplementary resources.

(continued)

(*continued*)

MONTH 3

Objective: Common instrumentation for geriatric assessment is established on both units.

Strategies

The APN will meet with the Geriatric Interest Group, the Advisory Committee, and the GRNs to present proposed tools for techniques and a more comprehensive geriatric assessment. The minimal domains to be considered will include mental status, functional assessment, and a depression index. The group will agree and select the instruments that are most applicable. The APN and the GRN will develop an educational program for the pilot unit(s) staff on the selected instrumentation and demonstrate geriatric-focused history taking and physical assessment.

MONTH 4

Objective: Unit-specific geriatric issues will emerge from the pilot unit data. Geriatric educational programs are implemented on each pilot unit and system-wide programs developed based on common issues across units.

Strategies

The SPICES card data from months 1 and 2 will be reviewed and analyzed for each of the pilot units by the APN and the GRNs. An analysis of the geriatric concerns that have been identified by the staff and the GRNs during rounds with the APN will be undertaken. The APN and the GRNs from each unit will develop unit-based protocols for addressing these concerns and the Geriatric Interest Group will identify and develop system-wide educational programs.

MONTH 5

Objective: Strategies for addressing the geriatric concerns that have been identified will be proposed under the unit-based and UVAMC quality improvement program(s) and are presented to the Advisory Committee for action and further direction.

Strategies

Unit-based protocols for addressing key geriatric care issues will be reviewed/modified/developed based on the unit data. Aggregate data from the two pilot units will be analyzed and presented to the Medical Center Quality Improvement staff for review and strategies. A summary will be presented to the Advisory Committee and priority areas will be targeted for action.

MONTH 6

Objective: Evaluate the effectiveness of the unit-based protocols in providing quality care to geriatric patients and their families.

(*continued*)

(continued)

Strategies

The unit quality improvement indicators demonstrate a high level of compliance with the established unit standard. Aggregate data from the two pilot units demonstrate the same.

MONTH 7

Objective: The effectiveness of the GRN model and the APN in Geriatrics will be determined.

Strategies

The GRNs from the two pilot units, the APN, and the Advisory Committee will review the effectiveness of the model and summarize the accomplishments of the defined objectives to date. The GRNs are becoming more confident in geriatrics and are initiating responsive educational programs with less consultation with the APN. The Patient Care Services management and staff of the two pilot units will be surveyed to determine satisfaction of the model. Modifications of the model will be proposed based on this data.

MONTHS 8 AND 9

Objective: Two additional units are added to the GRN model. The GIAP is completed again 1 year after NICHE participation to detect changes in perceptions of care.

Strategies

The model is implemented on two identified units with the modifications proposed by the pilot units. The information from the second GIAP is collected and analyzed for implications.

MONTHS 10 THROUGH 12

Objective: Two units are added to the GRN model monthly.

Strategies

A total of 10 units have successfully implemented the model within 14 months.

The goal for **Year 2** will be to implement the model on all inpatient units. How the model can be implemented in outpatient care (ambulatory and home care) will also be explored.

When staff feel that they are part of the change process and that their input is vital to the improvement process, they are more likely to be supportive of and assist with change.

An important aspect of the GIAP is the role it plays in signaling to staff that the organization is ready to make changes to improve geriatric care. The act of surveying staff also lets them know that the institution values their knowledge and opinions about what aspects of the care environment impede the provision of high-quality geriatric care. When staff feel that they are part of the change process and that their input is vital to the improvement process, they are more likely to be supportive of and assist with change.

GIAP EVOLUTION

The GIAP has evolved over the years, moving from a paper version to a scannable form, to a computerized assessment instrument. Further, the content has necessarily changed.

The original four constructs examined skin integrity, incontinence, restraint use, and sleep disorders; they were meant to serve as sentinel indicators of knowledge of best practice for older adults. In other words, if you were knowledgeable about these four, you were likely aware of additional key indicators of best practice for older adults. These four constructs were part of the original set of best practice protocols developed by the NICHE faculty in 1993 and today, the protocol book is in its fifth edition with 39 protocols to date (Boltz, Capezuti, Fulmer, & Zwicker, 2016). The sixth edition is in planning and will do much to move the protocol work forward with attention to application to all care settings.

Regular revision of the GIAP is required, but the principle remains that a baseline data set for geriatric care is essential to monitor and measure practice improvement.

Similar to other assessment instruments, regular revision of the GIAP is required, but the principle remains that a baseline data set for geriatric care is essential to monitor and measure practice improvement. It has been well documented that self-report is a valid way to garner practice information (Aguilar-Farías, Brown, Olds, & Peeters, 2015; Reuben, Siu, & Kimpau, 1992). However, self-report has limitations and competency-based assessment with observable demonstrations of best practice is a better way, where feasible, to understand improvement of care and is an important complement to self-report.

Today, GIAP version 8 continues in the tradition of previous versions. The new survey examines the environment of care, as well as nurses' knowledge of care for the syndromes that affect older adults during hospitalization. Some knowledge areas have been updated to reflect the changes in evidence-based practice, as well as the effects of the regulations, particularly those from the Centers for Medicare and Medicaid (CMS). The GIAP continues to be a survey provided to and completed by the newest NICHE-registered members and member organizations that are significantly expanding the NICHE program within the organization to establish a baseline for improving care and the environment of care, supporting changes in practice and perceptions of the practice environment. As with previous versions of the GIAP, it is not the only measure that organizations are urged to examine as a plan is developed to operationalize NICHE. During the formal NICHE Leadership Training Program, new member organizations and those expanding NICHE are guided to examine the institutional facilitators and obstacles and current quality data regarding syndromes associated with hospitalization for the purpose of establishing a plan for improving the care of the older adult. At the completion of The Leadership Training Program, the organization's NICHE team establishes an agreed-upon plan for initiating clinical practice changes necessary to improve care and the care environment. Sample work plans and newsletters are very helpful as NICHE programs get underway (Appendix 6.1 and 6.2).

It is important for those using the GIAP to determine exactly what data are being collected, who is completing the GIAP, and how the data will be used. Further, the institution needs to decide if follow-up data will be collected in the aggregate or matched on the same individual. Since the GIAP was initially designed to measure the environment in a specific care setting in the aggregate, it is not yet known if the results for other care settings with different care delivery models hold constant for reliability and validity. This is currently under analysis by NICHE staff.

PSYCHOMETRICS

Since its inception, there has been a continuous commitment to monitoring the psychometric properties of the GIAP (Abraham et al., 1999). Boltz et al. (2008a, 2008b) examined the repeated use of the GIAP to determine perceived changes in the care environment and to review responses for the changes in nurses' knowledge related to care of the older adult. A test–retest reliability measure was completed by Boltz, Capezuti, Kim, Fairchild, and Secic (2009). This examination of reliability using a test–retest strategy supported the GIAP as reliable for examining the knowledge, attitudes, and organizational attributes that support best practices in geriatric care. The GIAP was again determined to be a reliable instrument for determining the capacity of an acute care institution to improve care to older adults. The practice of readministration of the GIAP should be carefully planned. Repeating the GIAP might not be an accurate reflection of an individualized improvement in nursing knowledge or account for all aspects of a geriatric practice environment if staff and institutional changes are affecting practice (Boltz et al., 2009). In 2017, GIAP version 8 was piloted with 19 acute care institutions. This factor analysis will serve as a new basis for continuous improvement of the NICHE program.

GIAP AND NICHE MEMBERSHIP

Originally, NICHE participation was accessed by paying a flat fee for the program with GIAP data processing charges included. Over time, the sophistication of the membership model has evolved, and the accelerated change was especially notable under the leadership of Elizabeth Capezuti, with funding from The Atlantic Philanthropies (Capezuti, Bricoli, & Boltz, 2013). Organizations other than those providing acute care have had access to the wide range of educational materials and other references from NICHE. For example, the *Try This Series* as well as the *Solutions Series* have done much to assist nurses with practical approaches to improving care for older adults (Bricoli, 2016; Fulmer, 2007). Currently, the JAHF is funding NICHE Long-Term Care to further examine the utility and appropriateness of assessments and products that are best suited to those sites.

FUTURE DIRECTIONS

A current NICHE team goal is to finalize the development of a GIAP for long-term care by 2019. The intent of a long-term care GIAP is to examine and document the environment of care and the knowledge of the nursing staff in nonacute care settings to provide care for the same clinical syndromes that continue across care settings. The NICHE team supports the ideal that care and the care environment can and must be improved across the continuum of care settings.

CHAPTER SUMMARY

NICHE is an adaptive strategy for improving care of older adults and has evolved to keep up with contemporary strategies, tactics, and improvement science. The GIAP has served as an important protocol for understanding geriatric practice.

REFERENCES

Abraham, I., Bottrell, M. M., Dash, K., Fulmer, T., Mezey, M., O'Donnell, L., & Vince-Whitman, C. (1999). Profiling care and benchmarking best practice in care of hospitalized elderly: The Geriatric Institutional Assessment Profile. *Nursing Clinics of North America*, *34*(1), 237–255.

Aguilar-Farías, N., Brown, W. J., Olds, T. S., & Peeters, G. M. E. E. (2015). Validity of self-report methods for measuring sedentary behaviour in older adults. *Journal of Science and Medicine in Sport*, *18*(6), 662–666. doi:10.1016/j.jsams.2014.08.004

Boltz, M., Capezuti, E., Bowar-Ferres, S., Norman, R., Secic, M., Kim, H., . . . Fulmer, T. (2008a). Changes in the geriatric care environment associated with NICHE (Nurses Improving Care for HealthSystem Elders). *Geriatric Nursing*, *29*(3), 176–185. doi:10.1016/j.gerinurse.2008.02.002

Boltz, M., Capezuti, E., Bowar-Ferres, S., Norman, R., Secic, M., Kim, H., . . . Fulmer, T. (2008b). Hospital nurses' perception of the geriatric nurse practice environment. *Journal of Nursing Scholarship*, *40*(3), 282–289. doi:10.1111/j.1547-5069.2008.00239.x

Boltz, M., Capezuti, E., Fulmer, T. T., & Zwicker, D. (Eds.). (2016). *Evidence-based geriatric nursing protocols for best practice* (5th ed.). New York, NY: Springer Publishing.

Boltz, M., Capezuti, E., Kim, H., Fairchild, S., & Secic, M. (2009). Test—Retest reliability of the Geriatric Institutional Assessment Profile. *Clinical Nursing Research, 18*(3), 242–252. doi:10.1177/1054773809338555

Bricoli, B. (2016). NICHE solutions: Next in the series: Geriatric practice. *Geriatric Nursing, 37*(1), 80–81. doi:10.1016/j.gerinurse.2015.12.001

Capezuti, E. A., Bricoli, B., & Boltz, M. P. (2013). Nurses Improving the Care of Healthsystem Elders: Creating a sustainable business model to improve care of hospitalized older adults. *Journal of the American Geriatrics Society, 61*(8), 1387–1393. doi:10.1111/jgs.12324

de Almeida Tavares, J. P., & da Silva, A. L. (2013). Use of the Geriatric Institutional Assessment Profile: An integrative review. *Research in Gerontological Nursing, 6*(3), 209–220. doi:10.3928/19404921-20130304-01

Fletcher, K., Hawkes, P., Williams-Rosenthal, S., Mariscal, C. S., & Cox, B. A. (2007). Using nurse practitioners to implement best practice care for the elderly during hospitalization: The NICHE journey at the University of Virginia Medical Center. *Critical Care Nursing Clinics of North America, 19*(3), 321–337. doi:10.1016/j.ccell.2007.05.007

Francis, D., Fletcher, K., & Simon, L. J. (1998). The geriatric resource nurse model of care: A vision for the future. *Nursing Clinics of North America, 33*(3), 481–496.

Fulmer, T. (2007). How to try this: Fulmer SPICES. *American Journal of Nursing, 107*(10), 40–48; quiz 48–49. doi:10.1097/01.naj.0000292197.76076.e1

Reuben, D. B., Siu, A. L., & Kimpau, S. (1992). The predictive validity of self-report and performance-based measures of function and health. *Journal of Gerontology, 47*(4), M106–M110. doi:10.1093/geronj/47.4.M106

Turner, J. T., Lee, V., Fletcher, K., Hudson, K., & Barton, D. (2001). Measuring quality of care with an inpatient elderly population: The geriatric resource nurse model. *Journal of Gerontological Nursing, 27*(3), 8–9. doi:10.3928/0098-9134-20010301-04

Appendix 6.1

Finding Your NICHE . . .

SAMPLE WORK PLAN

1. Phase I Promotional Activities
   a. Article for staff newsletter
   b. Sample briefing to managers and other key staff
   c. Idea: general posting during Week of the Nurse

2. Conducting the GIAP
   a. Getting prepared to do the GIAP memo from New York University (NYU)
   b. Conference call with NYU to discuss sample, distribution, and return

3. Phase II Promotional Activities for the GIAP
   a. Memo to nursing staff—2 weeks before distribution (sample included)
   b. Alert posting—10 days before distribution
   c. Dates and channels (distribution and return) posting—3 days before distribution
   d. Reminder return date and channel posting—5 days after distribution
   Guidelines re: 1 and 2
   > Repeat key message(s)
   > Common/recognizable format
   > Consistency across messages
   > Contact person(s)

4. Distribution Channels
   a. Institution orders proper number of questionnaires from NYU
   b. NYU to mail proper number of questionnaires to site
   c. In-house distribution per suggestions made during preparation conference call

5. Return Channels
   a. In-house return per suggestions during preparation conference call
   b. Site will pick up after grace period at date to be announced (TBA)
   c. Site will mail completed surveys or data disk to NYU per conference call decisions

6. Help Desk (suggested for staff concerned about completing the GIAP)
   a. Site will make arrangements

7. Cover Letter for Survey
   a. Site to draft (see enclosed sample)

8. Dissemination
   a. Presentations (ideas for which to make)
      i. Nursing management group
      ii. Staff development days
      iii. Follow-up for nurses unable to attend staff development days
      iv. Administrative Executive Committee
      v. Medical Executive Committee
      vi. Board
   b. Publications (suggestions)
      i. Institutional reports or flyers
      ii. Mailings to patients or other interested parties

SAMPLE TIME TABLE

Start Date	End Date	Suggested Time Period	Activities
April 23	May 4	2 weeks	Develop work plan Design phases I and II promotional activities
May 5	May 18	2 weeks	Implement phase I promotional activities
May 19	May 25	1 week	Implement phase II promotional activities
May 26	June 6	3 weeks	Distribution of surveys with 6/6 return deadline Access to "help desk"
June 7	June 15	1 week	Grace period for survey returns Continued "help desk" access
June 16	July 6	3 weeks	Collection of surveys at institution Shipping of surveys to NYU Data entry
July 7	August 30	6–7weeks	Statistical analysis, tabulation, and graphics by NYU Outline dissemination activities
September 1			Dissemination activities at Site

Appendix 6.2

Draft Text for Newsletter 1993

FINDING OUR NICHE AT "INSTITUTION NAME"

Patients aged 65 and older make up about half of our admissions and about two-thirds of our hospital days. Caring for older adults is a major community responsibility of "Institution Name." We strive to provide the best possible care to older adults, and to achieve the highest possible patient satisfaction.

How prepared are we for this challenge? What are our strengths, and what are our weaknesses? How can we build on these strengths to improve our care? How can we empower our nursing staff in caring for older adults and their families?

In the next month or so, "Institution Name" will be conducting a survey on geriatric care among its nursing staff—part of Nurses Improving Care for Hospitalized Elderly (NICHE), a national initiative to assist healthcare organizations in meeting the needs of acutely ill elderly. The survey, the Geriatric Institutional Assessment Profile, assesses nurses':

> Attitudes toward caring for the elderly
>
> Knowledge of guidelines for care of the elderly
>
> Knowledge of common geriatric syndromes
>
> Perceptions of barriers to best nursing practice for elderly patients

The findings will be critical in our efforts to provide quality care to our older patients and their families. In addition, by linking our results to a national database, we will be able to assess how we compare to other healthcare providers. Where do we do better, and where do we not? What can we learn from other NICHE hospitals, and what can we teach them?

The survey will be another step in our CQI efforts. It will also help us plan for the future—an important task considering the changing demographics of this community and the local area.

We encourage all nursing staff to participate in this survey. We want to hear your voice!

We need your help in finding our NICHE at "Institution Name"!

The Geriatric Resource Nurse Model   III

The Origins of the Geriatric Resource Nurse Model

7

Terry Fulmer and Donna Marie Fick

The experience I had as a new geriatric clinical nurse specialist (CNS) working with Terry Fulmer and the geriatric resource nurse (GRN) model (and later Nurses Improving Care for Healthsystem Elders [NICHE]) profoundly influenced both my care and leadership as a health system CNS and laid the foundation for my National Institutes of Health (NIH)-funded research as a nurse scientist. . . . While practicing as a CNS in California, I continued to use this approach and the SPICES acronym while working as a care manager following older adults across all settings of care (home, assisted living, acute care, nursing home, and clinic) and it fostered continuity of care and strong gerontological principles regardless of the setting of care." . . . The NICHE model is person and staff centered, captures both the heart and science of good bedside care, engages and empowers staff, and improves the care of older adults and their families. This book is an important addition to gerontological nursing care.
—Donna Fick PhD, RN, FAAN, Elouise Ross Eberly Professor of Nursing, Professor of Medicine, Director, Center of Geriatric Nursing Excellence, Pennsylvania State University

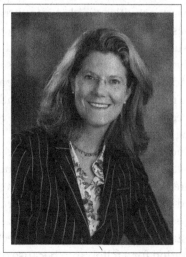

Donna Fick.

> ## CHAPTER OBJECTIVES
>
> 1. Discuss the genesis of the geriatric resource nurse (GRN) model
> 2. Appreciate the historical context and evolution of the role
> 3. Describe the way the GRN model adapts to different settings

INTRODUCTION

This chapter traces the origins of the geriatric resource nurse (GRN) model at Boston's Beth Israel Hospital (BIH) through the efforts of Joyce Clifford and Kate Reilly Morency and its early development at Yale through Terry Fulmer and Donna Birkenhauer Fick.

JOYCE CLIFFORD AND KATE REILLY MORENCY

The influence of the BIH professional nursing model (primary nursing) and the philosophy of the BIH Division of Geriatric Medicine on the evolution of the GRN model cannot be overstated. As early as 1982, Joyce Clifford saw the wisdom of launching the first "Gerontic Nurse Fellowship," which provided a 1-year, hospital-based, postmaster's fellowship in gerontic nursing. "Gerontic" was a term that combined gerontology and geriatric to represent the holistic nature of nursing care of older adults (Carter, 1982). While the term did not get adopted broadly, the work certainly did.

The program began officially in 1981 with the selection of the first fellow, Kate Reilly Morency, MS, RN. The fellowship training included clinical, educational, and research activities divided into three 4-month phases. Each phase had a specific emphasis with the first phase focused on learning the role of the gerontic nurse as a consultant to the nursing staff and as a member of the hospital-wide interdisciplinary geriatric consult team. The second phase was dedicated to caring for a caseload of elderly primary nursing patients and developing educational programs to the nursing staff. The final 4 months of the fellowship were meant to be devoted to deepening the fellow's practice, consultation, and educational skills and to analyzing research data.

Clifford and M. Patricia (Trish) Gibbons, the director for Medical Nursing at the BIH, felt that through this program, they would be able to retain master's-prepared clinicians at the bedside where patients would profit most from their specialized expertise both directly in terms of caring for the patients themselves as well as indirectly through role modeling educational and consultative activities with staff. Clifford and Gibbons selected care of older adults as the first area of concentration for a fellowship because of the willingness and interest of the geriatric medicine program.

Obviously, care of older adults is interdisciplinary and both the nursing and medical teams at the hospital understood that. Morency, formerly a staff nurse at the Beth Israel, completed her master's as a nurse practitioner from the University of Massachusetts Lowell and then transitioned into her fellowship at Beth Israel. Her article, "Primary Nursing and the Care and Management of the Elderly," appeared in the Summer 1981 issue of *Nursing Administration Quarterly* (Reilly, 1981). Reflecting on her first 4 months, she spoke about the hospital's geriatric consult team and said it was a wonderful experience to engage with a large number of patients with an interdisciplinary team and cited in particular "her ability to provide techniques that help in working with such nursing problems as incontinence, impaired mobility, and agitation among geriatric patients in informing how drugs affect the elderly" (Carter, 1982). Morency went on to say that she was especially struck by the lack of baseline information on older patients. She opined that "you can't really plan nursing interventions or assess change in a patient unless you know what it was like when he or she was admitted." One could lament that over 30 years later, we are still struggling with the same issues. Fortunately, today there are systematic approaches to meet the objectives that were laid out long ago. However, in general, nursing practice does not approach these clinical issues with reliability, which is why the Nurses Improving Care for Healthsystem Elders (NICHE) program is so important.

TERRY FULMER

Fulmer began her career at the BIH in 1975 and completed her master's in nursing at Boston College in 1977. She went on to join the faculty of Salem State College in the rehabilitation nursing track in 1977, which was most closely aligned to her passion in geriatrics. She joined the faculty of the Boston College School of Nursing in 1978. Throughout her master's program and for the entirety of her time in the Boston area, Fulmer retained an appointment as a practicing nurse at BIH. During the academic year she was able to schedule practice one day a week as well as every other weekend. In the summers, she worked full-time as a clinical advisor in nursing. The clinical advisor role, formerly referred to as a "nursing supervisor," gave her the opportunity to see older patients across a broad spectrum of health problems, from the emergency room to the intensive care unit (ICU), across surgical units, and all the medical units. Throughout this practice and along with her practice in the context of being a clinical instructor at Boston College where she precepted her students at the Massachusetts General Hospital every Thursday and Friday, there was extraordinary opportunity to observe nursing practice in the care of older adults and to apply concepts that were evolving at BIH (Fulmer, 1977, 1981, 1987b; Fulmer, Ashley, & Reilly, 1986). The gerontic nurse fellowship model was impressive but not scalable given financial demands and the necessary rigidity of who could apply and how the program was conducted. Fulmer noted this and spoke with Gibbons about more scalable models. It was agreed that Fulmer would use her summer months to develop geriatric nursing expertise on each of the appropriate units at BIH. She began by interviewing the nurse managers of units with elderly patients and requesting names of nurses who seemed to have a propensity for selecting and caring for older adults with complex care needs. This strategy worked. Fulmer soon headed a team of eight unit-based volunteer primary nurses who wanted to be responsible for improving care for the elderly. The term "geriatric resource nurse" was born.

In 1989, Fulmer moved to New York shortly after Gibbons transitioned to Yale New Haven Hospital (YNHH) as the chief nursing officer. Gibbons recruited Fulmer to Yale and the essential work of describing and refining the GRN model began. Fulmer had a joint appointment with the Yale School of Nursing (YSN) and YNHH and was responsible for the development of the new geriatric nursing master's program at YSN as well as the development of the geriatric nursing practice model at the hospital. With Gibbons's unfaltering support, the two strategized about the role and understood that for true spread and scale, the model Fulmer had started with staff nurses on the BIH units would be the preferable approach at YNHH (Fulmer, 1991a). Fulmer moved the GRN model across the medical units of the hospital and published the framework (Fulmer, 1987a, 1991a, 1991b).

Concomitantly, the Yale School of Medicine (YSM) was building a strong and reputable program in geriatric medicine. Led by Leo Cooney, MD, there was a strong geriatric medicine fellowship program along with outstanding geriatricians. The John A. Hartford Foundation, as previously noted in Chapter 3, was developing the plan for the Hospital Outcomes Project for the Elderly (HOPE) project and designated Yale as one of the sites. The GRN model was already in place and served to accelerate the Yale agenda.

DONNA BIRKENHAUER FICK AND THE GRN MODEL AT YNHH

By 1990, the HOPE project was underway and an important new recruit arrived as the first externally funded GRN: Donna Birkenhauer Fick. Fick had recently completed her master's degree in gerontological nursing at the University of Cincinnati and was certified by the American Nurses Credentialing Center (ANCC) in gerontological nursing. Fick arrived as a joint appointment clinical nurse specialist (CNS) and GRN on the orthopedic floor with responsibilities for assisting in the implementation of a $1.2 million grant newly awarded to Fulmer from the Kellogg Foundation: Better Elder Services Today (BEST). Fick's passion for the work and intuitive understanding of how to motivate staff nurses was a true catalyst for the program (Inouye et al., 1993).

The GRN model at YNHH had three key principles, which hold today: (a) the bedside nurse has the best knowledge of how the older patient is responding to

The GRN model at YNHH had three key principles, which hold today: (a) the bedside nurse has the best knowledge of how the older patient is responding to treatment and care, (b) is the one most likely to be engaged with the family, and (c) can apply key principles of geriatric nursing with the support and mentorship of a master's-prepared geriatric nurse specialist.

treatment and care, (b) is the one most likely to be engaged with the family, and (c) can apply key principles of geriatric nursing with the support and mentorship of a master's-prepared geriatric nurse specialist. Again, using a volunteer model, Fulmer met with nurse managers to determine their level of interest and willingness to allow staff to participate in the program, and to solicit names of nurses who demonstrated interest in care of complex older adults. Although there was not universal interest, especially in the ICU areas, there was a strong and positive response and the program implementation began in earnest.

A Geriatric Nursing Advisory Board (GNAB) was formed consisting of key leaders in the organization with similar interests. For example, the nurse manager of the geriatric outpatient clinic was a member as well as the geriatric social work director. This group met quarterly and was responsible for reviewing the goals of the GRN program, facilitating where possible, and helping communicate the goals to the broader YNHH community. At the same time, a geriatric nursing interest group (GNIG) was established for the purpose of educating GRNs and forming bonds among individual GRNs to ensure peer-to-peer support. Monthly brown bag meetings were held that consisted of presentations from GRN group members on key topics such as management of urinary incontinence, pressure ulcers, pain management, mobility problems, and nutritional challenges in older adults. Sometimes the meeting took the form of a journal club while other times guest speakers were invited. However, the predominant approach was to have the GRNs review the literature on a topic of their choice and come prepared to teach the group. This was most successful when tapping into the nursing staff's passion and allowing them to lead on topics they thought were knowledge gaps on their local unit or ones for which they had special interest and passion.

Fulmer formulated the acronym SPICES (skin problems, problems with eating and feeding, incontinence, confusion, evidence of falls, and sleep disorders) as a way of helping the GRNs organize their thinking around a simple framework that would resonate with the staff nurses (Fulmer, 2007). One example of this was a nurse at YNHH who was interested in the eating problems and nutrition part of SPICES who came to Fick asking to work on this issue on the unit. The nurse, Ophelia Empleo-Frazier, codeveloped the materials with the CNS Fick, including posters for the unit and educational programs that the nurse presented to her peers. With time, it became apparent that the GRN members of the group were developing deep expertise in their areas of interest and truly exceptional resources for the hospital. They further presented their work at the YNHH annual Nursing Research Day held by the hospital and competed to present regionally and nationally.

With time, it became apparent that the GRN members of the group were developing deep expertise in their areas of interest and truly exceptional resources for the hospital.

DEVELOPMENT OF THE GRN ROLE

The GRN model is easily adapted and implemented across settings of care and has a strong evidence base that supports the use of champions as GRNs. Fick has also used this model of GRN delirium champions in acute and long-term care with nursing staff in California and Pennsylvania and as a framework for interventions for delirium.

A key principle is to include in the GRN program any staff nurse who wishes to participate. Every nurse has something to offer to the program, and it is up to the leadership to determine how to best develop the passion and skills of each GRN.

One important caveat to carefully consider is how GRNs are encouraged, developed, and sustained. A key principle is to include in the GRN program any staff nurse who wishes to participate. Every nurse has something to offer to the program, and it is up to the leadership to determine how to best develop the passion and skills of each GRN. One way to sustain and reward GRNs is through a clinical care ladder program where participation as a GRN is used in the ladder. Conducting GRN rounds with the nurses on older adults with whom they have chosen to round is also a way to make a more lasting cultural change as nurses see the model making a difference in the lives of older adults and in improving the efficiency and quality of care at the bedside.

The GRN unit champions in Fick's intervention trials for delirium superimposed on dementia (DSD) engaged registered nurses to identify DSD along with the nurse manager, nurse educator, or advanced practice nurse on the unit. The GRN unit champion had at least 1 year nursing experience in the hospital, had a self-reported interest in geriatrics, and was willing to commit time each week to facilitation of delirium prevention and care. Intervention staff completed weekly rounds with the unit champion reviewing delirium cases and rounded on patients using the intervention pocket cards and rounding forms (see clinicaltrials.org for the study protocol). This model of rounding with nurses around delirium care was similar to using the SPICES cards (Fick, Steis, Mion, & Walls, 2011; Fulmer 2007; Yevchak et al., 2014).

Evidence has shown that improved care is best facilitated by direct care providers who are insiders in the setting and culture and are able to reinforce and individualize the care or intervention to their local setting of care (Kitson et al., 2008; Yevchak et al., 2017), thus the GRN model is easily applied across conditions and settings of care and has stood the test of time.

GRN PROGRAM EVOLUTION

There have been many places where the GRN model has been tested and where it is flourishing. Milisen and colleagues conducted a nurse-led interdisciplinary intervention focused on older persons with hip fractures who develop delirium. Their objective was to demonstrate the effect of using a GRN model to screen for delirium and determine whether the incidents and severity of delirium could be altered. While the incidence of delirium did not change, the intensity and duration was significantly less (Milisen et al., 2001). Others have written about the GRN model as a way to develop nurses' geriatric expertise (St. Pierre & Twibell, 2012). Outcomes from GRN model implementation have found that patients experience less pain, incontinence, and immobility on units where there are GRNs (Turner, Lee, Fletcher, Hudson, & Barton, 2001). Readmission rates are lower when a unit has GRNs and there is less use of vest restraints. Further reports have documented a decrease in rates of delirium as well as a reduction in indwelling catheter use, functional decline, and falls.

There have been further studies that report improvement in nurses' knowledge competence and attitudes as well as satisfaction when there is a GRN model in place. Further, GRNs are more likely to call for an appropriate geriatric care team consultation (Deschodt, Flamaing, Haentjens, Boonen, & Milisen, 2013; Deschodt et al., 2012). Common geriatric syndromes such as acute confusion and functional decline have shown improvement when a GRN model is in place. Nurses' knowledge and confidence in assessing acute confusion improved and led to more nurse-directed assessments (Rapp et al., 1998, 2001). Functional decline reduction was documented in two studies. The Yale Geriatric Care Program studied GRNs as a way to reduce functional decline in frail hospitalized elderly and documented that the GRN integrated into the geriatric care team intervention resulted in a beneficial effect with a relative risk of 0.82 (95% confidence interval 0.54 to 1.24) in patients ($n = 106$) with one of four geriatric target conditions at baseline (e.g., delirium, functional impairment, incontinence, and pressure sores; Inouye et al., 1993). Overall, they documented a decrease in functional decline in targeted elderly hospitalized patients. The NICHE model that uses the GRN as the intervention to improve care for health system elders is often cited as a successful approach to decreasing functional decline (Admi, Shadmi, Baruch, & Zisberg, 2015; Graf, 2006; Kleinpell, Fletcher, & Jennings, 2008). The NICHE website has a summary of published papers that document the success of the GRN model as the cornerstone of the NICHE intervention and we are learning daily about new ways the model can be enhanced for optimal care outcomes for older adults both in institutional settings and in primary care.

The GRN model is predicated on the theory that, given the knowledge and tools to assess and intervene in common geriatric syndrome care prevention and management, nurses readily take on and succeed in this work.

The GRN model is predicated on the theory that, given the knowledge and tools to assess and intervene in common geriatric syndrome care prevention and management, nurses readily take on and succeed in this work. Once they have the appropriate assessment tools (Table 7.1), such as those in the *Try This* series (Fulmer, 2007) along with evidence-based practice protocols (Boltz, Capezuti, Fulmer, & Zwicker, 2016) and administrative support for the role, there is ample evidence that nursing practice for older adults can and does improve along with staff satisfaction (Boltz et al., 2008).

TABLE 7.1 Commonly Used Geriatric Assessment Measures

INSTRUMENT	AREAS OF ASSESSMENT	REFERENCE
SPICES	Sleep, problems with eating or feeding, incontinence, confusion, evidence of falls, skin breakdown	Fulmer (1991a); Wallace and Fulmer (1998)
Geriatric Institutional Assessment Profile	Hospital staff knowledge of geriatric care principles, organizational environment	Abraham et al. (1999)
Hospital Admission Risk Profile (HARP)	ADL, IADL, cognitive status	Sager et al. (1996)
Lawton Instrumental Activities Daily Living Scale	IADL activities: medication management, housekeeping, food preparation, transportation, shopping, managing finances, laundry	Lawton and Brody (1996)
Functional Independence Measure (FIM)	Functional status in seven areas: self-care, locomotion, communication, social cognition, cooperation, problem solving, sphincter control	Kidd et al. (1995); Keith (1987)
Timed UP and Go Test	Mobility, balance, gait, transfer ability, walking	Podsiadlo and Richardson (1991)
2-Minute Walk Test	Exercise tolerance and exercise capacity	Brooks, Parsons, Hunter, Devlin and Walker (2001)
UB-2 CAM and 3D-CAM (www.hospitalelderlifeprogram.org)	For delirium quick screen: UB-2—has high > 90% sensitivity for delirium and if positive follow with the CAM or 3D-CAM.	Fick et al. (2015; 2018)

ADL, activities of daily living; IADL, instrumental activities of daily living scale.

Note: For additional geriatric assessment resources, the *Try This* series can be found at https://consultgeri.org/tools/try-this-series

CHAPTER SUMMARY

The GRN model is a straightforward, low-resource, high-value model that empowers nurses to use their education fully and to practice at the top of their license. The Institute of Medicine (IOM) report entitled The Future of Nursing *clearly outlines the need to reconceptualize the role of nurses in order to capitalize on their full potential (IOM, 2011). It is no surprise that key leaders, Joyce Clifford and Stuart Altman, worked closely together for years prior to this report and their understanding of the rich nature of nursing practice fully informed it. Dr. Clifford, who died in 2011, just as the report was fully in the public eye, would not live to see the dramatic response and affirmation of the report. However, Dr. Altman was invited to do a 5-year review for the Institute of Medicine (now the National Academy of Medicine) and his committee reported on the continuing need to remove barriers to practice in care (Altman, Butler, & Shern, 2016). While progress could be documented, barriers remain that limit the ability of nurses to fully practice to the top of their license. It is absolutely clear that education for nurses needs to be changed dramatically to ensure that the requisite leadership skills are in place that facilitate the way in which nurses assert their knowledge and practice. Further, nurses are fully recognized as highly collaborative healthcare team members, but they frequently lag in their capacity to lead in day-to-day practice given invisible health system forces and cultures that are strong and powerful. The GRN model is one approach to unleashing the full capacity, autonomy, authority, and requisite responsibility of nursing practice.*

REFERENCES

Abraham, I. L., Bottrell, M. M., Dash, K. R., Fulmer, T. T., Mezey, M. D., O'Donnell, L., & Vince-Whitman, C. (1999). Profiling care and benchmarking best practice in care of hospitalized elderly: The Geriatric Institutional Assessment Profile. *The Nursing Clinics of North America, 34*(1), 237–255.

Admi, H., Shadmi, E., Baruch, H., & Zisberg, A. (2015). From research to reality: Minimizing the effects of hospitalization on older adults. *Rambam Maimonides Medical Journal, 6*(2), e0017. doi:10.5041/RMMJ.10201

Altman, S. H., Butler, A. S., & Shern, L. (Eds.). (2016). *Assessing progress on the Institute of Medicine report* The Future of Nursing. Washington, DC: National Academies Press.

Boltz, M., Capezuti, E., Bowar-Ferres, S., Norman, R., Secic, M., Kim, H., . . . Fulmer, T. (2008). Hospital nurses' perception of the geriatric nurse practice environment. *Journal of Nursing Scholarship, 40*(3), 282–289. doi:10.1111/j.1547-5069.2008.00239.x

Boltz, M., Capezuti, E., Fulmer, T. T., & Zwicker, D. (Eds.). (2016). *Evidence-based geriatric nursing protocols for best practice* (5th ed.). New York, NY: Springer Publishing.

Brooks, D., Parsons, J., Hunter, J. P., Devlin, M., & Walker, J. (2001). The 2-minute walk test as a measure of functional improvement in persons with lower limb amputation. *Archives of physical medicine and rehabilitation, 82*(10), 1478–1483. doi:10.1053/apmr.2001.25153

Carter, K. (1982). *Gerontic Nurse Fellowship a first at BI.* Report on Professional Nursing at Boston's Beth Israel Hospital, newsletter, Vol. 1, pp. 1–3.

Deschodt, M., Flamaing, J., Haentjens, P., Boonen, S., & Milisen, K. (2013). Impact of geriatric consultation teams on clinical outcome in acute hospitals: A systematic review and meta-analysis. *BioMed Central Medicine, 11*, 48. doi:10.1186/1741-7015-11-48

Deschodt, M., Flamaing, J., Rock, G., Boland, B., Boonen, S., & Milisen, K. (2012). Implementation of inpatient geriatric consultation teams and geriatric resource nurses in acute hospitals: A national survey study. *International Journal of Nursing Studies, 49*(7), 842–849. doi:10.1016/j.ijnurstu.2011.11.015

Fick, D. M., Inouye, S. K., Guess, J., Ngo, L. H., Jones, R. N., Saczynski, J. S., & Marcantonio, E. R. (2015). Preliminary development of an ultrabrief two-item bedside test for delirium. *Journal of Hospital Medicine, 10*(10), 645–650. doi:10.1002/jhm.2418

Fick, D. M., Inouye, S. K., McDermott, C., Zhou, W., Ngo, L., Gallagher, J., … Marcantonio, E. R. (2018). Pilot study of a two-step delirium detection protocol administered by certified nursing assistants, physicians, and registered nurses. *Journal of Gerontological Nursing, 44*(5), 18–24. doi:10.3928/00989134-20180302-01

Fick, D. M., Steis, M. R., Mion, L. C., & Walls, J. L. (2011). Computerized decision support for delirium superimposed on dementia in older adults. *Journal of Gerontological Nursing, 37*(4), 39–47. doi:10.3928/00989134-20100930-01

Fulmer, T. (1977). On vitamins, calories, and help for the elderly. *American Journal of Nursing, 77*, 1614–1615. doi:10.1097/00000446-197710000-00026

Fulmer, T. (1981). Termination of life support systems in the elderly. Discussion: The registered nurse's role. *American Journal of Geriatric Psychiatry, 14*(1), 23–30.

Fulmer, T. (1987a). Lessons from a nursing home. *American Journal of Nursing, 87*(3), 332–333. doi:10.1097/00000446-198703000-00027

Fulmer, T. (1987b). Nursing care. The key to enhancing adaptation to long-term care. *Frontiers in Aging Series, 5*, 169–175.

Fulmer, T. (1991a). The geriatric nurse specialist role: A new model. *Nursing Management, 22*(3), 91–93. doi:10.1097/00006247-199103000-00025

Fulmer, T. (1991b). Grow your own experts in hospital elder care. *Geriatric Nursing, 12*(2), 64–66. doi:10.1016/s0197-4572(09)90116-1

Fulmer, T. (2007). How to try this: Fulmer SPICES. *American Journal of Nursing, 107*(10), 40–48; quiz 48–49. doi:10.1097/01.naj.0000292197.76076.e1

Fulmer, T., Ashley, J., & Reilly, C. (1986). Geriatric nursing in acute settings. *Annual Review of Gerontology and Geriatrics, 6*, 27–80.

Graf, C. (2006). Functional decline in hospitalized older adults: It's often a consequence of hospitalization, but it doesn't have to be. *American Journal of Nursing, 106*(1), 58–67. doi:10.1097/00000446-200601000-00032

Inouye, S. K., Acampora, D., Miller, R. L., Fulmer, T., Hurst, L. D., & Cooney, L. M., Jr. (1993). The Yale Geriatric Care Program: A model of care to prevent functional decline in hospitalized elderly patients. *Journal of the American Geriatrics Society, 41*(12), 1345–1352. doi:10.1111/j.1532-5415.1993.tb06486.x

Institute of Medicine. (2011). *The future of nursing: Leading change, advancing health.* Washington, DC: The National Academies Press.

Keith, R. A. (1987). The functional independence measure: A new tool for rehabilitation. *Advances in clinical rehabilitation, 2*, 6–18.

Kidd, D., Stewart, G., Baldry, J., Johnson, J., Rossiter, D., Petruckevitch, A., & Thompson, A. J. (1995). The functional independence measure: A comparative validity and reliability study. *Disability and Rehabilitation, 17*(1), 10–14. doi:10.3109/09638289509166622

Kitson, A. L., Rycroft-Malone, J., Harvey, G., McCormack, B., Seers, K., & Titchen, A. (2008). Evaluating the successful implementation of evidence into practice using the PARiHS framework: Theoretical and practical challenges. *Implementation Science, 3*(1), 1. doi:10.1186/1748-5908-3-1

Kleinpell, R. M., Fletcher, K., & Jennings, B. M. (2008). Reducing functional decline in hospitalized elderly. In R. G. Hughes (Ed.), *Patient safety and quality: An evidence-based handbook for nurses* (Chapter 11). Rockville, MD: Agency for Healthcare Research and Quality.

Lawton, M. P., & Brody, E. M. (1969). Assessment of older people: self-maintaining and instrumental activities of daily living. *The gerontologist, 9*(3_Part_1), 179–186. doi:10.1097/00006199-197005000-00029

Milisen, K., Foreman, M. D., Abraham, I. L., De Geest, S., Godderis, J., Vandermeulen, E., . . . Broos, P. L. (2001). A nurse-led interdisciplinary intervention program for delirium in elderly hip-fracture patients. *Journal of the American Geriatrics Society, 49*(5), 523–532. doi:10.1046/j.1532-5415.2001.49109.x

Podsiadlo, D., & Richardson, S. (1991). The timed "Up & Go": A test of basic functional mobility for frail elderly persons. *Journal of the American geriatrics Society, 39*(2), 142–148. doi: 10.1111/j.1532-5415.1991.tb01616.x

Rapp, C. G., Onega, L. L., Tripp-Reimer, T., Mobily, P., Wakefield, B., Kundrat, M., . . . Morrow-Howell, N. (1998). Unit-based acute confusion resource nurse: An educational program to train staff nurses. *The Gerontologist, 38*(5), 628–632. doi:10.1093/geront/38.5.628

Rapp, C. G., Onega, L. L., Tripp-Reimer, T., Mobily, P., Wakefield, B., Kundrat, M., . . . Waterman, J. (2001). Training of acute confusion resource nurses: Knowledge, perceived confidence, and role. *Journal of Gerontological Nursing, 27*(4), 34–40. doi:10.3928/0098-9134-20010401-08

Reilly, C. (1981). Primary nursing and the care and management of the elderly. *Nursing Administration Quarterly, 5*(4), 59–63.

Sager, M. A., Rudberg, M. A., Jalaluddin, M., Franke, T., Inouye, S. K., Landefeld, C. S., . . . & Winograd, C. H. (1996). Hospital admission risk profile (HARP): identifying older patients at risk for functional decline following acute medical illness and hospitalization. *Journal of the American Geriatrics Society, 44*(3), 251–257.

St. Pierre, J., & Twibell, R. (2012). Developing nurses' geriatric expertise through the geriatric resource nurse model. *Geriatric Nursing, 33*(2), 140–149. doi:10.1016/j.gerinurse.2012.01.005

Turner, J. T., Lee, V., Fletcher, K., Hudson, K., & Barton, D. (2001). Measuring quality of care with an inpatient elderly population: The geriatric resource nurse model. *Journal of Gerontological Nursing, 27*(3), 8–9. doi:10.3928/0098-9134-20010301-04

Wallace, M., & Fulmer, T. (1998). Fulmer SPICES An Overall Assessment Tool of Older Adults. *Journal of gerontological nursing, 24*(12), 3–13. doi: 10.3928/0098-9134-19981201-03

Yevchak, A., Fick, D. M., Kolanowski, A. M., McDowell, J., Monroe, T., LeViere, A., & Mion, L. (2017). Implementing nurse-facilitated person-centered care approaches for patients with delirium superimposed on dementia in the acute care setting. *Journal of Gerontological Nursing, 43*(12), 21–28. doi:10.3928/00989134-20170623-01

Yevchak, A. M., Fick, D. M., McDowell, J. A., Monroe, T., May, K., Grove, L., . . . Inouye, S. K. (2014). Barriers and facilitators to implementing delirium rounds in a clinical trial across three diverse hospital settings. *Clinical Nursing Research, 23*(2), 201–215. doi:10.1177/1054773813505321

Standardizing Geriatric Resource Nurse (GRN) Roles and Responsibilities: A Strategy for Sustaining NICHE in an Academic Medical Center

8

Marilyn Lopez

NICHE is all about being part of a network of like-minded individuals and health systems that thrive for age-friendly excellence. This book provides the context as well as concrete examples of how this is achieved in NICHE facilities.
—Elizabeth Capezuti, PhD, RN, FAAN, William Randolph Hearst Foundation Chair in Gerontology and Professor, Associate Dean of Research

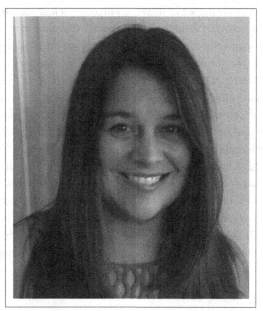

Marilyn Lopez.

CHAPTER OBJECTIVES

1. Discuss the roles and responsibilities of GRNs
2. Explain how an organization conducts GRN training
3. Describe the expectations of the GRN role
4. Describe implementation of the GRN role at New York University Langone Health

INTRODUCTION

It is estimated that the United States will require an additional 3.5 million healthcare workers by 2030 to maintain the current ratio of healthcare workers to the population (Centers for Disease Control and Prevention, 2018; Heimlich, 2010; Institute of Medicine [IOM], 2008; West, Cole, Goodkind, & He, 2010). This trend is consistent across all professions including physicians, nurses, social workers, and other disciplines (IOM, 2008). Adults 65 and older are predicted to grow twofold and people 85 and older mostly likely will require acute, primary, and long-term care, which is expected to increase fivefold (IOM, 2008; U.S. Census Bureau, 2008). The surge of aging older Americans will have a huge impact on the U.S. healthcare system and workforce needs over the coming decades. The demand for healthcare providers caring for older adults with competencies in geriatric care and gerontology will be felt across all settings (Colwill, Cultice, & Kruse, 2008).

New York University Langone Health (NYULH), similar to other academic medical centers, seeks strategies to improve outcomes while maintaining or reducing costs, issues germane to care of frail older adults who have complex needs that need to be quickly addressed. A core component to the Nurses Improving Care for Healthsystem Elders (NICHE) national program is the geriatric resource nurse (GRN) model, one of several clinical improvement models (Mezey et al., 2004; Mezey, Boltz, Esterson, & Mitty, 2005). The GRN model provides education and clinical training to prepare staff nurses as unit-based leaders, educators, and consultants to their peers in geriatric best practices (Fulmer et al, 2002). The GRN role and responsibilities differ between institutions and among specialty units within the same hospital (Boltz, Capezuti, & Shabbat, 2010; Boltz, Harrington, & Kuger, 2005; Bub, Boltz, Malsch, & Fletcher, 2015; Capezuti, Bricoli, & Boltz, 2013; Fulmer et al., 2002; Lopez et al., 2002; Mezey et al., 2004, 2005; Nickoley, 2013).

This chapter will discuss the roles and responsibilities of the GRN and illustrate how our NYULH organization conducts the GRN training program and the expectation for GRNs. The chapter will also address strategies used to strengthen the role of the GRN and how we have built upon the NICHE national program to address the challenges of an academic medical center.

NATIONAL NICHE/GRN MODEL

Before describing the history of our program and experiences at NYULH, it is instructive to summarize the national model. The GRN model has many variations

The principal goal of the GRN model is to enhance geriatric knowledge and expertise of registered nurses (RNs) providing direct patient care, which is key to successful implementation of geriatric best practice outcomes system wide.

and was not designed to be prescriptive, but rather to offer guidelines, tools, and resources to organizations committed to developing the GRN model (Capezuti, Bub, & Boltz, 2013; Francis, Fletcher, & Simon, 1998). Furthermore, the principal goal of the GRN model is to enhance geriatric knowledge and expertise of registered nurses (RNs) providing direct patient care, which is key to successful implementation of geriatric best practice outcomes system wide (Capezuti et al., 2012). The NICHE online Knowledge Center (KC), describes the roles and responsibilities of the GRN as:

- Demonstrating an interest in the care of older adults

- Enhancing skills in the care of older adults learned through education and training programs administered in the NICHE hospital by an advanced practice geriatric nurse (Fulmer, 1991)

- Advocating for patients, unit-based educators, role models, and elder care consultants

- Willingness to lead rounds and consult with an advanced practice nurse (APN) on patients identified as high risk

- Implementation of Fulmer's SPICES tool acronym, highly recommended as a systematic method to identify existing and potential problems common in hospitalized older adults (Fulmer, 2007, 1991; Wallace & Fulmer, 2003)

- Capacity to review all patients with an APN, geriatric physician, and primary nurses who present with geriatric issues, conditions, or syndromes during geriatric care rounds

- Utilization of clinical protocols as educational and management tools to assist primary nurses to care for patients during assessment and the management of common clinical problems

NICHE/GRN MODEL: THE EARLY DAYS (1997–2013) AT NYULH

As early pioneers in geriatric nursing, this academic medical center adopted the national NICHE training model in 1997. We worked closely with Drs. Mathy Mezey and Terry Fulmer, then faculty of the NYU Division of Nursing and initially focused on a 34-bed medical unit practice with a large diverse older population. RNs volunteered to train and this became the core group of GRNs. Their training focused on identifying care needs through systematic collection of clinical information, unit-based educational sessions, and case-by-case informal rounds presentations guided by the Geriatric Nurse Practitioner (GNP)-case manager (Lopez, 2006; Lopez et al., 2002). Through the institution's educational department we offered a supplemental monthly lecture series coordinated by GNP, which included

With the benefit of GNP expertise the GRNs were recognized as the first-line resources to advise and guide complex care with physicians, pharmacists, social workers, physical therapists, dietitians, and other specialty team members.

evidence-based geriatric care practices pertinent to the medical unit's needs. With the benefit of GNP expertise the GRNs were recognized as the first-line resources to advise and guide complex care with physicians, pharmacists, social workers, physical therapy, dietitians, and other specialty team members. NICHE leadership training conferences and the support of our chief nursing officer (CNO) were vitally important in the development of our GRN program. Training nurses to recognize and identify common concerns and needs of older patients was one of the key priorities and we introduced Fulmer's SPICES tool to assist RNs in their assessment of older adults. SPICES is an acronym for six areas of concern among older adults: sleep problems, problems with eating and feeding, incontinence, confusion, evidence of falls, and skin breakdown (Fulmer, 1991; Fulmer et al., 2002; Fulmer, 2019). To facilitate the utilization of the SPICES tool we designed a handy pocket card that accelerated the use of the card as standard practice for initial screening of older adults.

GRNs were trained to became familiar with and use tools and resources provided through the Hartford Institute for Geriatric Nursing found on Consult-GeriRN.org (with content formerly on GeroNurseOnline.org) a geriatric clinical nursing website with online resources such as the *Try This* assessment tools and *How to Try This* series. The *How to Try This* series comprises articles and videos demonstrating use of tools in areas of activities of daily living, mental status, orthostatic hypotension, predicting pressure injury risk, and other areas relevant to our medical unit patient population (Boltz, Capezuti, Mezey, & Fulmer, 2007; Hartford Institute for Geriatric Nursing, 2017). Informal lecture presentations, team rounds, and bedside consultation provided by GNPs and NYU faculty members were also integrated into the medical unit practice.

As our program matured from 1997 to 2000, we supplemented the training with informal lecture presentations and use of evidence-based assessment tools. Our explicit expectation was that GRNs would be first-line experts to assess the older adult for more complex patient needs and seek out the consult of geriatric experts. In short, RNs who became GRNs were regarded as providing their nursing colleagues direct access to unit-based geriatric expert nurses. The GRNs, for their part, developed their own expertise and increased their prospects for advancement through the clinical ladder program (American Nurses Association, 2015; Buyrket et al., 2010).

Over time the roles and responsibilities of NYULH GRNs were well aligned to meet the needs of practices on a medical unit. However, as their expertise matured GRNs became aware of other geriatric common concerns or syndromes in our older adults that had been identified through complex case studies and clinical rounds. For example, based on GRN observation, it became evident that hearing and vision issues and other geriatric conditions or syndromes were contributing to functional decline, cognitive impairment, and quality of life (Inouye, Studenski, Tinetti, & Kuchel, 2007; Lin, Niparko, & Ferrucci, 2011; Rogers & Langa, 2010). After several years of experience using the SPICES tool, we recognized that we needed to modify the tool to include vision and hearing and other geriatric concerns which were common among our patient population. Thus we created SHARING, a tool adapted from SPICES, with seven areas for assessment: skin breakdown, hearing and visual impairments, altered mental status, restraint alternatives, incontinence, nutritional needs, and gait needs (Lopez et al., 2002).

Aside from revisions to the SHARING tool, GRNs also recognized their need for palliative and end-of-life training to meet patient care needs. Thus, we adapted geriatric and palliative training of the End-of-Life Nursing Education Consortium (ELNEC) concepts and principles introduced through a nurse residency AgeWise project (Boltz et al., 2005; Ferrell et al., 2007). We provided GRNs educational training over a 6-month period assembled from established curricula from geriatric and palliative care.

Most recently, we have updated our SHARING tool to include a more holistic approach to ensure older adults with complex needs transition safely post-hospitalization. Currently, the SHARING tool also includes assessment of pain, medication reconciliation, health literacy, hearing loss, altered sleep patterns, poor vision, healthcare decisions, oral health, and hydration (Health in Aging Foundation, 2019; Berkman, Sheridan, Donahue, Halpern, & Crotty, 2011; El-Sharkawy, Sahota, Maughan, & Lobo, 2014; Isaia et al., 2011; Herr, Bjoro, & Decker, 2006; Lin et al., 2011; Rogers & Langa, 2010; Silveira, Kim, & Langa, 2010; Sjögren, Nilsson, Forsell, Johansson, & Hoogstraate, 2008; Villaire & Mayer, 2007). The revised SHARING tool is used today along with daily geriatric pearls on team rounds relevant to complex case studies in alignment with our organizational standards (see Figure 8.1). In short, the ongoing revisions and changes to GRN training, resource utilization, and education underscores the need to consistently innovate and revise the training program to reflect the clinical circumstances within the patient population.

The ongoing revisions and changes to GRN training, resource utilization, and education underscores the need to consistently innovate and revise the training program to reflect the clinical circumstances within the patient population.

NYULH is not alone in adopting national NICHE guidelines to meet organizational priorities or unique features of the local environment. Other NICHE sites

Identify Seniors ≥65 years of age
Exhibiting The Following Changes in Conditions ot Concerns:

- S – Skin integrity
- H – Hearing & vision/ Health Literacy / Healthcare decision making
- A – Altered memory / Altered sleep patterns
- R – Reconciliation of medications / Reassess pain
- I – Incontinence
- N – Nutrition, hydration & oral health
- G – Gait & function

"SHARING" tool is a mnemonic device used as a badge buddy on interprofessional safety rounds

FIGURE 8.1 *"SHARING" tool.*

have developed their own tools (e.g., SPPICEES, FANCAPES) to stimulate critical thinking during assessment of the older adult in various clinical settings (Ebersole, Hess, Touhy, Jett, & Luggen, 2007; Fletcher, Hawkes, Williams-Rosenthal, Mariscal, & Cox, 2007). In summary, the roles and responsibilities in our single medical unit NICHE program during the early years (1997–2013) included:

- Assess patients ≥65 years of age using the SHARING tool
- Utilize NICHE resources, *Try This* assessment tools, videos, and team expert consults
- Serve as a first-line resource and mentor to junior staff
- Conduct unit daily geriatric rounds with peers and team experts
- Teach unit staff, patients, and families about geriatric care issues
- Be active council member in falls, wound care, pain, or other councils
- Assist in the development, review, and revision of unit protocols
- Attain American Nurses Credentialing Center (ANCC) certification in Gerontological Nursing

During the early years from 1997 to 2013, 12 RNs were trained as GRNs; this group exhibited team camaraderie in providing geriatric best practices, leadership, and a commitment to our program. The majority of these nurses, 11 out of 12, obtained ANCC Gerontological Nursing certifications.

Beginning in 2012, we started using the national NICHE online, web-based system that covered essential curricula of geriatric practice, that is, training modules, tools, case examples, protocols, and other resources to prepare our GRNs. The 14 GRN content modules are now part of the NICHE core curriculum. The NICHE online KC expanded to provide information and resources for a wide range of users such as patients, families, clinicians, interdisciplinary teams, and organizations found on their website: www.nicheprogram.org (Boltz, Capezuti, Fulmer, & Zwicker, 2012; NICHE, 2016). Collectively, all the NICHE elements provide our organization a framework upon which we can build institution-specific programs focused on the older adult population (Boltz et al., 2008; Capezuti et al., 2012; Nickoley, 2013). At the close of our early years we had 12 GRNs, all of whom were ANCC certified in our medical unit. But things were about to change.

NICHE/GRN HYBRID MODEL AT NYULH: REDEFINING OUR PROGRAM (2014–2016)

As our program matured, we identified a range of areas for improvement and expansion. With changes at the national NICHE program, such as the introduction of 14 modules of online training and materials, and recent events in New York

City in the aftermath of Superstorm Sandy, nursing leadership at our organization saw opportunities to reconceptualize the NICHE program. As inpatient units were reconfigured, it became apparent that GRNs were needed not just in one medical unit but throughout the hospital. Additionally, as the organization's footprint in ambulatory care expanded, it was evident that GRNs could also be useful in outpatient settings.

As a result, the entire NICHE/GRN training program was reviewed and overhauled. A key decision was to examine effective learning strategies that were more sensitive to the needs of adult learners (Erwin-Toth, Stenger, Stricker, & Merlino, 2012; Sibbald, Alavi, Sibbald, Sibbald, & Goodman, 2012). Thus different learning strategies such as written, visual presentations, discussion groups, and interprofessional team rounds (learn-by-doing) coupled with other interactive learning methodologies were introduced with the expectation that clinicians are likely to process and incorporate new learned information into daily practice (D'Amour & Oandasan, 2005). With input from the GNP, nursing leaders, and members of the interprofessional advisory team, our NICHE/GRN program was reinforced in the following elements: (a) dedicated GNP NICHE coordinator; (b) in-house seminars and other specific training to supplement NICHE national online training; (c) creation of a GRN-specific nursing council to keep GRNs informed and to develop a sense of community; and (d) a process for ongoing interprofessional team education and evaluation of practice.

The GRN training program was transformed in several critical ways. First, with strong CNO support, a new dedicated fulltime GNP/NICHE coordinator was designated to manage, strengthen, and sustain the GRN training program, as well as to attend to the ongoing needs of GRNs practicing throughout the institution. Growing a larger GRN workforce required a wide range of considerations.

Among the earliest decisions was to change the training from a somewhat informal and organic process to a structured program offered twice a year with specific timelines and clear objectives. In addition, RNs were strategically recruited to the training program from areas outside medicine (intensive care unit [ICU], oncology, surgery, emergency department [ED], ambulatory sites). Opening recruitment of RNs from a variety of specialty units increased the likelihood of collaboration and opportunities to share knowledge and clinical experiences in care of the older adult across the institution. The dispersion of the growing GRN workforce made it necessary to create a sense of community of shared values and goals among the GRNs and so a monthly GRN Practice Council (GRNPC) led by GRNs was created. Recently we have expanded our GRNPC to include night staff to enhance geriatric best practices, by incorporating day and night shift handoffs and night team huddles to facilitate inpatient transitions of care to other specialty units.

The interprofessional geriatrics committee (IGC) led by the GNP/NICHE coordinator meets quarterly to brainstorm with clinical experts. GRNs and other key stakeholders target geriatric problems and how to effectively prioritize to work together

Opening recruitment of RNs from a variety of specialty units increased the likelihood of collaboration and opportunities to share knowledge and clinical experiences in care of the older adult across the institution.

for the same common goals. Finally, in summary, we developed a hybrid training program that combines the NICHE national program elements, such as self-paced modules, with unique homegrown, innovative, and interprofessional supplemental learning modalities to address our current older population needs. Additionally, we introduced several innovative educational components to the training and to ongoing programming intended to assist GRNs to stay current on geriatric nursing practices.

INNOVATIONS

To remain vital and responsive to changes in patient needs and organizational priorities, the NICHE/GRN program needs to be innovative and current. Recently we have introduced new elements of our NICHE/GRN program to strengthen our GRN training and practice.

The Geriatric Jeopardy Challenger Game (GJCG),[1] inspired by the TV show, is used in interprofessional GRN training seminars to advance knowledge from a novice clinician to an expert clinician level of geriatric practice experiences (Figure 8.2). NYULH GJCG adopts the format of the popular TV game show that allows GRNs and others to test their knowledge and engage in friendly competition with colleagues. Patricia Benner's conceptual framework from novice to expert is used with GJCG in advancing through five different levels of clinical experiences (Benner, 1984; Lopez, 2012). The clues get increasingly difficult as the point value increases and as the individual advances from novice to expert. The game is also being used in training of medical residents during their geriatric rotations and, from time to time, the GRNs compete with team members for top score. In contrast to traditional teaching where the instructor controls the learning, GJCG is learner centered and interactive (Kiili, 2005; Ricciardi & Tommaso De Paolis, 2014).

Given the current emphasis on data, metrics, and measurements, GRNs need to be competent in obtaining and analyzing data on their patient population. The advent of electronic health records offers many opportunities for GRNs to use clinical data to make informed decisions. Our EPIC system incorporates many of the well-known, reliable assessment tools such as the numeric visual and behavioral pain tools; Confusion Assessment Method (CAM) screen; Braden skin risk assessment; Mini Nutritional Assessment; Index of Independence in activities of daily living; and other evidence-based assessment tools (American Geriatrics Society [AGS], 2009; Ayello, 2004; Herr et al., 2006; Inouye, 2006; McCabe, 2019; Vellas et al., 2006).

Easy access to geriatric assessment tools increases the likelihood of their use. Moreover, once the tools are completed, the resulting data can be grouped with data from other similar patients to monitor trends, identify gaps, and so

---

[1] The Jeopardy template was created by Dr. Robert Pettis of the University of South Carolina, Spartanburg.

Physiological Changes	Pharmacology	Functional Assessment Tools	Geriatric Palliative Care	Psychosocial
100	100	100	100	100
200	200	200	200	200
300	300	300	300	300
400	400	400	400	400
Final Jeopardy 500	500	500	500	500

200 Points (Example) Pharmacology Q&A:

Question:
This drug is used to reverse overdose of benzodiazepines

Answer:
What is Flumazenil (Romazicon)

500 Points (Example) Functional Assesment Tools Q&A:

Question:
This is a pain assesment tool used to assess pain in older adults who have dementia or other cognitive impairment and are unable to reliably communicate their pain

Answer:
What is the Pain Assessment in Advanced Dementia (PAINAD) Scale

A fun method to strengthen and enhance geriatric education (adapted from Dr. Robert Pettis, An Adventure of the American Mind)

FIGURE 8.2 *Interprofessional innovations geriatric jeopardy challenger game.*

The creative use of Health Information Technology (HIT) has the potential to capture populated data from admission assessments, change over time, and real-time high-risk indicators for older adults.

on. The creative use of Health Information Technology (HIT) has the potential to capture populated data from admission assessments, change over time, and real-time high-risk indicators for older adults (Capezuti, 2010; Malone et al., 2010). For example, analysis of our fall data identified that falls are more likely to be associated with medications than age alone. The analysis also revealed that the falls risk tool being used was ineffective. This led to institutional improvement of the fall safety prevention bundle and GRN daily rounds with medication list review and interprofessional team experts—for example, application of Beers Criteria for inappropriate medications (Health in Aging Foundation, 2019; Boltz, Capezuti, Fulmer, & Zwicker, 2016).

Moreover, we recently introduced the Hospital Elder Life Program (HELP) delirium-risk reducing components in our revised SHARING tool that includes further focused assessment and interventions to prevent cognitive and functional decline in partnership with interprofessional team experts (Inouye, Baker, Fungal, & Bradley, 2006). GRNs are learning the skills and knowledge associated with HELP and sharing newfound knowledge with patient care technicians (PCTs), ancillary staff, and volunteers being trained in care of the older adult.

NICHE/GRN HYBRID MODEL: CURRENT STATUS

After reconceptualizing our NICHE program in 2014, the number of GRNs grew from 12 to 71 GRNs in 2015 and to 115 GRNs in 2017 (Figure 8.3). GRNs practice across 14 inpatient units and 12 specialty areas, which include the intensive care unit, medicine, oncology, ED, surgery, cardiac rehab, preadmission, and other specialty areas across our health system (Figure 8.4).

The structured GRN training program takes 5 months to complete. Admission to the GRN program requires a formal application process with eligibility and expectations criteria. Furthermore, the contract with GRNs is in alignment with ANCC exam requirements. Eligibility requirements include (a) approval of nurse manager (NM) or supervisor; (b) an impersonal statement and a resume; and (c) a minimum of 2 or more years or higher experience as an RN (ANCC exam requirement).

Once accepted to the program, trainees take the online GRN core curriculum comprising 14 modules and must achieve a score of 80% or higher for each post-test module. The core curriculum provides 21 continuing education contact hours to GRNs. In addition to the online training, our GRNs conduct a quality improvement (QI) project and present an oral presentation to their colleagues. After completing their training, GRNs are expected to continue providing support and guidance on aging-related QI projects on their units. GRN training has a strong interprofessional component covering a wide range of topics, for example skin pressure injury, delirium, health literacy, maintaining function, pain management, and other relevant current topics aligned with patient care needs. GRNs participate in afternoon interprofessional clinical rounds, for example, addressing the cognitively impaired older adult with a pressure injury and associated pain management with team experts in real time to complement seminar didactic

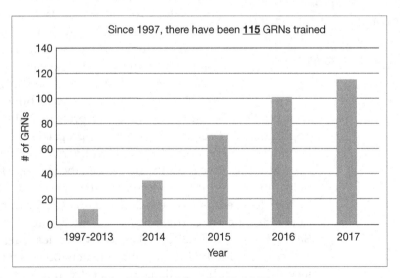

FIGURE 8.3 *Expansion of the GRN Workforce (1997–2017).*
Note: Table displays the cumulative total of GRNs trained since 1997.

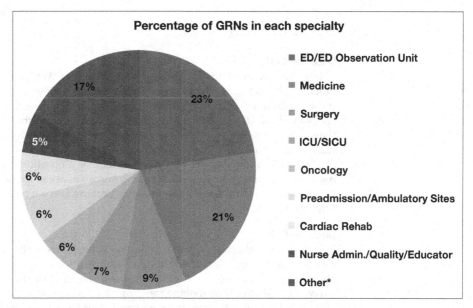

FIGURE 8.4 *Expansion of GRN Workforce by specialty (1997–2017).*
*Note: *Other specialty areas include psychiatry, alert team, venous access team, care management, epilepsy, MIUU/recovery, interventional radiology, noninvasive cardiology, same-day admit*

presentations (Lopez, 2017). In total, GRN training consists of five seminars (57.5 clinical hours), afternoon unit bedside rounds, and team discussions. GRNs are expected to complete ANCC Gerontological certification within 6 months of completing GRN training. They receive the credential RN-BC. Furthermore, GRNs receive an annual bonus for successfully completing this certification.

A successful NICHE coordinator is required to have strong advanced practice clinical skills as well as being a geriatric nurse expert in order to manage, strengthen, and sustain GRN training along with other specialty APNs. APNs are highly skilled (geriatrics, cardiology, orthopedics, neurology, intensive care) and care for the majority of patients 65 and older at our organization. The APN role in our new blended model is vital in meeting the unique needs of our older adults across specialties. They are frontline responders. Incorporating specialty APNs in our GRN training seminars creates opportunities to enhance geriatric knowledge and creates a forum for mutual exchange of clinical experiences. This assures that every APN counts in geriatric best practices at the bedside.

A GRNPC online community forum and graduate support group was formed to boost GRN to GRN collaboration and ANCC certifications. GRN postings on the GRNPC community homepage include GRN exam certification success insights, study tips, geriatric pearls, PowerPoint interactive polling questions, games, puzzles, a GRN newsletter with practice questions, and other certification exam prep resources (Box 8.1).

Commitment to scholarly QI project abstract writing for national conferences is challenging for bedside GRNs. In partnership with the Center for Innovations

> **BOX 8.1 GRN Insights**
>
> **Oncology GRN**
>
> "My mom saw me studying for the exam and asked 'Why is there a whole test on older adults? Is taking care of them really that much different?' And I shocked even myself with how much info I immediately began to rattle off about their needs for specialized care. If you are nervous about the ANCC exam, trust that you know more than you realize just from taking care of older adult patients, and we all definitely learned more than we thought possible during the GRN course. Taking 170 questions can be tough, but my advice is if you get stuck on a question, just mark it and come back to it, because you may get the answer somewhere else in the exam or you realize it's okay to be unsure about a few answers because you felt confident about so many other questions."
>
> **Medicine GRN**
>
> "I always remember a speech Martin Luther King, Jr. made about our life's blueprint. I am paraphrasing, but he said 'have a determination to achieve excellence in your chosen life's work' and 'If we can't fly to run, if we can't run to walk, if we can't walk to crawl but always keep moving forward.' My decision to become a nurse was made early in life but even though it was accomplished later in my life I am grateful for the chance to help others. The opportunity to take the GRN course and achieve certification is my commitment to moving forward so I can continue to help others."
>
> **Acute Cardiac Rehab GRN**
>
> "Just want to let everyone know I passed the ANCC Gerontological Nursing certification early this week. Thanks to the mentorship provided by the GRN course team, NICHE coordinator, and GRN colleagues—could not have done it without! Oh and of course I can't neglect to mention Geriatric Jeopardy."
>
> **ED Observation GRN**
>
> "Taking the NICHE course really helped me prepare for the GRN exam, especially having continued access to the modules and questions. I've posted numerous study tips and exam focused topics that were on my exam to the GRNPC community site early this week for GRN colleagues preparing to take ANCC exam."
>
> *Source:* Courtesy of NYULH NICHE Program 2017.

in the Advancement of Care (CIAC),[2] a research center within the NYULH Department of Nursing at our institution, we offer periodic Abstract Clinics to assist GRNs interested in submitting scholarly abstracts to conferences. The clinic sessions have been instrumental in our increased numbers of conference podium and poster presentations at the NICHE national conferences.

In 2016, with support from nursing leadership, we embarked on a formal program evaluation of our NICHE/GRN program. In collaboration with CIAC, a formal program evaluation was launched to examine the three components of

---

[2] CIAC supports a community of NYULH nurses and other researchers in studying patient care issues across the healthcare delivery spectrum.

our GRN program: (a) practice patterns of our GRN workforce, including their assessment of the strengths and weaknesses of their training; (b) the impact of GRNs on unit-level geriatric nursing practices to assess the extent to which GRNs are effective change leaders, resources, and mentors; and (3) the impact of GRNs on unit-based patient outcomes. Chapter 18 will discuss the program evaluation study and findings.

The NICHE coordinator is in constant liaison with the national program and seeks collaboration and communication in meeting our organization's priorities. It is essential to continue to raise NICHE awareness across our health system, in community outreach events, and national conference presentations. It has been invaluable to have strong connections to NICHE national headquarters to expand program initiatives through serving as an active member in the national conference committee as well as taking on other leadership appointments such as fellow advisor to the Hartford Institute for Geriatric Nursing at New York University's Rory Meyers College of Nursing. Furthermore, we remain informed through media and new research and by contributing to published scholarly work. These elements are required to make the NICHE champion and coordinator roles a success.

CHAPTER SUMMARY

The NYULH NICHE/GRN hybrid model is a reflection of our long-standing commitment to geriatric nursing care, strong CNO support, interprofessional team collaboration, and our historical relationship with national expert leaders in the colleges of nursing. Our restructured NICHE/GRN model is a culmination of years of experience and expertise to create something durable and sustainable. By infusing our NICHE/GRN program with homegrown innovations, use of HIT, and interprofessional collaboration in conjunction with NICHE materials, we have sustained a strong and reliable GRN workforce.

Sustaining our program with an infusion of innovative approaches reflects our commitment to responding to healthcare changes in our practice setting. In our fast-moving practice environment with growing numbers of older adults and advances in medicine, pharmacotherapies, and technology, it is anticipated that our institution will continue to strengthen GRN roles and responsibilities and sustain a strong workforce to produce favorable outcomes as expected from a NICHE exemplar site.

REFERENCES

American Geriatrics Society. (2009). Pharmacological management of persistent pain in older persons. *Journal of the American Geriatrics Society*, *57*, 1331–1346. doi:10.1111/j.1532-5415.2009.02376.x

American Nurses Association. (2015). *Nursing: Scope and Standards of Practice, Third Edition*. Silver Spring, MD: Nursesbooks.org

Ayello, E. A. (2017). Predicting pressure injury risk. In S. A. Greenberg (Ed.), *Try this: Best practices in nursing care to older adults. 1*(5). The Hartford Institute for Geriatric Nursing. Retrieved from https://consultgeri.org/try-this/general-assessment/issue-5.pdf

Benner, P. (1984). *From novice to expert: Excellence and power in clinical nursing practice.* Menlo Park, CA: Addison-Wesley.

Berkman, N. D., Sheridan, S. L., Donahue, K. E., Halpern, D. J., & Crotty, K. (2011). Low health literacy and health outcomes: An updated systematic review. *Annals of Internal Medicine, 155,* 97–107. doi:10.7326/0003-4819-155-2-201107190-00005

Boltz, M., Capezuti, E., Bower-Ferres, S., Norman, R., Secic, M., Kim, H., . . . Fulmer, T. (2008). Changes in the geriatric care environment associated with NICHE (Nurses Improving Care for HealthSystem Elders). *Geriatric Nursing, 29,* 176–185. doi:10.1016/j.gerinurse.2008.02.002

Boltz, M., Capezuti, E., Fulmer, T., & Zwicker, D. (Eds.). (2012). *Evidence-based geriatric nursing protocols for best practice* (4th ed.). New York, NY: Springer Publishing.

Boltz, M., Capezuti, E., Fulmer, T. T., & Zwicker, D. (Eds.). (2016). *Evidence-based geriatric nursing practice protocols for best practice* (5th ed.). New York, NY: Springer Publishing.

Boltz, M., Capezuti, E., Mezey, M., & Fulmer, T. (2007). *The NICHE implementation manual* (3rd ed). New York, NY: John A. Hartford Institute for Geriatric Nursing.

Boltz, M., Capezuti, E., & Shabbat, N. (2010). Building a framework for a geriatric acute care model. *Leadership in Health Services, 23*(4), 334–360. doi:10.1108/17511871011079029

Boltz, M., Harrington, C., & Kluger, M. (2005). Nurses Improving Care for Health System Elders (NICHE). *American Journal of Nursing, 105*(5), 101–102. doi:10.1097/00000446-200505000-00039

Bub, L., Boltz, M., Malsch, A., & Fletcher, K. (2015). The NICHE program to prepare the workforce to address the needs of older patients. In M. L. Malone, E. A. Capezuti, & R. M. Palmer (Eds.), *Geriatrics models of care* (pp. 57–70). New York, NY: Springer.

Buyrket, T., Felmlee, M., Greider, P. J., Hippensteel, D. M., Rohrer, E. A., & Shay, M. L. (2010). Clinical ladder program evolution: Journey from novice to expert to enhancing outcomes. *The Journal of Continuing Education in Nursing, 41*(8), 369–374. doi:10.3928/00220124-20100503-07

Capezuti, E. (2010). An electronic geriatric specialist workforce: Is it a viable option? *Geriatric Nursing, 31*(3), 220–222. doi:10.1016/j.gerinurse.2010.04.005

Capezuti, E., Boltz, E., Cline, D., Dickson, V. V., Rosenberg, M.-C., Wagner, L., . . . Nigolian, C. (2012). Nurses Improving the Care for Healthsystem Elders: A model for optimising the geriatric nursing practice environment. *Journal of Clinical Nursing, 21,* 3117–3125. doi:10.1111/j.1365-2702.2012.04259.x

Capezuti, E., Briccoli, B., & Boltz, M. (2013). Nurses Improving the Care of Healthsystem Elders: Creating a sustainable business model to improve care of hospitalized older adults. *Journal of the American Geriatrics Society, 61*(8), 1387–1393. doi:10.1111/jgs.12324

Capezuti, E., Bub, L., & Boltz, M. (2013). The NICHE guide: The geriatric resource nurse model. In L. Bub, M. Boltz, & E. Capezuti (Eds.), *NICHE planning and implementation guide* (pp. 1–34). New York, NY: University College of Nursing.

Centers for Disease Control and Prevention (2018). Adverse drug events in adults. Retrieved from http://www.cdc.gov/medicationsafety/adult_adversedrugevents.html

Colwill, J. M., Cultice, J. M., & Kruse, R. L. (2008). Will generalist physician supply meet demands of an increasing and aging population? *Health Affairs, 27*(3), 232–241. doi:10.1377/hlthaff.27.3.w232

D'Amour, D., & Oandasan, I. (2005). Interprofessionality as the field of interprofessional practice and interprofessional education: An emerging concept. *Journal of Interprofessional Care, 19*(Suppl 1), 8–20. doi:10.1080/13561820500081604

Ebersole, P., Hess, P., Touhy, T. A., Jett, K., & Luggen, A. S. (2007). *Toward healthy aging: Human needs and nursing response* (7th ed.). St. Louis, MO: Elsevier Science.

El-Sharkawy, A. M., Sahota, O., Maughan, R. J., & Lobo, D. N. (2014). The pathophysiology of fluid and electrolyte balance in the older adult surgical patient. *Clinical Nutrition, 33*, 6–13. doi:10.1016/j.clnu.2013.11.010

Erwin-Toth, P., Stenger, B., Stricker, L., & Merlino J. (2012). Teaching wound care to patients, families, and healthcare providers around the globe. In D. L. Krasner, G. T. Rodeheaver, R. G. Sibbald, & K. Y. Woo (Eds.), *Chronic wound care 5: A clinical source book for healthcare professionals* (5th ed., pp. 55–62). Malvern, PA: HMP Communications.

Ferrell, B. R., Dahlin, C., Campbell, M. L., Paice, J. A., Malloy, P., & Virani, R. (2007). End-of-life nursing education consortium (ELNEC) training program: Improving palliative care in critical care. *Critical Care Nursing Quarterly, 30*, 206–212. doi:10.1097/01.cnq.0000278920.37068.e9

Fletcher, K., Hawkes, P., Williams-Rosenthal, S., Mariscal, C. S., & Cox, B. A. (2007). Using nurse practitioners to implement best practice care for the elderly during hospitalization: The NICHE journey at the University of Virginia Medical Center. *Critical Care Nursing Clinics of North America, 19*, 321–337. doi:10.1016/j.ccell.2007.05.007

Francis, D., Fletcher, K., & Simon, L. F. (1998). The GRN model of care: A vision for the future. *Nursing Clinics of North America, 33*(3), 481–496.

Fulmer, T. (1991). Grow your own experts in hospital elder care. *Geriatric Nursing, 12*, 64–66. doi:10.1016/s0197-4572(09)90116-1

Fulmer, T. (2007). How to try this: Fulmer SPICES. *American Journal of Nursing, 107*(10), 40–48. doi:10.1097/01.naj.0000292197.76076.e1

Fulmer T. (2019). *How to try this: Best practices in nursing care to older adults.* Fulmer SPICES: An Overall Assessment Tool for Older Adults. Retrieved from https://consultgeri.org/try-this/general-assessment/issue-1.pdf

Fulmer, T., Mezey, M., Bottrell, M., Abraham, I., Sazant, J., Grossman, S., & Grisham, E. (2002). Nurses Improving Care for Healthsystem Elders (NICHE): Using outcomes and benchmarks for evidenced-based practice. *Geriatric Nursing, 23*(3), 121–127. doi:10.1067/mgn.2002.125423

Hartford Institute for Geriatric Nursing at New York University's Rory Meyers College of Nursing. (2017). *Try This* assessment tools. Retrieved from https://consultgeri.org/try this/general

Health in Aging Foundation. (2019). Medications & older adults: The 2019 American Geriatrics Society updated Beers criteria®: Medications that older adults should avoid or use with caution. Retrieved from http://www.healthinaging.org/medications-older-adults

Heimlich, R. (2010). Baby boomers retire. *Pew Research Center.* Retrieved from http://www.pewresearch.org/daily-number/baby-boomers-retire

Herr, K., Bjoro, K., & Decker, S. (2006). Tools for assessment of pain in nonverbal older adults with dementia: A state-of-the-science review. *Journal of Pain and Symptom Management 31*(2), 170–192. doi:10.1016/j.jpainsymman.2005.07.001

Inouye, S. K. (2006). Delirium in older persons. *New England Journal of Medicine, 354,* 1157–1165. doi:10.1056/nejmra052321

Inouye, S. K., Baker, D. I., Fugal, P., & Bradley, E. H. (2006). Dissemination of the Hospital Elder Life Program: Implementation, adaptation, and successes. *Journal of the American Geriatrics Society, 54,* 1492–1499. doi:10.1111/j.1532-5415.2006.00869.x

Inouye, S. K., Studenski, S., Tinetti, M. E., & Kuchel, G. A. (2007). Geriatric syndromes: Clinical, research, and policy implications of core geriatric concept. *Journal of the American Geriatrics Society, 55,* 780–791. doi: 10.1111/j.1532-5415.2007.01156.x

Institute of Medicine. (2008). *Committee on the Future Health Care Workforce for Older Americans. Retooling for an Aging America: Building the Health Care Workforce.* Washington, DC: National Academies Press.

Isaia, G., Corsinovi, L., Bo, M., Santos-Pereira, P., Michelis, G., Aimonino, N., & Zanocchi, M. (2011). Insomnia among hospitalized elderly: Prevalence, clinical characteristics and risk factors. *Archives of Gerontological and Geriatrics, 52*(2), 133–137. doi:10.1016/j.archger.2010.03.001

Kiili, K. (2005). Digital game-based learning: Towards an experiential gaming model. *The Internet and Higher Education, 8*(1), 13–24. doi:10.1016/j.iheduc.2004.12.001

Lin, F. R., Niparko, J. K., & Ferrucci, L. (2011). Hearing loss prevalence in the United States. *Archives of Internal Medicine, 171*(20), 1851–1853. doi:10.1001/archinternmed.2011.506

Lopez, M. (2006). Assessment at the time of hospitalization. In J. Gallo, H. R. Bogner, T. Fulmer, & G. J. Paveza (Eds.), *Handbook of geriatric assessment* (4th ed., pp. 399–418). Sudbury, MA: Jones & Bartlett.

Lopez, M. (2012). *Beyond traditional educational techniques: Building a Geriatric Jeopardy Challenger Game.* Paper presented at the NICHE Conference, New Orleans, LA.

Lopez, M. (2017). Pain in the cognitively impaired older adult with a wound. *World Council of Enterostomal Therapists Journal, 37*(2), 32–40.

Lopez, M., Delmore, B., Ake, J. M., Kim, Y. R., Golden, P., Bier, J., & Fulmer, T. (2002). Implementing a geriatric resource nurse model. *Journal of Nursing Administration, 32*(11), 577–585. doi:10.1097/00005110-200211000-00005

Malone, M. L., Vollbrecht, M., Stephenson, J., Burke, L., Pagel, P., & Goodwin, J. S. (2010). Acute Care for Elders (ACE) tracker and e-geriatrician: Methods to disseminate ACE concepts to hospitals with no geriatricians on staff. *Journal of the American Geriatrics Society, 58*, 161–167. doi:10.1111/j.1532-5415.2009.02624.x

McCabe, D. (2019). *How to try this: Best practices in nursing care to older adults. Monitoring functional status in hospitalized older adults.* (See Katz Index of Independence in Activities of Daily Living [ADL] section). Retrieved from https://consultgeri.org/try-this/general-assessment/issue-2

Mezey, M., Boltz, M., Esterson, J., & Mitty, E. (2005). Evolving models of geriatric nursing care. *Geriatric Nursing, 26*(1), 11–15. doi:10.1016/j.gerinurse.2004.11.012

Mezey, M., Kobayashi, M., Grossman, S., Firpo, A., Fulmer, T., & Mitty, E. (2004). Nurses Improving Care to Health System Elders (NICHE): Implementation of best practice models. *Journal of Nursing Administration, 34*(10), 451–457. doi:10.1097/00005110-200410000-00005

NICHE. (2016). NICHE program overview. Retrieved from https://nicheprogram.org/membership/benefits

Nickoley, S. (2010). Aligning NICHE and Magnet initiatives. In M. Boltz, J. Taylor, E. Capezuti, & T. Fulmer (Eds.), *NICHE Planning and Implementation Guide* (pp. 58–61). New York, NY: Hartford Institute for Geriatric Nursing.

Ricciardi, F., & Tommaso De Paolis, L. (2014). A comprehensive review of serious games in health professions. *International Journal of Computer Games Technology, 2014*, Article ID 787968. doi:10.1155/2014/787968

Rogers, M. A, & Langa, K. M. (2010). Untreated poor vision: A contributing factor to late-life dementia. *American Journal of Epidemiology, 171*(6), 728–735. doi:10.1093/aje/kwp453

Sibbald, R. G., Alavi, A., Sibbald, M., Sibbald, D., & Goodman L. (2012). Effective adult education principles to improve outcomes in patients with chronic wounds. In D. L. Krasner, G. T. Rodeheaver, R. G. Sibblad, & K. Y. Woo (Eds.), *Chronic wound care 5: A clinical source book for healthcare professionals* (5th ed., pp. 37–54). Malvern, PA: HMP Communications.

Silveira, M., Kim, S., & Langa, K. (2010). Advance directives and outcomes of surrogate decision making before death. *New England Journal of Medicine, 362*, 1211–1218. doi:10.1056/nejmsa0907901

Sjögren, P., Nilsson, E., Forsell, M., Johansson, O., & Hoogstraate, J. (2008). A systematic review of the preventive effect of oral hygiene on pneumonia and respiratory tract infection in elderly people in hospitals and nursing homes: Effect estimates and methodological quality of randomized controlled trials. *Journal of the American Geriatrics Society, 56*(11), 2124–2130. doi:10.1111/j.1532-5415.2008.01926.x

U.S. Census Bureau. (2008). *U.S. population projections: 2010 to 2050.* U.S. Department of Commerce: Washington, D.C.

Vellas, B., Villars, H., Abellan, G., Soto, M. E., Rolland, Y., Guigoz, Y., . . . Garry, P. (2006). Overview of the MNA®: Its history and challenges. *Journal of Nutrition, Health & Aging, 10*, 456–465.

Villaire, M, & Mayer, G. (2007). Low health literacy: The impact on chronic illness management. *Professional Case Management, 12*(4), 213–216. doi:10.1097/01. pcama.0000282907.98166.93

Wallace, M., & Fulmer, T. (2003). Fulmer SPICES: An overall assessment tool of older adults. *Alabama Nurse, 30*(3), 26.

West, L. A., Cole, S., Goodkind, D., & He, W. (2014). *65+ in the United States: 2010.* Washington, DC: U. S. Government Printing Office.

Evaluating Your Geriatric Resource Nurse (GRN) Workforce

9

Peri Rosenfeld

What do I think of when I think of Nurses Improving Care for Healthsystem Elders (NICHE)? The words that come to mind are: empowered, passionate, committed, visionary, innovative, forward-thinking, can-do attitude. I think of a group of empowered nurses and interdisciplinary healthcare professionals who lead the way to improving healthcare systems for older adults. Ahead of their time, NICHE was among the first organizations to embrace the importance of delirium, and to develop protocols and educational materials to address it. NICHE nurses were the earliest adopters and collaborators with the Hospital Elder Life Program (HELP). I had the tremendous honor and privilege of being a keynote speaker at the 25th anniversary NICHE conference and received a standing ovation: love, love, LOVE the NICHE nurses!

—Sharon Inouye, MD, Director, Aging Brain Center, Milton and Shirley F. Levy Family Chair, Professor of Medicine, Harvard Medical School, Beth Israel Deaconess Medical Center

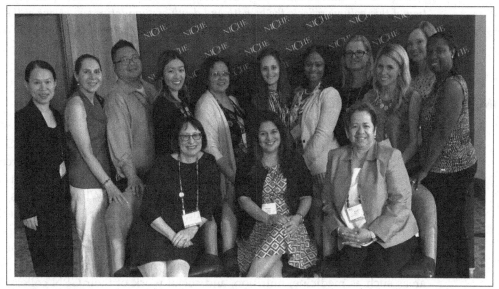

The NICHE program team at NYU Langone Health in New York City.

CHAPTER OBJECTIVES

1. Describe the program evaluation research study of the GRN workforce at one academic medical center
2. Describe the employment and demographic characteristics of the GRN workforce
3. Describe the utilization patterns of NICHE-related tools and materials among GRNs
4. Assess the unique GRN training program at this institution
5. Explore the perceptions, attitudes, and opinions of non-GRN registered nurses, nurse managers, and colleagues in other disciplines with respect to GRNs and the NICHE program

INTRODUCTION

Since its earliest days in the 1990s, a notable number of articles have been written about the Nurses Improving Care for Healthsystem Elders (NICHE) program and the geriatric resource nurse (GRN) model (Allen & Close, 2010; Boltz et al., 2008; Boltz, Capezuti, & Shabbat, 2010; Bub, Boltz, Malsch, & Fletcher, 2015; Capezuti, Briccoli, & Boltz, 2013; Fletcher, Hawkes, Williams-Rosenthal, Mariscal, & Cox, 2007; Fulmer et al., 2002; Guthrie, Edinger, & Schumacher, 2002; Hendrix, Matters, West, Stewart, & McConnell, 2011; Inouye et al., 1993; Kim, Capezuti, Boltz, & Fairchild, 2009; Lee & Fletcher, 2002; Lopez et al., 2002; Mezey et al., 2004; Mezey, Boltz, Esterson, & Mitty, 2005; Steele, 2010; Swauger & Tomlin, 2002; Turner, Lee, Fletcher, Hudson, & Barton, 2001). The publication of this volume reflects the breadth and depth of cumulative knowledge of the NICHE program—its history, its GRN and other practice models, and its significance to the development of geriatric nursing practices.

EVALUATING GRN TRAINING AND THE GRN WORKFORCE

To date, the literature has focused only on the potential benefits of the NICHE program from the institution's perspective. Yet, little is known about the perceptions, opinions, or attitudes of the individuals who are trained as GRNs. What types of registered nurses (RNs) make up the GRN workforce? What motivates them to become GRNs? How has NICHE training influenced their daily practices? What are their assessments of the NICHE training program?

In addition, little is known about the perceptions, attitudes, and opinions of non-GRN nurses, nurse managers (NMs) and interprofessional team members in areas such as medicine, nutrition, and social work of their GRN colleagues. For example, what is generally known about the NICHE program and GRNs? What perceived benefits (or disadvantages) does NICHE have to their institutions?

What do colleagues recommend to improve NICHE program contributions to the institution and/or to interdisciplinary collaboration?

This chapter describes the program evaluation research study conducted by New York University Langone Health (NYULH), a large, urban academic medical center, to study the GRN workforce at one academic medical center. The study was conducted in two phases: the first phase examined (a) the employment and demographic characteristics of the GRN workforce; (b) the utilization patterns of NICHE-related tools and materials among GRNs; and (c) assessment of the unique GRN training program at our institution. The second phase explored the perceptions, attitudes, and opinions of non-GRN RNs, NMs, and colleagues in other disciplines with respect to the GRNs and the NICHE program.

This is the first study to elicit information from individual RNs who completed GRN training and the perceptions and attitudes of their nursing colleagues, NMs, and members of the Interdisciplinary Advisory Group. We believe that this program evaluation methodology has relevance to other NICHE institutions interested in assessing their training programs and the practice patterns of their GRN workforces.

Given the institutional and financial commitments necessary to launch and maintain NICHE and sustain a GRN training program, it is important that institutions periodically evaluate their GRN programs to ensure that the program continues to perform at its optimum level.

Given the institutional and financial commitments necessary to launch and maintain NICHE and sustain a GRN training program, it is important that institutions periodically evaluate their GRN programs to ensure that the program continues to perform at its optimum level. Moreover, it is equally important to assess whether the size of the GRN workforce is adequate to achieve desired outcomes. These may be challenging issues for institutions interested in optimizing their nursing resources in an era of financial scrutiny.

BACKGROUND

Since its original designation in 1999, NYULH's NICHE program has evolved significantly. Initially, the NICHE program was implemented exclusively in one large, active medicine unit and training was informal and unstructured.[1] In the early years, faculty of the local college of nursing were deeply involved in educating RNs about geriatric syndromes and geriatric nursing practices. The charismatic leadership associated with those earlier years set in motion wide-ranging innovations in nursing care.

Over time, the national NICHE model changed and in 2010 the clinical and leadership training components were migrated to an online, web-based system. The availability of online training standardized the curriculum for GRN training, ensuring that all GRNs obtained education in the key areas of geriatric practice

---

[1] For a full description of our GRN training program, see Chapter 8, by Marilyn Lopez.

through the offering of 14 individual modules; this provided the impetus to formalize GRN training at the institution.

In 2014, under the leadership of a new NICHE Program Coordinator, NYULH'S NICHE program adopted more formalized processes and was significantly overhauled in several ways. First, GRN training was extended beyond the original medicine unit to other inpatient services and ambulatory settings. RNs from across the institution are now trained as cohorts (fall and spring) to increase synergy across clinical areas. To ensure that GRNs are distributed across the institution, recruitment to the program has become more strategic and competitive. Stringent admission criteria are used for admission to the program, including a minimal clinical ladder requirement (i.e., senior staff nurse or above),[2] personal statement, NM's approval, and admission interview. New cohorts of GRNs are expected to complete all 14 NICHE online modules as well as other components of the program, including a quality improvement (QI) project and attendance at seminars and workshops, within a prescribed amount of time (5 months). Thus, our hybrid model includes components of the national model as well as homegrown innovations.

The transition from charismatic leadership that focuses on personal interactions between leaders and their followers to more formal/institutional leadership is not unusual; it is seen as a natural progression as innovative ideas grow and spread, requiring administrative processes to realize and expand their desired objectives (Weber, Henderson, & Parsons, 1947).

PHASE I: SURVEY OF THE GRN WORKFORCE[3]

All RNs who completed the NICHE/GRN Program between 1997 and fall 2016 were eligible to participate in the online survey: 87 nurses were eligible to participate in the survey. A total of 74 completed surveys were received (85.1% response rate). Given this robust response rate, we can confidently presume the data do not contain any sampling bias.

Demographic, Educational, and Employment Characteristics of the GRN Workforce

As a group, the GRNs are, on average, 38 years old with 11.9 years of tenure at the institution, predominantly female and all with a minimum of baccalaureate-prepared nursing education (Table 9.1). Fewer than half have obtained American Nurses Credentialing Center (ANCC) certification in gerontological nursing

---

[2] The clinical ladder at *this* organization has four tiers: (a) staff nurse: advanced beginner (delivers care); (b) senior staff nurse: competent (directs care); (c) nurse clinician: proficient (innovates); and (d) senior nurse clinician: expert (designs and inspires).

[3] For a more detailed discussion of this study, see Rosenfeld, Kwok, and Glassman (2018).

TABLE 9.1 Summary Data on GRN Demographics, Education, and Employment Characteristics (N = 74)

Demographics	
Female, n (%)	52 (91.2)
Mean age, years (range)	38.13 (26–58)
Education	
Highest Education	
Bachelor's, n (%)	43 (74.1)
Master's, n (%)	11 (19.0)
Nurse Practitioner, n (%)	3 (5.2)
Other, n (%)	1 (1.7)
Certification in Geriatric Nursing, n (%)	24 (42.1)
Employment	
Current Title	
Senior Staff Nurse, n (%)	19 (27.9)
Nurse Clinician, n (%)	15 (22.1)
Senior Nurse Clinician, n (%)	23 (33.8)
Other, n (%)	11 (16.2)
Current Unit	
Med-Surg, n (%)	25 (39.7)
Emergency Department, n (%)	7 (11.1)
Cardiology & Cardiac Rehab, n (%)	6 (9.5)
Oncology & Radiation Oncology, n (%)	4 (6.4)
Administration/Leadership, n (%)	5 (7.9)
Other[a], n (%)	16 (25.4)
Cohort	
Prior to 2014, n (%)	8 (12.3)
Fall 2014, n (%)	14 (21.5)
Spring 2015, n (%)	13 (20.0)
Fall 2015, n (%)	11 (16.9)
Spring 2016, n (%)	19 (29.2)

[a]Other units include: MICU, NICU, Psychiatric, Surgery, Venous Access Team.

(42.1%) and more than one-third work on a medical–surgical unit (39.7%). ANCC certification is statistically significantly ($p < 0.001$) related to time since GRN training. Thus, 100% of GRNs trained prior to 2014 are ANCC certified; 73% of those trained in fall 2014 are certified and numbers diminish with newer cohorts. In other words, over time the proportion of GRNs with ANCC certification is likely to increase.

Measures

A specially designed survey instrument was developed, piloted, and distributed to GRNs via Qualtrics©, an online survey platform. The survey consists of 28 items in a variety of formats (e.g., Likert scale or nominal choices) and was vetted by several veteran and novice GRNs, as well as the NICHE Program Coordinator, to ensure that the survey items were understandable (e.g., do questions make sense?) and exhaustive (e.g., do the answers cover all possible options?). In addition to the demographic, educational, and employment characteristics described above, the survey included the following domains: (a) reasons for becoming a GRN; (b) utilization of evidence-based geriatric tools in practice; (c) GRNs' assessment of training components and roles preparation; and (d) NMs' support.

GRNs were invited to participate in the study via an email distribution list. In addition, research assistants (RAs) also attended monthly GRN council meetings to recruit participants and offered GRNs the use of an iPad with a survey link. The protocol was approved by the Institutional Review Board through expedited review. Recruitment and data collection occurred from October to November 2016.

Key Findings of the GRN Survey

Reasons for Becoming a GRN

Respondents were asked to rank their reason for becoming a GRN. More than half of the GRNs (53.7%) reported that they "want to provide better patient and family care." "Improve clinical competencies" garnered the second highest response at 19.4%. "Personal curiosity; interest/want to learn about geriatric care," "opportunity for professional growth," "tangible incentive associated with salary bonus," and "inspired by a particular person" trailed behind.

Utilization of Evidence-Based Geriatric Tools and Practices

A critical component of GRN/NICHE training focuses on knowledge and competence in utilizing geriatric evidence-based practice (EBP) assessment and other tools designed specifically for care of the elderly, such as the Confusion Assessment Method; the Braden Scale for predicting pressure injury risk; and the American Geriatrics Society Beers Criteria for Potentially Inappropriate Medication Use in Older Adults.

Participants were asked to estimate the frequency with which they used geriatric EBP tools as organized around the 14-module NICHE training. Using a 5-point Likert scale from "Never" (1) to "Always" (every day, every patient; = 5), respondents reported very frequent (between "usually" and "always") use of geriatric EBP tools and practices in a majority of domains (e.g., medication, falls, pain). It should be noted that several of these EBPs are integrated in NYULH's electronic health record and so the reported high frequency of utilization may be related to easy access to needed information rather than NICHE training. Less frequent usage of EBP tools was found in areas such as sleep, restraints, incontinence, and depression. It is difficult to ascertain whether the infrequent use of EBP in these areas is related to low prevalence of these issues among patients or provider issues. But overall, GRNs reported an average 4.08 (SD = 0.754, Min = 1.15, and

Max = 5) across all tools, which reflects a commitment to using geriatric EBP tools whenever they can in practice.

GRN Assessment of Training Components and Role Preparation

In contrast to earlier, informal training, our hybrid model provides a more formal training structure. GRN trainees are now expected to participate in specific activities and complete particular assignments as prescribed by the national NICHE program, plus homegrown activities developed at the institution. The hybrid training program uses a variety of teaching modalities such as clinical rounds with experts, daily huddles and pearls, and other methods described in Chapter 8. Respondents were asked to identify the two most useful teaching modules and as a group the top program components were (a) clinical rounds with experts and (b) presentations/lectures (Figure 9.1).

Our model distinguishes a range of potential roles that GRNs can play, so that at the completion of training, GRNs should be ready to advance beyond clinical expertise and perform leadership and other roles.

Our model distinguishes a range of potential roles that GRNs can play, so that at the completion of training, GRNs should be ready to advance beyond clinical expertise and perform leadership and other roles. Thus, we asked respondents to select the two GRN roles that were most valuable or important to them.[4] Not surprisingly, "enhancing geriatric nursing knowledge" was considered the most important role of the GRN (68.9%) followed by "serving as a resource to RNs and PCTs" (39.2%); the third

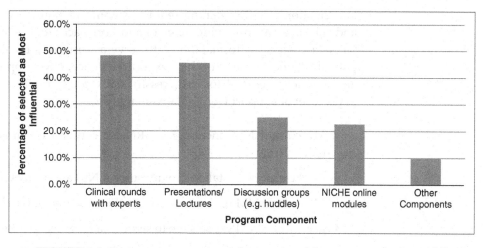

FIGURE 9.1 *Program components rated as most useful to your practice (n = 136).*

---

[4] The full list of GRN roles included: (a) enhance geriatric nursing knowledge; (b) master geriatric assessment tools; (c) serve as a resource to RNs and PCTs; (d) provide consultation/guidance to other providers, beyond RNs (e.g., residents and medical students); (e) expand GRN interdisciplinary collaboration; (f) encourage participation in the GRN council; (g) network with RNs across specialties; (h) improve effectiveness in patient and family advocacy; (i) provide access to online resources; and (j) present and publish scholarly work.

TABLE 9.2 GRN Rating: Two Roles Most Valuable to Your Practice ($N = 144$)	
GRN ROLES	**MOST VALUABLE, N (%)**
Enhance geriatric nursing knowledge	51 (68.9)
Serve as resource to RNs and PCTs	29 (39.2)
Improve effectiveness in patient and family advocacy	16 (21.6)
Master geriatric assessment tools	15 (20.3)
Provide consultation/guidance to other providers beyond RNs (e.g., residents and medical students)	10 (13.5)
Expand GRN interdisciplinary collaboration	7 (9.5)
Present and publish scholarly work	5 (6.8)
Other roles[a]	≤4%
GRN, geriatric resource nurse; PCT, patient care technician; RN, registered nurse. [a]Other roles include: network with RNs across specialties; encourage participation in GRN council; provide access to online resources.	

most important/valuable role reported was "improve effectiveness in patient and family advocacy" (21.6%; Table 9.2). The relatively low rating of "expand interprofessional collaboration," "presenting/publishing," and "network with RNs across specialties" suggests that GRNs may need encouragement to venture outside their units and expand contacts in other clinical and professional areas.

Nurse Manager Support

Participation in GRN training requires significant time away from patient units and clinical areas for a wide range of additional activities. In addition to training, GRNs are expected to make time to serve as resources for their colleagues and patient families in need of their expertise. Hence, NM support of GRN training and practice is critical for a successful GRN program. The key components of NMs' level of support were isolated in five areas:

- My current NM encourages GRNs to conduct QI projects specifically on older adults.

- I feel comfortable talking to my current NM about my GRN training.

- My current NM understands and values the role of GRNs and experience.

- My current NM expects me to serve as a resource to other nurses.

- My current NM supports my participation in the GRN program (e.g., taking time to attend GRN council meeting or training).

GRNs were asked to rate their current NMs on each of the items on a scale of 1 (lowest) to 5 (highest) level of support. Respondents reported high levels of support among their NMs, resulting in an overall average score of 22.76 (with a possible maximum of 25).

Summary of the Survey of GRNs

The findings of the GRN survey provide unique insights from the GRNs' perspective and have implications to both this institution's and the national program. In multiple items in the survey, GRNs repeatedly underscored their strong motivation to care for older adults and their families. Respondents reported high levels of satisfaction with the training program but preferred traditional learning modalities/skills development approaches such as lectures, clinical rounds, and huddles and were somewhat less enthusiastic about the online training and other modalities. Nonetheless, contemporary workforce training typically includes use of online and digital learning, which are more cost effective and time efficient than traditional lecture-style teaching. From the perspective of adult education, the GRNs are most eager to increase knowledge in areas that are directly relevant to their practice.

Respondents report very positive attitudes toward the multifaceted GRN role at NYULH. However, certain aspects of the GRN roles and responsibilities were considered less valuable than others. Interprofessional collaborations, networking, presenting/publishing scholarly work, and being active on the GRN council—all areas outside the comfort zone of many GRNs—were viewed less positively than elements focused on patients and their families. These data suggest that GRNs perceive their primary role as providers of care to patients and colleagues to RNs on their units, rather than reaching beyond their local units, disciplines, and clinical specialties to improve care for all older patients to a wider audience. Finally, GRNs reported strong support from their NMs. This support undoubtedly reflects long-standing commitment to geriatric nursing care at the institution and its historical relationship with the NYU Rory Meyers College of Nursing.

Although the program received overall positive feedback, in an open-ended survey item GRNs identified several structural barriers to their ability to implement the knowledge and skills they learned in NICHE training. The hectic nature of the work environment was seen as a barrier to implementing NICHE-related innovative geriatric practices. Respondents also identified lack of collaboration, in the form of resistance and avoidance from staff and colleagues in other disciplines, as a barrier. Addressing this impediment may require more training in leadership development to enable GRNs to be effective change agents, communicators, and collaborators, particularly with colleagues in disciplines other than nursing.

The structured training program at NYULH has led to a steady, predictable increase in our GRN workforce and allows targeted recruitment to specific clinical areas that could benefit from GRN talents and knowledge.

The structured training program at NYULH has led to a steady, predictable increase in our GRN workforce and allows targeted recruitment to specific clinical areas that could benefit from GRN talents and knowledge. Regardless of where each GRN is found, they all have had unitary and standardized training. This is particularly relevant in an era that emphasizes high reliability organizations (HROs).

PHASE II: QUALITATIVE STUDY OF NURSE MANAGERS, RNS, AND OTHERS

In order to better understand the level of awareness and knowledge of the NICHE programs and GRNs, we conducted a qualitative study that included focus groups and one-to-one interviews. Using a purposive sampling we recruited (a) nurse colleagues of GRNs; (b) NMs of GRNs; and (c) members of the Interprofessional Advisory Group (IAG), all of whom had lectured at GRN training sessions. Focus groups were conducted with RNs who worked on units that had a large number of GRNs. Face-to-face semi-structured interviews were conducted with NMs and IAG members. In the final analysis, we interviewed four NMs and three members of the IAG. To the extent possible, questions to the focus groups paralleled the semi-structured interview questions posed to other study participants. All interviews and focus groups were recorded and transcribed by RAs. The protocol was approved by the NYULH Institutional Review Board and the study was conducted in July to September 2017.

Each transcription was coded by the principal investigator (PI) and three trained independent researchers using a thematic analysis approach, which was best suited for answering the specific set of questions we had about the program at NYULH (Braun & Clarke, 2006). First, each researcher independently coded the data based on each question, a process called "open coding" (Strauss, 1987) or "generating initial codes" (Braun & Clarke, 2006). After the initial coding and theme creation, the researchers met and talked about the findings and came to a consensus about the themes found. In the meeting, the research team tried to reconcile the codes; the PI would settle disagreements, if any. Ultimately the team would meet one last time to settle on central themes (Braun & Clarke, 2006).

Key Findings

The research team has not completed a comprehensive analysis of the focus groups and interview data and so preliminary findings are presented here. This summary highlights many insightful observations and perceptions of individuals who work closely with the NICHE program and GRNs at our organization.

Focus Group of RNs

RNs who work on units with large numbers of GRNs readily and fairly accurately stated the overall purpose of NICHE program, as these two illustrative comments demonstrate: "A program to bring awareness about needs of elderly in hospitals" and "Provides specific information for caring for and improving care of geriatric patients."

They were aware of the annual conference and recognized that GRNs were involved in "projects." However, they expressed confusion about GRNs, geriatric nurse practitioners (GNPs), and nurses on specialty services such as the geriatric consult team or on the palliative care council at NYULH. Some thought GRN training resulted in certification. As a group, they were unaware of the training and other requirements to become a GRN. Few RNs could confidently name the GRNs on their units. RNs were dubious that GRNs were more expert at caring for the elderly than a typical RN who has years of experience caring for older adults. One RN explained that the majority of patients on her units are elderly and so "everyone on this unit is a GRN one way or another."

Interviews With Nurse Managers

Interviews were conducted with NMs on four units with the largest number of GRNs. NMs were universally supportive of the NICHE program and the GRNs on their unit. Unanimously, they all saw the value of geriatric training for RNs and believed that any and all educational programs could benefit patient care. However, NMs were not able to identify concrete examples of how GRNs have impacted patient care nor could they recommend any particular metric or approaches for measuring outcomes of their GRNs.

NMs held accurate perceptions about the objectives of the NICHE program, could articulate many of the roles GRNs might play, and could identify the GRNs on their unit, as well as the Program Coordinator at NYULH. NMs were aware of GRN participation in projects and expressed mixed feelings about the topics being examined and the amount of time spent on projects. Two NMs held very positive perceptions of the ability of GRNs to advocate for geriatric patients and their families and influence practices of patient care technicians (PCTs) and RNs on their units. The other two expressed support for the program but were uncertain that there was evidence that GRNs improve patient care and outcomes on their units. There was consensus among the NMs that GRNs and the NICHE program needed more visibility in the organization and one suggested that all NMs throughout the organization have periodic workshops to learn about the value of NICHE program for the institution, expectations of GRNs, and possible measures of their impact.

Members of the Interprofessional Advisory Group

Three members of the IAG were interviewed and they were well versed in the objectives of the NICHE program and had detailed knowledge of GRN training, each having served as a lecturer for the training program. The NICHE program coordinator was highly praised for her superior interpersonal style and geriatric expertise. All three noted that the program had value for the organization and recommended that GRNs should not be associated exclusively with their particular units and should be more engaged in institution-wide initiatives and projects. This would increase their visibility and offer opportunities to use their knowledge and experiences more expansively. Strong nursing leadership was considered vital to the success of NICHE and there was consensus that increasing the membership of the IAG to include other disciplines would be desirable. Two participants strongly recommended that the NICHE program at our institution develop and monitor geriatric-specific metrics in a dashboard or scorecard. The specifics of what those metrics would look like and who would be responsible were not so obvious.

Summary of Focus Groups and Interviews

The feedback received from RNs, NMs, and members of the IAGs are eye-opening, instructive, and exceptionally important. Basic familiarity of the NICHE program and recognition of the NICHE program coordinator and the presence of GRNs in the institutions were universal across the groups. However, misperceptions and confusion abound among RN colleagues of GRNs, indicating a need to better inform the nursing workforce as to the presence and benefits of the institution's GRNs. NM support for GRN training is widespread and strong. Yet, some NMs expressed reservations about the amount of time GRNs spend off the unit and questioned the value of unit-based projects, favoring instead projects that were institution-wide. NMs and members of the IAG voiced concern that GRNs (and the NICHE program) did not have concrete, empirical evidence of their contributions to patient outcomes. Though no specific recommendations were made, this is an area that would require additional, more concentrated efforts. Nonetheless, these data will be instrumental in developing action plans to address these concerns.

Basic familiarity of the NICHE program and recognition of the NICHE program coordinator and the presence of GRNs in the institutions were universal across the groups. However, misperceptions and confusion abound among RN colleagues of GRNs, indicating a need to better inform the nursing workforce as to the presence and benefits of the institution's GRNs.

CHAPTER SUMMARY

This chapter provides details on the methodology and findings of the first research study to examine the attitudes, opinions, and perceptions of GRNs about their training and current practices, as well as the perceptions and opinions of RNs, NMs, and IAG members who work alongside them. The hybrid NICHE training course offered at NYULH effectively prepares GRNs with a variety of teaching modalities covering a wide range of topics and issues. The hybrid institution-tailored training model has demonstrated value in effectively training GRNs.

We found that several of our strategies have been particularly effective in developing and sustaining our hybrid model. First, the involvement and support of nursing leadership—from the chief nursing officer to the unit-based NM—sends a clear message that geriatric care is a priority for the organization. The fact that nursing leadership requested this program evaluation indicates their commitment to the GRN workforce and improvements in their training and practice.

Another form of leadership support is evident in the visibility and recognized expertise of the NICHE program coordinator. A strong program coordinator, especially one with formal geriatric nurse practitioner training, can recruit high-level experts for seminars and clinical rounds and is able to facilitate communication with physicians and hospital administration. The presence of a program coordinator who has access to important stakeholders throughout the organization can raise awareness of the value of the GRN workforce. Relatedly, an effective IAG enables the NICHE coordinator to negotiate solutions to barriers to practice. Creating a sense of community among GRNs has been challenging but produces desirable outcomes. The cohort approach for GRN training brings individuals from different areas to train together and each acquires a better appreciation of nursing practices across clinical areas. In addition, after training is completed, a social network emerges so that GRNs have colleagues they can call upon throughout the organization.

There is always room for improvement in any program and the survey results indicate areas for reinforcement of the program. Incorporating leadership development in GRN training is a clear area for improvement. This can allow GRNs to be more effective communicators and change agents and increase their visibility throughout the organization beyond nursing. The focus groups and interviews provide a clarion call that, while efforts and resources have been invested in the GRN training program, more needs to be done to promote and disseminate a coherent portrayal of the NICHE program and our GRN workforce to nurses and other providers at our institution. Undoubtedly, clear and consistent messages would reinforce the generally positive attitudes providers have of the program. With the benefit of quantitative and qualitative data, our evaluation study provides important feedback to develop action plans to continue refining and improving our GRN training and NICHE program.

REFERENCES

Allen, J., & Close, J. (2010). The NICHE geriatric resource nurse model: Improving the care of older adults with Alzheimer's disease and other dementias. *Geriatric Nursing, 31*(2), 128–132. doi:10.1016/j.gerinurse.2010.02.006

Boltz, M., Capezuti, E., Bowar-Ferres, S., Norman, R., Secic, M., Kim, H., . . . Fulmer, T. (2008). Hospital nurses' perception of the geriatric nurse practice environment. *Journal of Nursing Scholarship, 40*(3), 282–289. doi:10.1111/j.1547-5069.2008.00239.x

Boltz, M., Capezuti, E., & Shabbat, N. (2010). Building a framework for a geriatric acute care model. *Leadership in Health Services, 23*(4), 334–360. doi:10.1108/17511871011079029

Braun, V., & Clarke, V. (2006). Using thematic analysis in psychology. *Qualitative Research in Psychology, 3*(2), 77–101. doi:10.1191/1478088706qp063oa

Bub, L., Boltz, M., Malsch, A., & Fletcher, K. (2015). The NICHE program to prepare the workforce to address the needs of older patients. In M. Malone, E. Capezuti, & R. Palmer (Eds.), *Geriatrics models of care* (pp. 57–70). Cham, Switzerland: Springer International. doi:10.1007/978-3-319-16068-9

Capezuti, E., Briccoli, B., & Boltz, M. (2013). Nurses Improving the Care of Healthsystem Elders: Creating a sustainable business model to improve care of hospitalized older adults. *Journal of the American Geriatrics Society, 61*(8), 1387–1393. doi:10.1111/jgs.12324

Fletcher, K., Hawkes, P., Williams-Rosenthal, S., Mariscal, C. S., & Cox, B. A. (2007). Using nurse practitioners to implement best practice care for the elderly during hospitalization: The NICHE journey at the University of Virginia Medical Center. *Critical Care Nursing Clinics of North America, 19*(3), 321–337. doi:10.1016/j.ccell.2007.05.007

Fulmer, T., Mezey, M., Bottrell, M., Abraham, I., Sazant, J., Grossman, S., & Grisham, E. (2002). Nurses Improving Care for Healthsystem Elders (NICHE): Using outcomes and benchmarks for evidenced-based practice. *Geriatric Nursing*, 23(3), 121–127. doi:10.1067/mgn.2002.125423

Guthrie, P. F., Edinger, G., & Schumacher, S. (2002). Twice: A NICHE program at North Memorial Health Care. *Geriatric Nursing*, 23(3), 133–138. doi:10.1067/mgn.2002.125409

Hendrix, C. C., Matters, L., West, Y., Stewart, B., & McConnell, E. S. (2011). The Duke-NICHE Program: An academic-practice collaboration to enhance geriatric nursing care. *Nursing Outlook*, 59(3), 149–157. doi:10.1016/j.outlook.2011.02.007

Inouye, S. K., Acampora, D., Miller, R. L., Fulmer, T., Hurst, L. D., & Cooney, L. M., Jr. (1993). The Yale Geriatric Care Program: A model of care to prevent functional decline in hospitalized elderly patients. *Journal of the American Geriatrics Society*, 41, 1345–1352. doi:10.1111/j.1532-5415.1993.tb06486.x

Kim, H., Capezuti, E., Boltz, M., & Fairchild, S. (2009). The nursing practice environment and nurse-perceived quality of geriatric care in hospitals. *Western Journal of Nursing Research*, 31(4), 480–495. doi:10.1177/0193945909331429

Lee, V. K., & Fletcher, K. R. (2002). Sustaining the geriatric resource nurse model at the University of Virginia. *Geriatric Nursing*, 23(3), 128–132. doi:10.1067/mgn.2002.125410

Lopez, M., Delmore, B., Ake, J. M., Kim, Y. R., Golden, P., Bier, J., & Fulmer, T. (2002). Implementing a geriatric resource nurse model. *Journal of Nursing Administration*, 32(11), 577–585. doi:10.1097/00005110-200211000-00005

Mezey, M., Boltz, M., Esterson, J., & Mitty, E. (2005). Evolving models of geriatric nursing care. *Geriatric Nursing*, 26(1), 11–15. doi:10.1016/j.gerinurse.2004.11.012

Mezey, M., Kobayashi, M., Grossman, S., Firpo, A., Fulmer, T., & Mitty, E. (2004). Nurses Improving Care to Health System Elders (NICHE): Implementation of best practice models. *Journal of Nursing Administration*, 34(10), 451–457. doi:10.1097/00005110-200410000-00005

Rosenfeld, P., Kwok, G., and Glassman, K. (2018). Assessing the perceptions and attitudes of geriatric resource nurses: Evaluating the NICHE program at a large academic medical center. *Gerontology & Geriatrics Education*, 39(3), 268–282. doi:10.1080/02701960.2018.1428577

Steele, J. S. (2010). Current evidence regarding models of acute care for hospitalized geriatric patients. *Geriatric Nursing*, 31(5), 331–347. doi:10.1016/j.gerinurse.2010.03.003

Strauss, A. L. (1987). *Qualitative analysis for social scientists*. Cambridge, England: Cambridge University Press.

Swauger, K., & Tomlin, C. (2002). Best care for the elderly at Forsyth Medical Center. *Geriatric Nursing*, 23(3), 145–150. doi:10.1067/mgn.2002.125413

Turner, J. T., Lee, V., Fletcher, K., Hudson, K., & Barton, D. (2001). Measuring quality of care with an inpatient elderly population. The geriatric resource nurse model. *Journal of Gerontological Nursing*, 27(3), 8–18. doi:10.3928/0098-9134-20010301-04

Weber, M., Henderson, A. M., & Parsons, T. (1947). *The theory of social and economic organization* (1st American ed.). New York, NY: Oxford University Press.

Geriatric Care Models for Intervention

10

Elizabeth Capezuti and Marie Boltz

As a high school student in the summertime, I would work on the Nurses Improving Care for Healthsystem Elders (NICHE) project at the New York University (NYU) College of Nursing. We scanned Geriatric Institutional Assessment Profiles (GIAPs) and I had great fun working with Susan Fairchild. All these years later, I am a geriatric nurse practitioner. I guess you can call that real impact!
—Holly Fulmer, MSN, RN, AGPCNP-BC, Nurse Practitioner, The Hebrew Home for the Aged in Riverdale

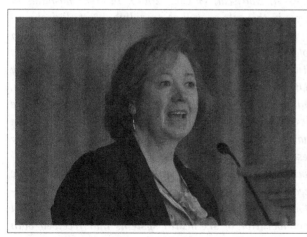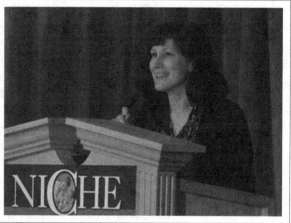

From left: Marie Boltz, Elizabeth Capezuti.

CHAPTER OBJECTIVES

1. Identify the objectives common to all geriatric care models
2. Describe the most common types of care models used in NICHE health systems
3. Describe the specialty care models used in NICHE health systems

INTRODUCTION

The system-level approach of Nurses Improving Care for Healthsystem Elders (NICHE) provides a structure for nurses to collaborate with other disciplines and to actively participate in or coordinate multiple geriatric acute care models (Capezuti, Bricoli, & Boltz, 2013). The geriatric resource nurse (GRN) model is foundational to NICHE implementation. Guided by a geriatric advanced practice nurse (GAPN) and/or NICHE coordinator, staff nurses are educated as clinical resources nurses (Capezuti et al., 2012; Fulmer et al., 2002; Mezey, Boltz, Esterson, & Mitty, 2005).

> *A NICHE coordinator acts in a leadership role by facilitating, teaching, and mentoring others and changing systems of care. In some hospitals, a GAPN functions in this role as well as providing direct clinical consultation for evaluating and managing patients.*

A NICHE coordinator acts in a leadership role by facilitating, teaching, and mentoring others and changing systems of care (Fletcher, Hawkes, Williams-Rosenthal, Mariscal, & Cox, 2007). In some hospitals, a GAPN functions in this role as well as providing direct clinical consultation for evaluating and managing patients. (For a full description of the GRN role, see Chapter 8.)

In addition to the GRN model, NICHE health systems employ multiple geriatric models in a portfolio approach (Capezuti, Boltz, Tejada, & Malone, 2018). NICHE is often paired with Acute Care of the Elderly (ACE) program and the Hospital Elder Life Program (HELP) or part of a larger geriatric consultation service or department. The GAPN may serve as coordinator of these multiple models. In an effort to reduce the potential duplicative activities involved with implementing multiple models, the Medicare Innovations Collaborative utilized a portfolio or service line approach to model integration (Leff et al., 2012). With a focus on improving inpatient hospital and transitional care, they brought together a collaborative of six health systems that received both peer-to-peer guidance and advice from model innovators through a central technical assistance program. These systems implemented two or more models simultaneously while customizing their healthcare organizations' local circumstances. The models included NICHE, ACE, and HELP as well as the care transitions intervention, the palliative care consultation, and the Hospital at Home® models. The Medicare Innovations Collaborative demonstrated that this approach is feasible and their findings suggest the potential for expansion across the care continuum. This program also demonstrated the essential role of nursing and NICHE for successful system-level integration (Boltz et al., 2013).

More recently, the John A. Hartford Foundation partnered with the Institute for Healthcare Improvement (IHI) to spearhead a "Creating Age-Friendly Health Systems" initiative. The ambition for this project is to develop an Age-Friendly Health Systems portfolio model and implement the model in 20% of U.S. health systems by 2020 (Fulmer & Berman, 2016; Fulmer & Li, 2018; Mate, Berman, Laderman, Kabcenell, & Fulmer, 2017).

Since the development of the comprehensive geriatric assessment (CGA) programs first developed in the 1970s (Palmer, 2014), geriatric care models have addressed the unique needs of older hospitalized patients.

Since the development of the comprehensive geriatric assessment (CGA) programs first developed in the 1970s (Palmer, 2014), geriatric care models have addressed the unique needs of older hospitalized patients. These models were driven by advances in geriatric science, the increasing older adult patient population, and the recognition of older patients' vulnerability to complications during their hospitalization.

The primary aim of geriatric care models is to facilitate improved overall outcomes. This is accomplished by promoting a rehabilitative approach while preventing adverse events that occur more commonly in older patients. The latter include geriatric syndromes, which are clinical conditions in older persons that do not fit into discrete disease categories (Palmer, 2014) and include frailty, functional decline, pressure ulcers, fall-related injury, undernutrition or malnutrition, urinary tract infection, and delirium. These syndromes or complications often lead to prolonged hospital stays and are highly associated with rehospitalization, institutionalization, emergency department (ED) usage, and post-acute rehabilitation therapy services. These complications rarely occur alone and the interrelationships among these are well recognized (Flood et al., 2015; Inouye, Studenski, Tinetti, & Kuchel, 2007; Palmer, 2014).

In addition to attending to age-specific vulnerabilities, these models also address the role of institutional factors, which determine staff practices, and the physical environment, which can contribute to iatrogenic complications. Thus, the overall goals of geriatric models of care include both (a) prevention of complications that occur more commonly in older adults and (b) minimization of hospital factors that contribute to complications (Capezuti, Boltz, & Kim, 2011).

This chapter provides a summary of the overlapping objectives these models share, a succinct description of geriatric models of care in the hospital setting, and various combinations of geriatric models of care.

MODEL OBJECTIVES

Although each geriatric care model utilizes its own approach to prevent complications and address institutional/staff practices that can contribute to complications, they all share a common set of general objectives (Capezuti & Boltz, 2014; Capezuti, Parks, Boltz, Malone, & Palmer, 2016; Hickman, Newton, Halcomb,

Chang, & Davidson, 2007; Hickman, Rolley, & Davidson, 2010). The following are the general objectives of geriatric care models.

Employ Geriatric Specialists

The expert knowledge of clinicians with specific geriatric preparation such as geriatricians, geriatric psychiatrists, GAPNs, social workers, pharmacists, and others (some disciplines provide only continuing education without recognized specialty expertise) are needed to facilitate the integration of geriatric care principles into practice (Conley et al., 2012; Maxwell, Mion, & Minnick, 2013).

Educate Healthcare Providers in Core Geriatric Principles

Many healthcare providers have not been exposed to basic or continuing education to core geriatric care principles such as recognition of age-specific factors that increase the risk of complications (Berman et al., 2005; Wald, Huddleston, & Kramer, 2006). All acute care models require a coordinator with advanced geriatric education; however, successful implementation also depends on direct care staff with the knowledge and competencies to deliver evidence-based geriatric care to older patients. Thus, the coordinator or a provider with geriatric specialization will facilitate staff learning by role modeling (e.g., individual patient consultation, unit rounds), encouraging use of geriatric protocols (see Chapter 2 and Mezey, Fulmer, & Abraham, 2003), education (group lectures, grand rounds, journal clubs, web-based discussion groups, and other internal institutional educational venues), and supporting attendance at conferences (Fletcher et al., 2007; Smyth, Dubin, Restrepo, Nueva-Espana, & Capezuti, 2001).

Incorporate Patient or Family Choices and Treatment Goals

Informed patients' choices are essential—not only for complex issues such as advance directives but also decisions about activity level and medication use. Staff and providers need to attend to outcomes that matter most to patients. When patients can no longer participate in decision making, family members must often deal with the complicated balance between quality-of-life considerations and potential length of life. Unfortunately, the decision regarding life-sustaining treatments consistent with patients' preferences is often considered only when the patient is hospitalized (Somogyi-Zalud, Zhong, Hamel, & Lynn, 2002). For this reason, many geriatric models work collaboratively or in conjunction with palliative care programs (Saracino, Bai, Blatt, Solomon, & McCorkle, 2018).

Promote Intraprofessional Communication

Detection and management of geriatric syndromes are not limited to medical intervention but require other disciplines such as nursing, pharmacy, social work, and physical and occupational therapy to address the complex interaction of medical, functional, psychological, and social issues contributing to these complications.

Detection and management of geriatric syndromes are not limited to medical intervention but require other disciplines such as nursing, pharmacy, social work, and physical and occupational therapy to address the complex interaction of medical, functional, psychological, and social issues contributing to these complications. Communication among the various disciplines is often facilitated by geriatric care providers to support informed participation by older patients and their family members.

Target Risk Factors for Complications

Timely screening of potential geriatric syndromes, early identification, and subsequent reduction of contributing risk factors are the ideal methods to prevent complications. Some of the models focus on a particular syndrome; however, because of the interrelationship of shared risk factors, reduction of one complication will involve the prevention of other geriatric syndromes. Standardized assessment tools with documented validity and reliability are recommended to properly identify individuals who are at an increased risk of geriatric syndromes. The Portal of Geriatrics Online Education (www.pogoe.org) and the Hartford Institute for Geriatric Nursing (www.hartfordign.org) websites provide assessment instruments. To facilitate staff uptake, healthcare systems need to incorporate these risk assessment tools into the workflow of everyday practice. This requires hospital policies, procedures, and protocols that will support usability such as embedding these tools within the electronic health record.

Emphasize Proactive Discharge Planning

Older hospitalized patients are more likely to experience delays in discharge, greater emergency service use, hospital readmission, and rehabilitation in an institution or at home (Coleman, Min, Chomiak, & Kramer, 2004). Hospital readmission for older patients is associated with medical errors in medication continuity (Coleman, Smith, Raha, & Min, 2005; Foust, Naylor, Boling, & Cappuzzo, 2005), diagnostic workup, or test follow-up (Forster, Murff, Peterson, Gandhi, & Bates, 2003). Geriatric care models emphasize early recognition of limited home resources or an overreliance on family for care at home. The models focus on the transition between hospital discharge and the posthospital care environment by promoting coordination among healthcare providers, facilitating medication reconciliation, preparing patients and their caregivers to carry out discharge instructions, and making appropriate home care referrals

(Bowles, Naylor, & Foust, 2002; Flacker, Park, & Sims, 2007; Moore, McGinn, & Halm, 2007). Two of the six models consider the care transition the primary focus of their programs.

Embed Geriatric Care Principles Within the Organization

Common complications in older hospitalized patients can be partly attributed to the lack of evidence-based geriatric care practices. The adoption of geriatric protocols is highly variable (Neuman, Speck, Karlawish, Schwartz, & Shea, 2010). Issues with polypharmacy or inappropriate medications (e.g., overuse of psychoactive drugs), unnecessary restraints, inadequate detection of cognitive or affective changes (e.g., delirium, depression), lack of consideration of frailty, and poor pain control are examples of system-level factors that can lead to adverse outcomes. Thus, geriatric care models promote the use of the highest level of evidence-based practices. These models are not consistently adopted in hospital practice.

To be effective, geriatric models of care cannot be limited to a few individuals or a team but most work within institutional committees to embed evidence-based geriatric care processes within the organizational structure of the health system.

Thus, to be effective, geriatric models of care cannot be limited to a few individuals or a team but most work within institutional committees to embed evidence-based geriatric care processes within the organizational structure of the health system. For example, this may include incorporating these geriatric-specific screening tools in the electronic medical record (Khan, Malone, Pagel, Vollbrecht, & Baumgardner, 2012) as well as in hospital policies, procedures, and protocols (Capezuti et al., 2012, 2013).

Support a Senior-Friendly Physical Environment

The built environment is meant to reduce physical obstacles for transferring and ambulating, and to promote cognitive orientation and socialization (Boltz, Capezuti, Shabbat, & Hall, 2010; Fox et al., 2013; Palmer, Landefeld, Kresevic, & Kowal, 1994). Physical modifications in the typical hospital setting include grab bars, furniture (chairs and bed) that adjusts height to facilitate mobility, carpeted flooring, clocks, and calendars (Fox et al., 2013). Most of these are now considered universal design elements to promote patient safety. Other environmental interventions are not typically used (Parke et al., 2016), such as a communal dining space to reduce isolation, which can promote intake and reduce incontinence, falls, and cognitive decline (Singh, Subhan, Krishnan, Edwards, & Okeke, 2016). Others include shock-absorbing flooring (Latimer, Dixon, Drahota, & Servers, 2013), therapeutic use of lighting to reduce agitation (Barrick et al., 2010) and promote nighttime sleep (Patel, Baldwin, Bunting, & Laha, 2014).

GENERAL CARE MODEL TYPES

Most geriatric models target medical inpatients by addressing the aforementioned care delivery issues. Most consider all geriatric syndromes, whereas others target specific ones such as delirium. The models are implemented in various degrees from a hospital-wide to a unit-based approach, while others focus on specific processes of hospitalization such as discharge planning.

Acute Care for Elders (ACE) Units

These discrete geriatric units provide CGA delivered by a multidisciplinary team with a focus on the rehabilitative aspects of care management. Team rounds and patient-centered team conferences are essential for communication among the core team (usually a geriatrician, GAPN, and social worker) as well as specialists from other disciplines providing consultation—occupational and physical therapy, nutrition, pharmacy, audiology, and psychiatry/psychology. Geriatric evaluation and management (GEM) units were first developed in the U.S. Department of Veterans Affairs (VA) system. ACE units were also tested in the John A. Hartford Foundation HOPE project (see Chapter 2). GEM units have documented significant reductions in functional decline and suboptimal medication use as well as decreased rate of nursing home placement among hospitalized veterans on GEM units compared to general medical units (Phibbs et al., 2006).

Since the 1990s, ACE units have been implemented in non-VA hospitals. Most ACE units have made physical environment adaptations to address age-related changes (e.g., flooring to reduce glare), support orientation (white boards indicating staff names, discharge goals), and promote staff observation (e.g., alarmed exit doors, communal space for meals). Led by geriatricians and/or GAPNs, the interdisciplinary team facilitates care coordination and identification of modifiable risk factors for geriatric syndromes (Flood et al., 2015; Fox et al., 2013; Malone, Capezuti, & Palmer, 2014). This is linked to reduced costs due to shorter hospital stays (Barnes et al., 2012; Fox et al., 2012) and fewer 30-day readmissions (Flood et al., 2013).

Compared with other medical units, patients hospitalized on ACE units maintain prehospital or demonstrate improved functional status at discharge without increases in hospital or post-discharge costs and are less likely to be discharged to nursing homes (Fox et al., 2012; Landefeld, Palmer, Kresevic, Fortinsky, & Kowal, 1995). Moreover, ACE units are associated with improved drug prescribing (Spinewine et al., 2007), fewer falls (Fox et al., 2012), less delirium (Bo et al., 2009; Fox et al., 2012), and reduced mortality (Saltvedt, Mo, Fayers, Kaasa, & Sletvoide, 2002).

Processes of care (minimal restraint use, early mobilization, fewer days to discharge planning, and less use of high-risk medications) found in ACE units are the mediating drivers to these positive outcomes (Counsell et al., 2000). Fox et al.'s (2012) systematic review reported that the most desirable outcomes from ACE programs were those that included patient-centered care, medical review, and early mobilization. More hospitals are currently using ACE units for those at highest risk for age-related complications with ACE staff also providing consultation, based on ACE principles, throughout the health system to reach more older hospitalized patients. These "ACE without walls" consultation teams work similar to a geriatric consultation service, except that there is also an inpatient ACE unit within the hospital or health system.

Geriatric Consultation Service/Mobile ACE Unit

A geriatric consultation team may include a geriatrician, a geropsychiatrist, a GAPN, or an interdisciplinary team of geriatric healthcare providers to conduct a CGA or evaluate a specific condition (delirium), symptom (new-onset verbal agitation), or situation (adequacy of spouse to care for patient at home). Some hospitals require that patients who are deemed frail or are screened at high risk for geriatric-related complications or are admitted from a homebound program or a nursing home receive a geriatric consult, whereas most are requested by another primary service for an individual patient (Hung, Tejada, Soryal, Akbar, & Bowman, 2015). A meta-analysis of geriatric consult studies did not find a statistically significant reduction in functional decline, readmissions, or length of stay but did report fewer consult patients dying at 6 and 8 months following discharge (Deschodt, Flamaing, Haentjens, Boonen, & Milisen, 2013). It should be noted, however, that it is difficult to evaluate any consultation service because their recommendations may not be followed or the hospital may not have the resources or staff to adequately implement the recommendations (C. M. Allen et al., 1986).

The Mobile Acute Care for Elders (MACE) service is a model that aims to provide continuity of care across settings. It consists of an outpatient geriatric team (attending geriatrician hospitalist, geriatric medicine fellow, social worker, and clinical nurse specialist) who provide primary care to their patients when hospitalized (Hung, Ross, Farber, & Siu, 2013). An evaluation of this model in one hospital reported that MACE-serviced patients, compared to similar older patients cared for on medical units, experienced fewer adverse events (catheter-associated urinary tract infection, pressure ulcers, restraint use, and falls) and had shorter hospital stays (Hung et al., 2013).

The Hospital Elder Life Program

The HELP utilizes evidence-based protocols implemented by an interdisciplinary team that includes trained volunteers and geriatric specialists. The protocols target risk factors for delirium (mental orientation, therapeutic activities, early mobilization, vision and hearing adaptations, hydration and feeding assistance, and sleep enhancement). Positive HELP outcomes include less incidence of delirium and, among those who did develop delirium, a decrease in the total number of episodes and days with delirium, as well as less functional decline, lower hospital costs, and less use of long-term nursing home services (Babine, Farrington, & Wierman, 2013; Inouye et al., 1999; Inouye, Baker, Fugal, & Bradley, 2006; Reuben et al., 2000; Yue, Kshieh, & Inouye, 2015). The HELP program has been successfully disseminated in diverse hospital settings and units, including those that serve older surgery patients who have a high occurrence of delirium (Chen et al., 2014; Zaubler et al., 2013). Currently, the HELP protocols also incorporate the National Institute for Clinical Excellence (NICE) guidelines (National Clinical Guideline Centre, 2010).

The HELP program is coordinated by an Elder Life Specialist who trains, supervises, and coordinates the hospital volunteers who implement HELP interventions (Bradley, Webster, Schlesinger, Baker, & Inouye, 2006b). The Elder Life Nurse Specialist typically has advanced geriatric nursing education and is often responsible for overseeing nursing assessments and quality initiatives related to delirium and other geriatric syndromes.

Transitional Care Models

Transitional care models address the needs of older adult patients with complex medical and social needs and their caregivers as they navigate the healthcare system from hospital to post-acute care. There are numerous transitional care programs and the strength of the evidence to reduce postdischarge negative outcomes varies considerably. Two models with demonstrated positive outcomes include the advanced practice nurse (APN) transitional care model (Naylor & Keating, 2008) and the care transitions coaching or care transitions intervention (Coleman, Parry, Chalmers, & Min, 2006; Coleman et al., 2004).

In the transitional care model, APNs aim to influence the hospital course and plan for the discharge of high-risk, cognitively intact older adults with a variety of medical and surgical conditions. The focus is on designing and overseeing the plan for follow-up care following discharge. The APN works collaboratively with the older adult, family caregiver, physician, and other health team members to enact an evidence-based transitional plan of care. The same APN implements this plan after discharge by providing customary home care services and phone availability 7 days a week.

Care transitions coaching or care transitions intervention utilizes a registered nurse or "transitions coach" to encourage older patients and their family caregivers to assume more active roles during care transitions by facilitating self-management and collaborative communication between the patient/caregiver and the primary care provider.

COMBINATION MODELS

In some NICHE sites, a combination of other geriatric models is implemented such as a geriatric consultation team and transitional care (Arbaje et al., 2010) or inpatient geriatric assessment and intensive home care (Buurman, Parlevliet, van Deelen, de Haan, & de Rooij, 2010). In others, the geriatric interdisciplinary team provides direct consultation as well as screens patients for other related services such as palliative care, rehabilitative services, or pain management programs. Some hospitals have units with a dual function such as merging an ACE unit with a palliative care (Gelfman, Meier, & Morrison, 2008; Tomasović, 2005), stroke (K. R. Allen et al., 2003), or oncology (Flood, Brown, Carroll, & Locher, 2011) unit. Others have incorporated a room or several rooms for specific purposes, such as a "delirium room" within an ACE unit for those actively delirious (Flaherty et al., 2003) or rooms with environmental features and trained staff to prevent delirium (Chong et al., 2011). Others incorporate geriatric comanagement with other specialties such as rehabilitation, orthopedics, trauma, and oncology (K. R. Allen et al., 2003; Gelfman et al., 2008; Kammerlander et al., 2010; Mendelson & Friedman, 2014). Such programs have demonstrated improved detection of and decreased incidence of delirium, as well as reduced length of stay, readmission rates, morbidity, and mortality (Flaherty et al., 2003; Flood et al., 2011; Kates, 2014; Milisen et al., 2001).

Virtual Approaches

Geriatric care models require clinicians and coordinators with geriatric expertise; however, there is a significant shortage of fellowship-trained geriatricians, geriatric psychiatrists, and GAPNs as well as specialists in other disciplines.

Geriatric care models require clinicians and coordinators with geriatric expertise; however, there is a significant shortage of fellowship-trained geriatricians, geriatric psychiatrists, and GAPNs as well as specialists in other disciplines (Committee on the Future Health Care Workforce for Older Americans, 2008). Most NICHE hospitals that use a variety of other geriatric care models are teaching hospitals located in urban/suburban areas. It is difficult for hospitals located in rural areas and small hospitals since they lack the access and financial capacity to employ geriatric specialists (Jayadevappa, Bloom, Raziano, & Lavizzo-Mourey, 2003). One solution is for hospitals to work with other hospitals in their health system or in their region to create learning collaboratives or "knowledge networks" incorporating web-based and other long-distance communication strategies. A geriatrician (Malone et al., 2010) or a GAPN (Capezuti, 2010) can participate in "virtual" rounds with staff in another location (Friedman, Mendelson, Kates, & McCann, 2008; Pallawala & Lun, 2001). This is meant to foster communication so that the e-geriatrician or e-APN has access to a system-wide electronic health record such as the ACE Tracker and the TeleGeriatric system (Pallawala & Lun, 2001) or a similar web-based assessment tool (Gray & Wootton, 2008;

Martin-Khan et al., 2012; Meyer, 2011; Vollbrecht et al., 2015). This not only provides geriatric expertise to enhance care provided to older adults but also serves to mentor professional colleagues.

Hospitalist Collaborative Models

Hospitalists provide care for an increasing number of older acutely ill Medicare patients (Welch, Stearns, Cuellar, & Bindman, 2014).

In response, some hospitals have started a proactive geriatrics consultation service to collaborate with hospitalists (Sennour, Counsell, Jones, & Weiner, 2009). A 4-year evaluation of over 1,500 consults using this service demonstrated a high level of satisfaction among hospitalists, and patients receiving a geriatrics consultation experienced a shorter hospital stay and lower hospital costs (Sennour et al., 2009).

In the Better Outcomes for Older adults through Safer Transitions (BOOST) program, hospitalists are trained to lead transitional care teams. Preliminary results suggest prevention of postdischarge complications and readmissions within 30 days and increased confidence in self-management (Dedhia et al., 2009). In the project evaluation of the initial hospitals participating in the quality improvement program, BOOST was associated with a modest but significant reduction in 30-day hospital readmissions from 14.7% at baseline to 12.7% after the intervention (Hansen et al., 2013). The BOOST program is administered by the Society of Hospital Medicine, which provides fee-based training as well as technical support to optimize the hospital discharge process and diminish discontinuity and fragmentation of care (Williams & Coleman, 2009).

SPECIALTY CARE MODELS

Senior Emergency Department Care

Organizational models have emerged to address the specialized needs of older adults utilizing the ED and their families. Core components of these models include nurse-led, interdisciplinary teams (including a geriatric physician specialist, nurse practitioner, rehabilitation therapists, and social worker) and the use of evidence-based protocols. The interdisciplinary team evaluates high-risk patients in the ED and typically follows them throughout the hospital stay (Gold & Bergman, 1997). A prospective, randomized, controlled trial conducted in a medical school–affiliated urban public hospital in Sydney, Australia found that CGA provided for older adults sent home from the ED demonstrated positive outcomes. Although there was no difference in admission to nursing homes or mortality, patients randomized to the intervention group maintained a greater degree of physical and mental function (Caplan, Williams, Daly, & Abraham, 2004). In the SIGNET randomized controlled trial, CGA of high-risk patients conducted in the ED by an APN was associated with a shorter hospital length of stay and less risk of 90-day admission of older adults (Mion et al., 2003).

Mobile interdisciplinary teams in the ED conduct a brief geriatric assessment and develop a comprehensive plan. These teams make recommendations for (a) diagnosis and treatment of the presenting illnesses, (b) management of geriatrics syndromes, and (c) accessing social and home needs. Outcomes reported include shortened hospital stay and early discharge from the ED (Launay, Decker, Hureaux-Huynh, Annweiler, & Beauchet, 2012).

Geriatric emergency management (GEM) nurses provide targeted geriatric assessment and intervention for older adult patients (ages 65+) in the ED. At-risk patients are identified through the Triage Risk Factor Screening Tool (TRST) and the Identification of Seniors at Risk (ISAR) tool. Interventions include training and operational support for staff to implement geriatric care strategies in the ED; linkage to community support services and specialized geriatric services; and collaboration with the family physician. GEM nurses have provided timely development of care plans and initiation of needed referrals (Rogers, 2009).

The first senior-friendly ED, a self-contained unit within a larger ED, was created by Holy Cross Hospital in Maryland in 2008. The physical environment is adapted to age-related changes (warm colors with select use of color contrast, thick mattresses, indirect light, glare-free floors, large easy-to-use call light/TV remotes, and telephones, clocks, and documents with larger print). Dedicated, gerontologically prepared nursing staff, a nurse practitioner, and social workers staff the unit and volunteers provide comfort measures. Evidence-based clinical protocols are utilized. A geriatric pharmacist reviews the medications of seniors who receive seven or more medications. The staff provides follow-up calls or home visits after discharge from the ED and care coordination is provided as indicated. The trend of senior-friendly EDs is growing and future research is planned to evaluate clinical and organizational effectiveness (Hwang & Morrison, 2007). The elder-friendly hospital conceptual framework offered by Parke and Brand (2004) provides guidance to efforts to develop a senior-friendly ED. This framework includes four major components to consider when developing a senior-friendly ED:

- Physical design and architectural features (including equipment, furnishings, and décor) that enable an older person's independent functioning. Examples include levered door handles, handrails, rest areas at regular intervals, and the appropriate use of languages, graphics, symbols, clocks, and calendars to support orientation and wayfinding.

- A social climate in the ED environment that reflects respectful, adapted communication and information. Information should be offered on common conditions and treatments, in "plain language" and an easy to read format. Volunteers are recommended to provide nutrition and mobility, wayfinding, emotional support, and information seeking.

- Policies and procedures that reflect senior-friendly principles in the hospital vision, mission, and strategic plan. Interdisciplinary educational programs for staff ideally address gerontologically best practices in relevant areas including advance directives, communication skills, community services, dementia care, medication, and elder abuse.

- Healthcare system approaches that promote communication between ED staff and community providers and services as well as collaboration on regional initiatives to improve the health of older adults.

Surgical Specialty Models

Although most geriatric care models target medical patients, there has been a growing trend for surgical programs to consult or integrate geriatrics. The latter are developing geriatric comanagement programs in both general surgery and other surgical specialties (urology, vascular surgery, cardiothoracic surgery, and neurosurgery). A VA hospital with these multiple comanagement surgical units reported higher rates of discharge back to the community (Walke et al., 2014). A urology comanagement program utilizing geriatrician-led unit rounds resulted in reduced inpatient stay by patients and lowered total postoperative complications (Braude et al., 2017).

Orthogeriatric Models

The American College of Surgeons Trauma Quality Improvement Program (TQIP) Geriatric Trauma Management Guidelines (www.facs.org/quality-programs/trauma/tqip/best-practice) support specialized geriatric surgical care including criteria for early geriatric consultation and geriatric expertise on the multidisciplinary trauma care team. During the last 30 years, orthopedic programs have emerged that incorporate geriatric input into hip surgery care. The goal is to reduce the incidence of iatrogenic complications and streamline flow in hospital care, including early discharge that will improve survival, clinical, and cost outcomes (Giusti et al., 2015).

The organization of orthogeriatrics programs varies considerably but generally fits within one of these three types: (a) a geriatrician and/or geriatric interdisciplinary team consistently consults older patients admitted to an orthopedic hospital unit; (b) a geriatric or ACE unit with the orthopedic surgeon provides consultation; or (c) comanagement in which the responsibility for care of the older patient on an orthopedic unit is shared between the surgeon and the geriatrician/geriatric team (Grigoryan, Javedan, & Rudolph, 2014). The latter has become the more frequently employed approach.

The components of care including the outcome criteria also differ considerably among orthogeriatric programs (Grigoryan et al., 2014). Some focus on minimizing time to surgery and employment of standardized orders and protocols (Friedman et al., 2008) while some deliver daily geriatrics recommendations for older patients who are receiving care for hip fractures. The latter demonstrated reduction of delirium by over one-third and severe delirium by over one-half, as well as decreased predicted length of stay, readmission rates, complication rates, and mortality (Marcantonio, Flacker, Wright, & Resnick, 2001). Another approach is having a geriatrician and GAPN evaluate all older trauma patients and share recommendations in weekly multidisciplinary rounds and performance improvement meetings of the trauma service. Fallon et al. (2006) reported that nearly all (91%) geriatric recommendations were followed including advanced care planning, disposition decisions to promote function, a decrease in inappropriate medications, and pain management.

The difference among orthogeriatric programs in terms of overall organization, personnel, and interventions employed makes it challenging to compare outcomes among these programs. A systematic review and meta-analysis of 18 orthogeriatric programs (Grigoryan et al., 2014) reported that the 10 programs utilizing routine geriatric consultation resulted in significant decreases in long-term mortality, in-hospital mortality, and time to surgery, compared with controls receiving usual orthopedic care. There were only three studies examining the geriatric unit approach but it was not possible to report conclusions due to low quality methodology and sample size. The five studies of orthogeriatric comanagement found patients experienced shortened length of stay, compared with controls. Other positive outcomes among the 18 studies in this review included reduced postoperative complications such as decreased incidence of delirium and functional decline.

Since 2012, three other reviews of comanaged care have reported reductions in hospital complications (Giusti et al., 2015; Martinez-Reig, Ahmad, & Duque, 2012; Van Grootven et al., 2017) while two demonstrate decreased occurrence of short- and long-term mortality (Giusti et al., 2015; Martinez-Reig et al., 2012). In particular, two well-executed, randomized control trials have shown that orthogeriatric care is positively associated with improved mobility at 4 months postsurgery compared to controls (Prestmo et al., 2015; Watne et al., 2014).

The increased uptake of orthogeriatric comanagement demonstrates the feasibility of easily integrating this care. Fortunately, there has been a considerable amount of outcome data from these programs. The evidence supports that consistent geriatric input embedded into the orthopedic service is ideal since "as needed" geriatric consultation is often too late to prevent common complications of older patients (Giusti et al., 2015). The outcome reporting, however, needs to be consistent. In response, the AO trauma network of Europe recommends that the following should be collected at admission: quality of life, pain, satisfaction, function, falls, medication use, and place of residence. At discharge, the following should also be collected: mortality, length of stay, time to surgery, complications (medical and surgical), and costs (Liem et al., 2013). Depending on the type of surgery, readmission rates should also be collected 30 days, 90 days, and 1 year postsurgery.

Surgical Oncogeriatrics

Most (60%) persons with cancer are over 65 years of age and older cancer patients account for 70% of annual cancer deaths. The high complication rate, such as delirium (Korc-Grodzicki et al., 2015), with oncologic treatment has prompted the integration of geriatric assessment into standard oncology practice in cancer centers (McEvoy & Cope, 2012) and oncology units of general hospitals (Burhenn, Perrin, & McCarthy, 2016; Lynch, DeDonato, & Kutney-Lee, 2016). Functional status, comorbidity, and frailty are the most predictive factors associated with post-oncology surgery complications according to a systematic review of nine systematic reviews (Huisman, Kok, de Bock, & van Leeuwen, 2017). Moreover, older oncology patients, in general, have more complex medical and social needs than adult oncology patients. This has spurred the development of oncogeriatric consultation teams or geriatric oncology units, some of which are part of an existing ACE unit, to address prevention or reduction of these complications (Flood et al., 2006, 2011; Retornaz et al., 2007; Retornaz, Seux, Pauly, & Soubeyrand, 2008).

Medical Gero-Oncology

The complexity of nursing care for older cancer patients has led to many cancer centers educating nurses in comprehensive geriatric screening and assessments.

The complexity of nursing care for older cancer patients has led to many cancer centers educating nurses in comprehensive geriatric screening and assessments (Burhenn et al., 2016; Lynch et al., 2016). These efforts are often led by APNs (Morgan & Tarbi, 2016) and many are conducted within their NICHE implementation. This is also being integrated in medical oncology (Magnuson et al., 2016). An innovative pilot program that embedded a medical oncologist within an ED did not reduce hospital admissions among those with solid tumor malignancies but the overall length of stay was lower, suggesting the positive effect of care coordination beginning in the ED (Brooks et al., 2016).

CHAPTER SUMMARY

Geriatric care models differ in their approach or foci; however, all models share common goals. The choice of model for a health system is based on the individual features of that hospital's patient population, resource availability (geriatric clinicians, bed size, volunteers, etc.), and especially the senior/corporate administrator's commitment to geriatric programming (Chodosh & Weiner, 2018). There is currently no direct reimbursement for many components of these models, thus administrators are motivated by the model's alignment to the institution's strategic plan or mission, consumer or community satisfaction, and cost savings (e.g., reduced costly and non-reimbursable complications; Adunsky et al., 2005; Boult et al., 2009; Bradley, Webster, Schlesinger, Baker, & Inouye, 2006a;

Capezuti et al., 2013; Hart, Frank, Hoffman, Dickey, & Kristjansson, 2006; Kammerlander et al., 2010; Leff et al., 2012; Siu, Spragens, Inouye, Morrison, & Leff, 2009).

As indicated in this review, all geriatric models have demonstrated positive outcomes; however, only a small proportion (approximately 750) has been implemented in U.S. hospitals with most in academic or teaching hospitals. The aim of the current "Creating Age-Friendly Health Systems" initiative is to reach at least 20% of U.S. health systems with a portfolio model (Fulmer & Berman, 2016; Fulmer & Li, 2018; Mate et al., 2017). An integrated model such as this is needed to enhance the hospital experience of older patients (Capezuti & Brush, 2009; Chodosh & Weiner, 2018; Leff et al., 2012; Marcantonio et al., 2001).

REFERENCES

Adunsky, A., Arad, M., Levi, R., Blankstein, A., Zeilig, G., & Mizrachi, E. (2005). Five-year experience with the 'Sheba' model of comprehensive orthogeriatric care for elderly hip fracture patients. *Disability and Rehabilitation, 27,* 1123–1127. doi:10.1080/09638280500056030

Allen, C. M., Becker, P. M., McVey, L. J., Saltz, C., Feussner, J. R., & Cohen, H. J. (1986). A randomized, controlled clinical trial of a geriatric consultation team: Compliance with recommendations. *The Journal of the American Medical Association, 255,* 2617–2621. doi:10.1001/jama.1986.03370190101032

Allen, K. R., Hazelett, S. E., Palmer, R. R., Jarjoura, D. G., Wickstrom, G. C., Weinhardt, J. A., . . . Counsell, S. R. (2003). Developing a stroke unit using the acute care for elders intervention and model of care. *Journal of the American Geriatrics Society, 51,* 1660–1667. doi:10.1046/j.1532-5415.2003.51521.x

Arbaje, A. I., Maron, D. D., Yu, Q., Wendel, V. I., Tanner, E., Boult, C., . . . Durso, S. C. (2010). The geriatric floating interdisciplinary transition team. *Journal of the American Geriatrics Society, 58,* 364–370. doi:10.1111/j.1532-5415.2009.02682.x

Babine, R.L., Farrington, S., & Wierman, H.R. (2013). HELP© prevent falls by preventing delirium. *Nursing 2013, 43,* 18–21. doi:10.1097/01.nurse.0000428710.81378.aa

Barnes, D. E., Palmer, R. M., Kresevic, D. M., Fortinsky, R. H., Kowal, J., Chren, M.-M., & Landefeld, C. S. (2012). Acute care for elders units produced shorter hospital stays at lower cost while maintaining patients' functional status. *Health Affairs, 31,* 1227–1236. doi:10.1377/hlthaff.2012.0142

Barrick, A. L., Sloane, P. D., Williams, C. S., Mitchell, C. M., Connell, B. R., Wood, W., . . . Zimmerman, S. (2010). Impact of ambient bright light on agitation in dementia. *International Journal of Geriatric Psychiatry, 25,* 1013–1021. doi:10.1002/gps.2453

Berman, A., Mezey, M., Kobayashi, M., Fulmer, T., Stanley, J., Thornlow, D., & Rosenfeld, P. (2005). Gerontological nursing content in baccalaureate nursing programs: Comparison of findings from 1997 and 2003. *Journal of Professional Nursing, 21,* 268–275. doi:10.1016/j.profnurs.2005.07.005

Bo, M., Martini, B., Ruatta, C., Massaia, M., Ricauda, N. A., Varetto, A., . . . Torta, R. (2009). Geriatric ward hospitalization reduced incidence delirium among older medical inpatients. *The American Journal of Geriatric Psychiatry, 17,* 760–768. doi:10.1097/jgp.0b013e3181a315d5

Boltz, M., Capezuti, E., Shabbat, N., & Hall, K. (2010). Going home better not worse: Older adults' views on physical function during hospitalization. *International Journal of Nursing Practice, 16,* 381–388. doi:10.1111/j.1440-172x.2010.01855.x

Boltz, M., Capezuti, E., Shuluk, J., Brouwer, J., Carolan, D., Conway, S., . . . Galvin, J. E. (2013). Implementation of geriatric acute care best practices: Initial results of the NICHE SITE self-evaluation. *Nursing & Health Sciences. 15*(4), 518–524. doi:10.1111/nhs.12067

Boult, C., Green, A. F., Boult, L. B., Pacala, J. T., Snyder, C., & Leff, B. (2009). Successful models of comprehensive care for older adults with chronic conditions: Evidence for the Institute of Medicine's "retooling for an aging America" report. *Journal of the American Geriatrics Society, 57,* 2328–2337. doi:10.1111/j.1532-5415.2009.02571.x

Bowles, K. H., Naylor, M. D., & Foust, J. B. (2002). Patient characteristics at hospital discharge and a comparison of home care referral decisions. *Journal of the American Geriatrics Society, 50,* 336–342. doi:10.1046/j.1532-5415.2002.50067.x

Bradley, E. H., Webster, T. R., Schlesinger, M., Baker, D., & Inouye, S. K. (2006a). Patterns of diffusion of evidence-based clinical programmes: A case study of the Hospital Elder Life Program. *BMJ Quality & Safety, 15,* 334–338. doi:10.1136/qshc.2006.018820

Bradley, E. H., Webster, T. R., Schlesinger, M., Baker, D., & Inouye, S. K. (2006b). The roles of senior management in improving hospital experiences for frail older adults. *Journal of Healthcare Management, 51,* 323–336. doi:10.1097/00115514-200609000-00009

Braude, P., Goodman, A., Elias, T., Babic-Illman, G., Challacombe, B., Harari, D., & Dhesi, J. K. (2017). Evaluation and establishment of a ward-based geriatric liaison service for older urological surgical patients: Proactive care of Older People undergoing Surgery (POPS)-urology. *BJU International, 120,* 123–129. doi:10.1111/bju.13526

Brooks, G. A., Chen, E. J., Murakami, M. A., Giannakis, M., Baugh, C. W., & Schrag, D. (2016). An ED pilot intervention to facilitate outpatient acute care for cancer patients. *The American Journal of Emergency Medicine, 34,* 1934–1938. doi:10.1016/j.ajem.2016.06.076

Burhenn, P. S., Perrin, S., & McCarthy, A. L. (2016). Models of care in geriatric oncology nursing. *Seminars in Oncology Nursing, 32,* 24–32. doi:10.1016/j.soncn.2015.11.004

Buurman, B. M., Parlevliet, J. L., van Deelen, B. A., de Haan, R. J., & de Rooij, S. E. (2010). A randomised clinical trial on a comprehensive geriatric assessment and intensive home follow-up after hospital discharge: The Transitional Care Bridge. *BMC Health Services Research, 10,* 296. doi:10.1186/1472-6963-10-296

Capezuti, E. (2010). An electronic geriatric specialist workforce: Is it a viable option? *Geriatric Nursing, 31*(3), 220–222. doi:10.1016/j.gerinurse.2010.04.005

Capezuti, E., & Boltz, M. (2014). An overview of hospital-based models of care. In M. L. Malone, E. Capezuti, & R. Palmer. (Eds.), *Acute Care for Elders: A model for interdisciplinary care* (pp. 49–68). Cham, Switzerland: Springer International.

Capezuti, E., Boltz, E., Cline, D., Dickson, V., Rosenberg, M., Wagner, L., . . . Nigolian, C. (2012). Nurses Improving Care for Healthsystem Elders: A model for optimizing the geriatric nursing practice environment. *Journal of Clinical Nursing, 21,* 3117–3125. doi:10.1111/j.1365-2702.2012.04259.x

Capezuti, E., Boltz, M., & Kim, H. (2011). Geriatric models of care. In R. A. Rosentahl, M. E. Zenilman, & M. R. Katlic (Eds.), *Principles and practice of geriatric surgery* (2nd ed., pp. 253–266). New York, NY: Springer-Verlag.

Capezuti, E., Boltz, M., Shuluk, J., Denysyk, L., Brouwers, J., Roberts, M.-C., . . . Secic, M. (2013). Utilization of a benchmarking database to inform NICHE implementation. *Research in Gerontological Nursing, 6*, 198–208. doi:10.3928/19404921-20130607-01

Capezuti, E., Boltz, M., Tejada, J. A. M., & Malone, M. (2018). Models of care. In R. A. Rosentahl, M. E. Zenilman, & M. R. Katlic (Eds.), *Principles and practice of geriatric surgery* (3rd ed., pp. 1–19). Cham, Switzerland: Springer International. doi:10.1007/978-3-319-20317-1_24-1

Capezuti, E., Bricoli, B., & Boltz, M. (2013). Nurses Improving the Care of Healthsystem Elders: Creating a sustainable business model to improve care of hospitalized older adults. *Journal of the American Geriatrics Society, 61*, 1387–1393. doi:10.1111/jgs.12324

Capezuti, E., & Brush, B. L. (2009). Implementing geriatric care models: What are we waiting for? *Geriatric Nursing, 30*, 204–206. doi:10.1016/j.gerinurse.2009.03.003

Capezuti, E., Parks, A. J., Boltz, M., Malone, M., & Palmer, M. (2016). Acute care models. In M. Boltz, E. Capezuti, D. Zwicker, & T. Fulmer (Eds.), *Evidence-based geriatric nursing protocols for best practice* (5th ed., pp. 621–631). New York, NY: Springer Publishing.

Caplan, G. A., Williams, A. J., Daly, B., & Abraham, K. (2004). A randomized, controlled trial of comprehensive geriatric assessment and multidisciplinary intervention after discharge of elderly from the emergency department—The DEED II study. *Journal of the American Geriatrics Society 52*, 1417–1423. doi:10.1111/j.1532-5415.2004.52401.x

Chen, C. C., Chen, C.-N., Lai, I.-R., Huang, G.-H., Saczynski, J. S., & Inouye, S. K. (2014). Effects of a modified Hospital Elder Life Program on frailty in individuals undergoing major elective abdominal surgery. *Journal of the American Geriatrics Society, 62*, 261–268. doi:10.1111/jgs.12651

Chodosh, J., & Weiner, M. (2018). Implementing models of geriatric care—Behind the scenes. *Journal of the American Geriatrics Society, 66*(2), 364–366. doi:10.1111/jgs.15183

Chong, M. S., Chan, M. P., Kang, J., Han, H. C., Ding, Y. Y., & Tan, T. L. (2011). A new model of delirium care in the acute geriatric setting: Geriatric monitoring unit. *BMC Geriatrics, 11*(1), 41. doi:10.1186/1471-2318-11-41

Coleman, E. A., Min, S.-J., Chomiak, A., & Kramer, A. M. (2004). Posthospital care transitions: Patterns, complications, and risk identification. *Health Services Research, 39*, 1449–1465. doi:10.1111/j.1475-6773.2004.00298.x

Coleman, E. A., Parry, C., Chalmers, S., & Min, S.-J. (2006). The Care Transitions Intervention: Results of a randomized controlled trial. *Archives of Internal Medicine, 166*, 1822–1828. doi:10.1001/archinte.166.17.1822

Coleman, E. A., Smith, J. D., Frank, J. C., Min, S.-J., Parry, C., & Kramer, A. M. (2004). Preparing patients and caregivers to participate in care delivered across settings: The Care Transitions Intervention. *Journal of the American Geriatrics Society, 52*, 1817–1825. doi:10.1111/j.1532-5415.2004.52504.x

Coleman, E. A., Smith, J. D., Raha, D., & Min, S.-J. (2005). Posthospital medication discrepancies: Prevalence and contributing factors. *Archives of Internal Medicine, 165*, 1842–1847. doi:10.1001/archinte.165.16.1842

Committee on the Future Health Care Workforce for Older Americans. (2008). *Retooling for an aging America: Building the health care workforce.* Washington, DC: National Academies Press.

Conley, D. M., Burket, T. L., Schumacher, S., Lyons, D., DeRosa, S. E., & Schirm, V. (2012). Implementing geriatric models of care: A role of the gerontological clinical nurse specialist—part I. *Geriatric Nursing, 33*, 229–234. doi:10.1016/j.gerinurse.2012.03.009

Counsell, S. R., Holder, C. M., Liebenauer, L. L., Palmer, R. M., Fortinsky, R. H., Kresevic, D. M., . . . Landefeld, C. S. (2000). Effects of a multicomponent intervention on functional outcomes and processes of care in hospitalized older patients: A randomized controlled trial of Acute Care for Elders (ACE) in a community hospital. *Journal of the American Geriatrics Society, 48*, 1572–1581. doi:10.1111/j.1532-5415.2000.tb03866.x

Dedhia, P., Kravet, S., Bulger, J., Hinson, T., Sridharan, A., Kolodner, K., . . . Howell, E. (2009). A quality improvement intervention to facilitate the transition of older adults from three hospitals back to their homes. *Journal of the American Geriatrics Society, 57*, 1540–1546. doi:10.1111/j.1532-5415.2009.02430.x

Deschodt, M., Flamaing, J., Haentjens, P., Boonen, S., & Milisen, K. (2013). Impact of geriatric consultation teams on clinical outcomes in acute hospitals: A systematic review and meta-analysis. *BMC Medical, 11*, 48. doi:10.1186/1741-7015-11-48

Fallon, W. F., Jr., Rader, E., Zyzanski, S., Mancuso, C., Martin, B., Breedlove, L., . . . Campbell, J. (2006). Geriatric outcomes are improved by a geriatric trauma consultation service. *Journal of Trauma and Acute Care Surgery, 61*, 1040–1046. doi:10.1097/01.ta.0000238652.48008.59

Flacker, J., Park, W., & Sims, A. (2007). Hospital discharge information and older patients: Do they get what they need? *Journal of Hospital Medicine, 2*, 291–296. doi:10.1002/jhm.166

Flaherty, J. H., Tariq, S. H., Raghavan, S., Bakshi, S., Moinuddin, A., & Morley, J. E. (2003). A model for managing delirious older inpatients. *Journal of the American Geriatrics Society, 51*, 1031–1035. doi:10.1046/j.1365-2389.2003.51320.x

Fletcher, K., Hawkes, P., Williams-Rosenthal, S., Mariscal, C. S., & Cox, B. A. (2007). Using nurse practitioners to implement best practice care for the elderly during hospitalization: The NICHE journey at the University of Virginia Medical Center. *Critical Care Nursing Clinics of North America, 19*, 321–337. doi:10.1016/j.ccell.2007.05.007

Flood, K. L., Booth, E. P., Pierluissi, E., Danto-Nocton, E. S., Kresevic, D. M., & Palmer, R. M. (2015). Acute care for elders. In M. L. Malone, E. Capezuti, & R. M. Palmer (Eds.), *Geriatrics models of care: Bringing 'best practice' to an aging America* (1st ed., pp. 3–23). Cham, Switzerland: Springer International.

Flood, K. L., Brown, C. J., Carroll, M. B., & Locher, J. L. (2011). Nutritional processes of care for older adults admitted to an oncology-acute care for elders unit. *Critical Reviews in Oncology/Hematology, 78*, 73–78. doi:10.1016/j.critrevonc.2010.02.011

Flood, K. L., Carroll, M. B., Le, C. V., Ball, L., Esker, D. A., & Carr, D. B. (2006). Geriatric syndromes in elderly patients admitted to an oncology-acute care for elders' unit. *Journal of Clinical Oncology, 24,* 2298–2303. doi:10.1200/jco.2005.02.8514

Flood, K. L., MacLennan, P. A., McGrew, D., Green, D., Dodd, C., & Brown, C. J. (2013). Effects of an acute care for elders unit on costs and 30-day readmissions. *Journal of the American Medical Association Internal Medicine, 173,* 981–987. doi:10.1001/jamainternmed.2013.524

Forster, A. J., Murff, H. J., Peterson, J. F., Gandhi, T. K., & Bates, D. W. (2003). The incidence and severity of adverse events affecting patients after discharge from the hospital. *Annals of Internal Medicine, 138,* 161–167. doi:10.7326/0003-4819-138-3-200302040-00007

Foust, J. B., Naylor, M. D., Boling, P. A., & Cappuzzo, K. A. (2005). Opportunities for improving post-hospital home medication management among older adults. *Home Health Care Services Quarterly, 24,* 101–122. doi:10.1300/j027v24n01_08

Fox, M. T., Persaud, M., Maimets, I., O'Brien, K., Brooks, D., Tregunno, D., & Schraa, E. (2012). Effectiveness of acute geriatric unit care using acute care for elders components: A systematic review and meta-analysis. *Journal of the American Geriatrics Society, 60,* 2237–2245. doi:10.1111/jgs.12028

Fox, M. T., Sidani, S., Persaud, M., Tregunno, D., Maimets, I., Brooks, D., & O'Brien, K. (2013). Acute care for elders components of acute geriatric unit care: Systematic descriptive review. *Journal of the American Geriatrics Society, 61,* 939–946. doi:10.1111/jgs.12282

Friedman, S. M., Mendelson, D. A., Kates, S. L., & McCann, R. M. (2008). Geriatric co-management of proximal femur fractures: Total quality management and protocol-driven care result in better outcomes for a frail patient population. *Journal of the American Geriatrics Society, 56,* 1349–1356. doi:10.1111/j.1532-5415.2008.01770.x

Fulmer, T., & Berman, A. (2016). Age-friendly health systems: How do we get there? Retrieved from http://healthaffairs.org/blog/2016/11/03/age-friendlyhealth-systems-how-do-we-get-there

Fulmer, T., & Li, N. (2018). Age-friendly health systems for older adults with dementia. *The Journal for Nurse Practitioners, 14*(3), 160–165. doi:10.1016/j.nurpra.2017.09.001

Fulmer, T., Mezey, M., Bottrell, M., Abraham, I., Sazant, J., Grossman, S., & Grisham, E. (2002). Nurses Improving Care for Healthsystem Elders (NICHE): Using outcomes and benchmarks for evidenced-based practice. *Geriatric Nursing 23*(3), 121–127. doi:10.1067/mgn.2002.125423

Gelfman, L. P., Meier, D. M., & Morrison, R. S. (2008). Does palliative care improve quality? A survey of bereaved family members. *Journal of Pain and Symptom Management, 36,* 22–28. doi:10.1016/j.jpainsymman.2007.09.008

Giusti, A., Barone, A., Razzano, M., Raiteri, R., Del Rio, A., Bassoli, V., . . . Pilotto, A. (2015). Optimal setting and care organization in the management of older adults with hip fracture: A narrative review. *Geriatric Care, 1*(1), 9–16. doi:10.4081/gc.2015.5602

Gold, S., & Bergman, H. (1997). A geriatric consultation team in the emergency department. *Journal of the American Geriatrics Society, 45,* 764–767. doi:10.1111/j.1532-5415.1997.tb01485.x

Gray, L., & Wootton, R. (2008). Comprehensive geriatric assessment 'online.' *Australasian Journal on Ageing, 27*, 205–208. doi:10.1111/j.1741-6612.2008.00309.x

Grigoryan, K. V., Javedan, H., & Rudolph, J. L. (2014). Orthogeriatric care models and outcomes in hip fracture patients: A systematic review and meta-analysis. *Journal of Orthopaedic Trauma, 28*, e49–e55. doi:10.1097/BOT.0b013e3182a5a045

Hansen, L. O., Greenwald, J. L., Budnitz, T., Howell, E., Halasyamani, L., Maynard, G., . . . Williams, M. V. (2013). Project BOOST: Effectiveness of a multihospital effort to reduce rehospitalization. *Journal of Hospital Medicine, 8*, 421–427. doi:10.1002/jhm.2054

Hart, B., Frank, C., Hoffman, J., Dickey, D., & Kristjansson, J. (2006). Senior friendly health services. *Perspectives, 30*, 18–21.

Hickman, L., Newton, P., Halcomb, E. J., Chang, E., & Davidson, P. (2007). Best practice interventions to improve the management of older people in acute care settings: A literature review. *Journal of Advanced Nursing, 60*, 113–126. doi:10.1111/j.1365-2648.2007.04417.x

Hickman, L. D., Rolley, J. X., & Davidson, P. M. (2010). Can principles of the Chronic Care Model be used to improve care of the older person in the acute care sector? *Collegian, 17*, 63–69. doi:10.1016/j.colegn.2010.05.004

Huisman, M. G., Kok, M., de Bock, G. H., & van Leeuwen, B. L. (2017). Delivering tailored surgery to older cancer patients: Preoperative geriatric assessment domains and screening tools—A systematic review of systematic reviews. *European Journal of Surgical Oncology, 43*, 1–14. doi:10.1016/j.ejso.2016.06.003

Hung, W. W., Ross, J. S., Farber, J., & Siu, A. L. (2013). Evaluation of the Mobile Acute Care for the Elderly (MACE) service. *Journal of the American Medical Association Internal Medicine, 173*, 990–996. doi:10.1001/jamainternmed.2013.478

Hung, W. W., Tejada, J. A. M., Soryal, S., Akbar, S. T., & Bowman, E. H. (2015). The acute care for elders consult program. In M. L. Malone, E. Capezuti, & R. M. Palmer (Eds.), *Geriatrics models of care: Bringing 'best practice' to an aging America* (1st ed., pp. 39–49). Cham, Switzerland: Springer International.

Hwang, U., & Morrison, R. S. (2007). The geriatric emergency department. *Journal of the American Geriatrics Society 55*, 1873–1876. doi:10.1111/j.1532-5415.2007.01400.x

Inouye, S. K., Baker, D. I., Fugal, P., & Bradley, E. H. (2006). Dissemination of the hospital elder life program: Implementation, adaptation, and successes. *Journal of the American Geriatrics Society, 54*, 1492–1499. doi:10.1111/j.1532-5415.2006.00869.x

Inouye, S. K., Bogardus, S. T., Jr., Charpentier, P. A., Leo-Summers, L., Acampora, D., Holford, T. R., & Cooney, L. M., Jr. (1999). A multicomponent intervention to prevent delirium in hospitalized older patients. *The New England Journal of Medicine, 340*, 669–676. doi:10.1056/nejm199903043400901

Inouye, S. K., Studenski, S., Tinetti, M. E., & Kuchel, G. A. (2007). Geriatric syndromes: Clinical, research, and policy implications of a core geriatric concept. *Journal of the American Geriatrics Society, 55*, 780–791. doi:10.1111/j.1532-5415.2007.01156.x

Jayadevappa, R., Bloom, B. S., Raziano, D. B., & Lavizzo-Mourey, R. (2003). Dissemination and characteristics of acute care for elders (ACE) units in the United States.

International Journal of Technology Assessment in Health Care, 19, 220–227. doi:10.1017/s0266462303000205

Kammerlander, C., Roth, T., Friedman, S. M., Suhm, N., Luger, T. J., Kammerlander-Knauer, U., . . . Blauth, M. (2010). Ortho-geriatric service—A literature review comparing different models. *Osteoporosis International, 21*(Suppl. 4), S637–S646. doi:10.1007/s00198-010-1396-x

Kates, S. L. (2014). Lean business model and implementation of a geriatric fracture center. *Clinics in Geriatric Medicine, 30,* 191–205. doi:10.1016/j.cger.2014.01.002

Khan, A., Malone, M. L., Pagel, P., Vollbrecht, M., & Baumgardner, D. J. (2012). An electronic medical record-derived real-time assessment scale for hospital readmission in the elderly. *Wisconsin Medical Journal, 111,* 119–123.

Korc-Grodzicki, B., Sun, S. W., Zhou, Q., Iasonos, A., Lu, B., Root, J. C., . . . Tew, W. P. (2015). Geriatric assessment as a predictor of delirium and other outcomes in elderly cancer patients. *Annals of Surgery, 261,* 1085–1090. doi:10.1097/sla.0000000000000742

Landefeld, C. S., Palmer, R. M., Kresevic, D. M., Fortinsky, R. H., & Kowal, J. (1995). A randomized trial of care in a hospital medical unit especially designed to improve the functional outcomes of acutely ill older patients. *The New England Journal of Medicine, 332,* 1338–1344. doi:10.1056/nejm199505183322006

Latimer, N., Dixon, S., Drahota, A. K., & Severs, M. (2013). Cost–utility analysis of a shock-absorbing floor intervention to prevent injuries from falls in hospital wards for older people. *Age and Ageing, 42,* 641–645. doi:10.1093/ageing/aft076

Launay, C., Decker, L., Hureaux-Huynh, R., Annweiler, C., & Beauchet, O. (2012). Mobile geriatric team and length of hospital stay among older inpatients: A case-control pilot study. *Journal of the American Geriatrics Society, 60,* 1593–1594. doi:10.1111/j.1532-5415.2012.04088.x

Leff, B., Spragens, L. H., Morano, B., Powell, J., Bickert, T., Bond, C., . . . Siu, A. L. (2012). Rapid reengineering of acute medical care for Medicare beneficiaries: The Medicare innovations collaborative. *Health Affairs, 31,* 1204–1215. doi:10.1377/hlthaff.2011.1187

Liem, I. S., Kammerlander, C., Suhm, N., Blauth, M., Roth, T., Gosch, M., . . . Kates, S. L. (2013). Identifying a standard set of outcome parameters for the evaluation of orthogeriatric co-management for hip fractures. *Injury, 44,* 1403–1412. doi:10.1016/j.injury.2013.06.018

Lynch, M. P., DeDonato, D. M., & Kutney-Lee, A. (2016). Geriatric oncology program development and gero-oncology nursing. *Seminars in Oncology Nursing, 32,* 44–54. doi:10.1016/j.soncn.2015.11.006

Magnuson, A., Canin, B., van Londen, G. J., Edwards, B., Bakalarski, P., & Parker, I. (2016). Incorporating geriatric medicine providers into the care of the older adult with cancer. *Current Oncology Reports, 18,* 65. doi:10.1007/s11912-016-0550-9

Malone, M. L., Capezuti, E., & Palmer, R. (Eds.). (2014). *Acute Care for Elders: A model for interdisciplinary care.* Cham, Switzerland: Springer International.

Malone, M. L., Vollbrecht, M., Stephenson, J., Burke, L., Pagel, P., & Goodwin, J. S. (2010). Acute Care for Elders (ACE) tracker and e-Geriatrician: Methods to disseminate ACE concepts to hospitals with no geriatricians on staff. *Journal of the American Geriatrics Society, 58*, 161–167. doi:10.1111/j.1532-5415.2009.02624.x

Marcantonio, E. R., Flacker, J. M., Wright, R. J., & Resnick, N. M. (2001). Reducing delirium after hip fracture: A randomized trial. *Journal of the American Geriatrics Society, 49*, 516–522. doi:10.1046/j.1532-5415.2001.49108.x

Martin-Khan, M., Flicker, L., Wootton, R., Loh, P., Edwards, H. E., Varghese, P., . . . Gray, L. C. (2012). The diagnostic accuracy of telegeriatrics for the diagnosis of dementia via video conferencing. *Journal of the American Medical Directors Association, 13*, 487. e19–487.e24. doi:10.1016/j.jamda.2012.03.004

Martinez-Reig, M., Ahmad, L., & Duque, G. (2012). The orthogeriatrics model of care: Systematic review of predictors of institutionalization and mortality in post-hip fracture patients and evidence for interventions. *Journal of the American Medical Directors Association, 13*, 770–777. doi:10.1016/j.jamda.2012.07.011

Mate, K. S., Berman, A., Laderman, M., Kabcenell, A., & Fulmer, T. (2017). Creating age-friendly health systems: A vision for better care of older adults. *Healthcare, 6*(1), 4–6. doi:10.1016/j.hjdsi.2017.05.005

Maxwell, C. A., Mion, L. C., & Minnick, A. (2013). Geriatric resources in acute care hospitals and trauma centers: A scarce commodity. *Journal of Gerontological Nursing, 39*, 33–42. doi:10.3928/00989134-20130731-01

McEvoy, L. K., & Cope, D. G. (Eds.). (2012). *Caring for the older adult with cancer in the ambulatory setting*. Pittsburgh, PA: Oncology Nursing Society.

Mendelson, D. A., & Friedman, S. M. (2014). Principles of comanagement and the geriatric fracture center. *Clinics in Geriatric Medicine, 30*, 183–189. doi:10.1016/j.cger.2014.01.016

Meyer, H. (2011). Using teams, real-time information, and teleconferencing to improve elders' hospital care. *Health Affairs, 30*, 408–411. doi:10.1377/hlthaff.2011.0073

Mezey, M., Boltz, M., Esterson, J., & Mitty, E. (2005). Evolving models of geriatric nursing care. *Geriatric Nursing, 26*(1), 11–15. doi:10.1016/j.gerinurse.2004.11.012

Mezey, M. D., Fulmer, T., & Abraham, I. L. (Eds.). (2003). *Geriatric nursing protocols for best practice* (2nd ed.). New York, NY: Springer Publishing.

Mion, L. C., Palmer, R. M., Meldon, S. W., Bass, D. M., Singer, M. E., Payne, S. M. C., . . . Emerman, C. (2003). Case finding and referral model for emergency department elders: A randomized clinical trial. *Annals of Emergency Medicine, 41*, 57–68. doi:10.1067/mem.2003.3

Milisen, K., Foreman, M. D., Abraham, I. L., De Geest, S., Godderis, J., Vandermeulen, E., . . . Broos, P. L. (2001). A nurse-led interdisciplinary intervention program for delirium in elderly hip-fracture patients. *Journal of the American Geriatrics Society, 49*, 523–532. doi:10.1046/j.1532-5415.2001.49109.x

Morgan, B., & Tarbi, E. (2016). The role of the advanced practice nurse in geriatric oncology care. *Seminars in Oncology Nursing, 32*, 33–43. doi:10.1016/j.soncn.2015.11.005

Moore, C., McGinn, T., & Halm, E. (2007). Tying up loose ends: Discharging patients with unresolved medical issues. *Archives of Internal Medicine, 167*(12), 1305–1311. doi:10.1001/archinte.167.12.1305

National Institute for Health and Care Excellence. (2010). Delirium: Prevention, diagnosis and management. Retrieved from https://www.nice.org.uk/guidance/cg103

Naylor, M., & Keating, S. A. (2008). Transitional care. *American Journal of Nursing, 108,* 58–63. doi:10.1097/01.naj.0000336420.34946.3a

Neuman, M. D., Speck, R. M., Karlawish, J. H., Schwartz, J. S., & Shea, J. A. (2010). Hospital protocols for the inpatient care of older adults: Results from a statewide survey. *Journal of the American Geriatrics Society, 58,* 1959–1964. doi:10.1111/j.1532-5415.2010.03056.x

Pallawala, P. M. D. S., & Lun, K. C. (2001). EMR based telegeriatric system. *International Journal of Medical Informatics, 61,* 229–234. doi:10.1016/s1386-5056(01)00144-7

Palmer, R. (2014). Geriatric evaluation and management units. In E. Capezuti, M. Malone, P. Katz, & M. Mezey (Eds.), *The encyclopedia of elder care* (3rd ed., pp. 337–339). New York, NY: Springer Publishing.

Palmer, R. M., Landefeld, C. S., Kresevic, D., & Kowal, J. (1994). A medical unit for the acute care of the elderly. *Journal of the American Geriatrics Society, 42,* 545–552. doi:10.1111/j.1532-5415.1994.tb04978.x

Parke, B., Boltz, M., Hunter, K. F., Chambers, T., Wolf-Ostermann, K., Adi, M. N., . . . Gutman, G. (2016). A scoping literature review of dementia-friendly hospital design. *The Gerontologist, 57,* e62–e74. doi:10.1093/geront/gnw128

Parke, B., & Brand, P. (2004). An elder-friendly hospital: Translating a dream into reality. *Nursing Leadership, 17,* 62–77. doi:10.12927/cjnl.2004.16344

Patel, J., Baldwin, J., Bunting, P., & Laha, S. (2014). The effect of a multicomponent multidisciplinary bundle of interventions on sleep and delirium in medical and surgical intensive care patients. *Anaesthesia, 69,* 540–549. doi:10.1111/anae.12638

Phibbs, C. S., Holty, J.-E., Goldstein, M. K., Garber, A. M., Wang, Y., Feussner, J. R., & Cohen, H. J. (2006). The effect of geriatrics evaluation and management on nursing home use and health care costs: Results from a randomized trial. *Medical Care, 44,* 91–95. doi:10.1097/01.mlr.0000188981.06522.e0

Prestmo, A., Hagen, G., Sletvold, O., Helbostad, J. L., Thingstad, P., Taraldsen, K., . . . Saltvedt, I. (2015). Comprehensive geriatric care for patients with hip fractures: A prospective, randomised, controlled trial. *Lancet, 385,* 1623–1633. doi:10.1016/s0140-6736(14)62409-0

Retornaz, F., Seux, V., Pauly, V., & Soubeyrand, J. (2008). Geriatric assessment and care for older cancer inpatients admitted in acute care for elders unit. *Critical Reviews in Oncology-Hematology, 68,* 165–171. doi:10.1016/j.critrevonc.2008.04.001

Retornaz, F., Seux, V., Sourial, N., Braud, A.-C., Monette, J., Bergman, H., & Soubeyrand, J. (2007). Comparison of the health and functional status between older inpatients with and without cancer admitted to a geriatric/internal medicine unit. *Journals of*

Gerontology Series A-Biological Sciences & Medical Sciences, 62, 917–922. doi:10.1093/gerona/62.8.917

Reuben, D. B., Inouye, S. K., Bogardus, S. T., Jr., Baker, D. I., Leo-Summers, L., & Cooney, L. M., Jr. (2000). The Hospital Elder Life Program: A model of care to prevent cognitive and functional decline in older hospitalized patients. *Journal of the American Geriatrics Society, 48*, 1697–1706. doi:10.1111/j.1532-5415.2000.tb03885.x

Rogers, J. A. (2009). Emergency care: A new model. Softer surroundings meet seniors' special needs. *Health Progress, 90*, 36–39.

Saltvedt, I., Mo, E.-S., Fayers, P., Kaasa, S., & Sletvold, O. (2002). Reduced mortality in treating acutely sick, frail older patients in a geriatric evaluation and management unit. A prospective randomized trial. *Journal of the American Geriatrics Society, 50*, 792–798. doi:10.1046/j.1532-5415.2002.50202.x

Saracino, R. M., Bai, M., Blatt, L., Solomon, L., & McCorkle, R. (2018). Geriatric palliative care: Meeting the needs of a growing population. *Geriatric Nursing, 39*(2), 225–229. doi:10.1016/j.gerinurse.2017.09.004

Sennour, Y., Counsell, S. R., Jones, J., & Weiner, M. (2009). Development and implementation of a proactive geriatrics consultation model in collaboration with hospitalists. *Journal of the American Geriatrics Society, 57*, 2139–2145. doi:10.1111/j.1532-5415.2009.02496.x

Singh, I., Subhan, Z., Krishnan, M., Edwards, C., & Okeke, J. (2016). Loneliness among older people in hospitals: A comparative study between single rooms and multi-bedded wards to evaluate current health service within the same organisation. *Gerontology & Geriatrics: Research, 2*, 1–5. Retrieved from http://austinpublishinggroup.com/gerontology/fulltext/ggr-v2-id1015.php

Siu, A. L., Spragens, L. H., Inouye, S. K., Morrison, R. S., & Leff, B. (2009). The ironic business case for chronic care in the acute care setting. *Health Affairs, 28*, 113–125. doi:10.1377/hlthaff.28.1.113

Smyth, C., Dubin, S., Restrepo, A., Nueva-Espana, H., & Capezuti, E. (2001). Creating order out of chaos: Models of GNP practice with hospitalized older adults. *Clinical Excellence for Nurse Practitioners, 5*, 88–95.

Somogyi-Zalud, E., Zhong, Z., Hamel, M. B., & Lynn, J. (2002). The use of life-sustaining treatments in hospitalized persons aged 80 and older. *Journal of the American Geriatrics Society, 50*, 930–934. doi:10.1046/j.1532-5415.2002.50222.x

Spinewine, A., Swine, C., Dhillon, S., Lambert, P., Nachega, J. B., Wilmotte, L., & Tulkens, P. M. (2007). Effect of a collaborative approach on the quality of prescribing for geriatric inpatients: A randomized, controlled trial. *Journal of the American Geriatrics Society, 55*, 658–665. doi:10.1111/j.1532-5415.2007.01132.x

Tomasović, N. (2005). Geriatric-palliative care units model for improvement of elderly care. *Collegium Antropologicum, 29*, 277–282. Retrieved from https://pdfs.semanticscholar.org/0bd9/ddb9ae94296a8a440d03703fff3b23a04ea5.pdf

Van Grootven, B., Flamaing, J., Dierckx de Casterlé, B., Dubois, C., Fagard, K., Herregods, M.-C., . . . Deschodt, M. (2017). Effectiveness of in-hospital geriatric co-management: A systematic review and meta-analysis. *Age and Ageing, 46,* 903–910. doi:10.1093/ageing/afx051

Vollbrecht, M., Malsch, A., Hook, M. L., Simpson, M. R., Khan, A, & Malone, M. (2015). Acute care for elders tracker, e-geriatrician telemedicine programs. In M. L. Malone, E. Capezuti, & R. M. Palmer (Eds.), *Geriatrics models of care: Bringing 'best practice' to an aging America* (1st ed., pp. 51–56). Basel, Switzerland: Springer International.

Wald, H., Huddleston, J., & Kramer, A. (2006). Is there a geriatrician in the house? Geriatric care approaches in hospitalist programs. *Journal of Hospital Medicine, 1,* 29–35. doi:10.1002/jhm.9

Walke, L. M., Rosenthal, R. A., Trentalange, M., Perkal, M. F., Maiaroto, M., Jeffery, S. M., & Marottoli, R. A. (2014). Restructuring care for older adults undergoing surgery: Preliminary data from the Co-Management of Older Operative Patients En Route Across Treatment Environments (CO-OPERATE) model of care. *Journal of the American Geriatrics Society, 62,* 2185–2190. doi:10.1111/jgs.13098

Watne, L. O., Torbergsen, A. C., Conroy, S., Engedal, K., Frihagen, F., Hjorthaug, G. A., . . . Wyller, T. B. (2014). The effect of a pre- and postoperative orthogeriatric service on cognitive function in patients with hip fracture: Randomized controlled trial (Oslo Orthogeriatric Trial). *BMC Medicine, 12,* 63. doi:10.1186/1741-7015-12-63

Welch, W. P., Stearns, S. C., Cuellar, A. E., & Bindman, A. B. (2014). Use of hospitalists by Medicare beneficiaries: A national picture. *Medicare & Medicaid Research Review, 4,* E1–E8. doi:10.5600/mmrr.004.02.b01

Williams, M. V., & Coleman, E. (2009). BOOSTing the hospital discharge. *Journal of Hospital Medicine, 4,* 209–210. doi:10.1002/jhm.525

Yue, J., Kshieh, T. T., & Inouye, S. K. (2015). Hospital Elder Life Program (HELP). In M. L. Malone, E. Capezuti, & R. M. Palmer (Eds.), *Geriatrics models of care: Bringing 'best practice' to an aging America* (1st ed., pp. 25–37). Basel, Switzerland: Springer International.

Zaubler, T. S., Murphy, K., Rizzuto, L., Santos, R., Skotzko, C., Giordano, J., . . . Inouye, S. K. (2013). Quality improvement and cost savings with multicomponent delirium interventions: Replication of the Hospital Elder Life Program in a community hospital. *Psychosomatics, 54,* 219–226. doi:10.1016/j.psym.2013.01.010

NICHE in Long-Term Care

Inna Popil, Sherry Greenberg, and Amy Berman

*The stunning national success of the Nurses Improving Care for Healthsystem
Elders (NICHE) program was the inspiration for the Center to Advance
Palliative Care's transition to a membership model. NICHE proved that there is
sustained demand for training and technical assistance
that improves the care of our most vulnerable and frail patients.*

—Diane Meier, MD, Director of the Center to Advance
Palliative Care(CAPC), Geriatrician

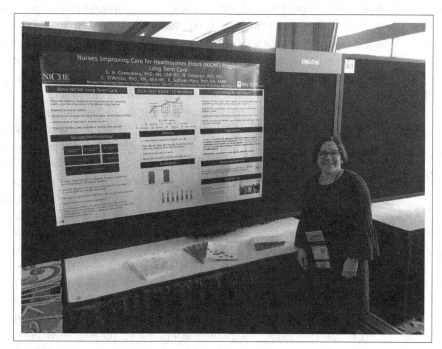

Sherry Greenberg.

CHAPTER OBJECTIVES

1. Provide the rationale for the development of NICHE long-term care (NICHE-LTC)
2. Present the NICHE-LTC core curriculum and educational resources
3. Discuss the specific NICHE-LTC content and materials developed for certified nursing assistants
4. Review the challenges in recruiting and retaining nursing homes into the NICHE-LTC program

INTRODUCTION

The most frail and vulnerable older adults in the United States reside in one of the nearly 16,000 long-term care (LTC) facilities (Harris-Kojetin et al., 2016). The majority of LTC facilities are nursing homes, serving more than 1.4 million residents (Harris-Kojetin et al., 2016). The majority of nursing home residents are older adults; 84.9% are age 65 and over with 41.6% age 85 and older (Harris-Kojetin et al., 2016). Nursing homes provide round-the-clock nursing care to people with multiple chronic conditions who cannot be cared for at home, and complex skilled care needs, including wound care or physical therapy following a fall. While some nursing home residents may return home following short-term rehabilitation, others may reside in a nursing home for years, some through the end of their lives, needing the ongoing management of complex medical or nursing care that cannot be managed safely at home. Nursing homes are also an important site for hospice care, with some people entering LTC facilities as they approach the end of life.

The number of older adults who will need LTC services will only increase in the future, while at the same time, the number of caregivers and healthcare professionals prepared to provide this care is decreasing.

As residents of nursing homes are among the most vulnerable population (Murray & Laditka, 2010), they need and deserve evidence-based, safe, quality care to ensure health, function, and quality of life. The number of older adults who will need LTC services will only increase in the future, while at the same time, the number of caregivers and healthcare professionals prepared to provide this care is decreasing (Deschodt, Zúñiga, & Wellens, 2017). Residents of LTC facilities typically have multiple chronic conditions, functional issues, mobility challenges, cognitive impairment, and urinary incontinence. Yet, despite the high complexity of care of their older adult residents, nursing home staff often lack adequate training in geriatric evidence-based practice. There are no national standards or requirements for geriatric-related training or experience for the LTC workforce. As a result, care in nursing homes may be subpar and even harmful to older adults.

LTC has been charged with implementing multiple healthcare initiatives to improve transitions in care, provide person-centered care, and prevent avoidable hospitalizations of residents, to name a few. Consumers, advocates, and governmental agencies are increasing their demand for accountability and quality through national and local initiatives. Some of the organizations setting standards and monitoring outcomes in long-term healthcare organizations across the United States include the Centers for Medicare and Medicaid Services (CMS), Agency for Healthcare Research and Quality (AHRQ), National Quality Forum (NQF), and Joint Commission, to name a few. Implementation of evidence-based initiatives in LTC has been difficult due to multiple challenges while working under limited budgetary resources. Challenges include frequent turnover of leadership and frontline staff; use of agency staff who are unfamiliar with residents and facility policies and procedures; employment of licensed practical nurses (LPNs) who have limitations in their scope of practice as compared to registered nurses (RNs); and staff at all educational levels that lack training in the unique aspects of care for older adults.

Implementation of evidence-based initiatives in LTC has been difficult due to multiple challenges while working under limited budgetary resources.

There is a crucial need for education related to transitional care issues and prevention of avoidable hospital readmissions, assessment and management of older adults with dementia, and how to best communicate and collaborate with interprofessional team members to enhance evidence-based quality care and promote positive outcomes. The purpose of this chapter is to describe the expansion of the Nurses Improving Care for Healthsystem Elders (NICHE) hospital model into LTC settings.

EXPANDING NICHE INTO LONG-TERM CARE

NICHE is the leading nurse-driven membership program designed to help healthcare organizations improve the care of older adults. In 2016, New York University Rory Meyers College of Nursing's (NYU Meyers) NICHE program received a $1.5 million grant from The John A. Hartford Foundation to fund the expansion and adaptation of the successful NICHE hospital program into long-term care (NICHE-LTC). The aim of NICHE-LTC is to further develop and improve treatment outcomes, older adult person-centered care, and geriatric workforce capacity in nursing homes, assisted living facilities, and other postacute institutional settings. This project is led by Eileen Sullivan-Marx, PhD, RN, FAAN, principal investigator; Dean and Erline Perkins McGriff Professor, NYU Meyers. This builds on The John A. Hartford Foundation's previous investment in NICHE, the expertise and leadership at NYU Meyers, and the existing set of high quality geriatric resources produced by NICHE and the Hartford Institute for Geriatric Nursing.

The aim of NICHE-LTC is to further develop and improve treatment outcomes, older adult person-centered care, and geriatric workforce capacity in nursing homes, assisted living facilities, and other postacute institutional settings.

NICHE LONG-TERM CARE PROGRAM

Developing the nursing workforce in LTC settings is key to achieving improvements in the overall quality of care for older adults in nursing homes and other LTC facilities. The goal of the NICHE-LTC program is to provide clinical, organizational change and quality improvement content pertinent to LTC organizations, managers, direct care providers, and interprofessional staff to improve health outcomes for LTC residents. Building upon NICHE's successful hospital-based model, NICHE-LTC provides support for nursing homes and other LTC facilities in meeting the changing federal quality and regulatory mandates by developing the geriatric expertise of nursing staff and other members of the interdisciplinary team. NICHE-LTC promotes the use of evidence-based clinical interventions and equips nurses with the necessary leadership skills to bring about changes in the quality of care delivered to older adults in LTC facilities. NICHE's expansion into LTC is extremely important, essential, and timely. Developing the nursing workforce in LTC settings is crucial to achieving improvements in the overall quality of care.

The NICHE-LTC program emphasizes education and practice development through two complementary initiatives during the first year of NICHE-LTC membership, namely the Leadership Training Program for nurse managers and clinical leaders in participating member organizations, and the geriatric resource nurse (GRN) and geriatric certified nursing assistant (GCNA) educational curriculum designed for frontline clinical staff. By joining the NICHE program, members gain access to evidence-based clinical education resources, nursing practice models, and clinical guidelines in the NICHE Knowledge Center, which is designed to improve the knowledge, skills, and abilities to provide person-centered care for older adults.

NICHE-LTC CORE CURRICULUM AND EDUCATIONAL RESOURCES

Leadership Training Program

NICHE's Long-Term Care Leadership Training Program provides tools, strategies, and resources to help organizations think critically and strategize about how to develop a system-wide program to improve care for older adults.

NICHE's Long-Term Care Leadership Training Program provides tools, strategies, and resources to help organizations think critically and strategize about how to develop a system-wide program to improve care for older adults, and also gives an introduction to the NICHE community overall. The program is designed to be an 8-week, blended learning program that consists of online modules with corresponding readings and articles, group conference calls with faculty mentors, live and recorded webinars, instructional videos, and assignments. It provides clinical leaders a roadmap to implement necessary changes and achieve desirable outcomes in their facilities. The program helps leaders develop a vision; evaluate strengths, weaknesses, opportunities, and threats; target priorities; identify a pilot unit(s) to implement the NICHE model; and develop an action plan change project with measurable outcomes and specific timeframes. During the program, participants are guided by NYU Meyers faculty mentors, who come from well-established NICHE participating sites. NICHE mentors discuss and share their experiences with program participants and review submitted assignments. NYU Meyers faculty mentors offer suggestions and provide feedback to participants during conference calls, webinars, and through communications via the online discussion forum, emails, and calls.

The educational materials for NICHE-LTC build on NICHE's robust and successful resources in acute care. *Evidence-Based Geriatric Nursing Protocols for Best Practice* (5th ed.) by Boltz, Capezuti, Fulmer, and Zwicker (editors), published in 2016 by Springer Publishing Company, LLC, though first used only in the NICHE Acute Care program, is now also used for the Long-Term Care program for its important, relevant, clinical content. Online access to the evidence-based protocols from this book is readily available, with permission from Springer Publishing Company, on the Hartford Institute for Geriatric Nursing's clinical website at consultgeri.org. Another core text for the NICHE-LTC program is *Leadership and Management Skills for Long-Term Care* by Sullivan-Marx and Gray-Miceli (editors), published by Springer Publishing Company, LLC in 2008. The purpose of this book, funded by a Comprehensive Geriatric Education Program grant from the U.S. Health and Resource Services Administration (HRSA), is to provide nurses with evidence-based information about leadership and management in LTC to help improve quality of care. The book addresses commonly seen issues in LTC including workforce shortages, time constraints, and nursing staff retention. Book chapters from this text are used as the foundation for the individual teaching sessions in the LTC Leadership Training Program. Teaching modules include the topics of cultural competence and adult teaching and learning principles. Leadership content focuses on team building, communication, power and negotiation, change theory and process, and management techniques such as directing and delegating as well as shifting from conflict to collaboration. The text chapters include learning objectives, pre- and post-tests (with answers), topic content, case studies, handouts, and evaluation. The book may be used for self-learning or in group training.

Educational Development

The GRN course is foundational and a critical component of the NICHE program. The nurse plays a central role in bridging the quality chasm by facilitating prompt detection and treatment of common geriatric syndromes, promoting health, and preventing functional decline (Capezuti et al., 2012). The GRN model promotes best practice utilizing a systematic and interdisciplinary approach to address common conditions and issues among older adults in all healthcare settings (see Chapter 8). Implementing this model becomes an initial step in developing system-wide improvements and changes in care for older adults. As a clinical intervention, the GRN model features education, coaching, and mentorship by the "expert" GRN to peers and colleagues. The multidimensional GRN model addresses the complex care and advocacy needs of older adults in all healthcare settings. Caring for older adults requires a team approach. Because many healthcare professionals are not educated in geriatric evidence-based care, the GRN must mentor colleagues as well. The GRN model is supported by the NICHE curriculum (Table 11.1) and many educational resources. GRN educational resources include specific education for RNs and LPNs in a LTC setting.

In addition to topics specific to geriatric care, new topics were developed based on demands and initiatives specific to LTC. A variety of interactive educational resources were developed including person-centered care; reducing preventable hospitalizations; change leadership; medication management and reconciliation; effective communication with situation, background, assessment, recommendation (SBAR); quality assurance and performance improvement (QAPI); and documentation essentials (for RNs and LPNs in LTC). Clinical topics include fall prevention; nutrition and hydration; pressure injuries and skin tears; function; dementia; pain; advanced directives and palliative care; and decision making. Educational resources include interactive PowerPoints, case studies, video clips, clinical practice guidelines, posters, and diagrams.

Certified nursing assistants (CNAs) are the providers of direct patient care in LTC (Cramer et al., 2014). Many of the outcomes of care in LTC settings are related to the work of nursing assistants, such as maintaining function and mobility, encouraging self-care, providing hydration, feeding, and improving nutritional intake. Spending the most time with older adults, nursing assistants may be the first care providers to detect subtle changes that might signal the onset of a geriatric syndrome, such as delirium, early signs of skin changes, and/or acute illness. Educational modules and resources have been completed to educate CNAs in the interdisciplinary care of the older adult and family in LTC. CNAs are provided with information from the NICHE curriculum, which is easy for them to understand and apply clinically. Topics include age-related sensory loss, function, feeding and

Spending the most time with older adults, nursing assistants may be the first care providers to detect subtle changes that might signal the onset of a geriatric syndrome.

TABLE 11.1 Long-term Care Curriculum: Leadership Training Program	
Professional levels	GRN-RN
	GRN-LPN
	GCNA
Resources	Medication management guidelines
	SBAR poster
	Webinars
	Case studies
GCNA, geriatric certified nursing assistant; GRN, geriatric resource nurse; LPN, licensed practical nurse; RN, registered nurse; SBAR, situation, background, assessment, recommendation.	

TABLE 11.2 NICHE Long-term Care Content Alignment With CMS Five-Star Quality Measures	
CMS FIVE-STAR QUALITY MEASURES	**NICHE EDUCATIONAL RESOURCES**
Activities of daily living	Function
Ability to move independently	Function
High-risk residents with pressure ulcers	Pressure injuries and skin tears
Residents physically restrained	Restraints
Moderate-to-severe pain	Pain management
Falls with major injury	Fall prevention
Residents receiving antipsychotic medications	Medication management (including management of antipsychotics)
CMS, Centers for Medicare and Medicaid Services.	

nutrition, falls, pressure injuries and skin tears, frailty, pain, sleep, palliative care, dementia, delirium, and depression.

NICHE-LTC educational resources are aligned with the CMS Five-Star Quality Rating System. This system was created to help persons and their caregivers compare nursing homes to help identify areas about which people may want to inquire further. The Nursing Home Compare website details a quality rating system rating nursing homes between one and five stars. Nursing homes with five stars are considered to have well above average quality and nursing homes with one star are considered to have quality well below average. The quality measure rating has information on 11 different physical and clinical measures for nursing home residents. NICHE resources include education on these quality measures (Table 11.2).

Person and Caregiver Resources

Person, family, and caregiver educational resources, including "Need to Know" materials, have been updated to include LTC-specific language and topics. "Need to Know" handouts include useful information for residents and families on various topics, such as care after hip fracture surgery, communicating with the healthcare team, delirium, depression, functional decline, hearing, managing medications, meals and nutrition, pain, palliative care, patient environment, restraint use, safety and falls, skin care, sleep, vaccines, and vision. NICHE open resources provide links to leading resources and include assessment and operational tools, interprofessional education and practice eBooks, covering a variety of topics such as vaccinations, safety, and making end-of-life decisions.

Webinars

In order for LTC staff to learn at their own pace and at their convenience, NICHE webinars are offered in live and recorded formats, offering continuing education contact hours completion. Leading expert faculty and researchers from the field of gerontological nursing and health services research present webinars on cutting-edge topics to advance nurse-led care in member organizations. Topics presented are relevant to the care of older adults across the continuum of care. NICHE-LTC members are invited and encouraged to participate. The webinar library housed in the NICHE Knowledge Center contains over 60 webinars. Selected webinar topics include Steps to H.O.P.E.: Building Health, Optimism, Purpose and Endurance in Palliative Care for Family Caregivers of Persons with Dementia; Reducing Fall Rates Using an Interdisciplinary Approach; Decreasing Falls: Interventions Aimed at Sensory Impairments; Preventing Functional Decline With Simple Mobility; Caution! CAUTI-Free Zone: Improving Outcomes in Heart Failure Patients; and American Nurses Credentialing Center's (ANCC) Pathway to Excellence® Program.

EVALUATION

Evaluation methods for NICHE-LTC facilities include (a) completion of a postleadership training program satisfaction survey; (b) a 1-year follow-up report; and (c) organizational progress with achieving action plan change project goals and implementing the educational model on selected units. The Geriatric Institutional Assessment Profile (GIAP), a core measure used by the NICHE members to assess the geriatric nursing practice environment and to plan clinical improvement projects, is being adapted for use in LTC. The GIAP LTC builds on the original survey designed for hospital work environments and will be specific to the needs of the LTC environment.

Individual sites measure their own quality outcomes based on a template provided. NICHE suggests collecting the following data per measurable outcome: future tasks needed to achieve next steps, timeframe by when task(s) should be completed, resources needed to complete tasks, method(s) of measuring outcome, method(s) of evaluation, and the outcomes. NICHE-LTC member organization outcomes have included fall reduction, pressure injury reduction, increased mobility, decreased hospitalizations, integrating palliative care into daily practice, and improving resident satisfaction.

DISSEMINATION

A market for the NICHE-LTC program exists, though identifying and recruiting LTC sites willing and able to invest in NICHE membership is a challenge. Since the start of NICHE-LTC, 54 new LTC sites have become NICHE members. Efforts continue to recruit and retain sites. In order to attract new LTC sites, marketing materials describing NICHE-LTC were developed and shared with staff at the ANCC's Pathway to Excellence® program and at regional and national conferences designed for nurse leaders and other decision makers responsible for clinical services in the LTC sector. The goal of attending these conferences is to raise awareness of the NICHE-LTC program, cultivate sales leads, and establish the NICHE program brand in the LTC market. Conferences attended since the start of NICHE-LTC include those of the Gerontological Advanced Practice Nurses Association (GAPNA), National Council of Post-Acute Care Practitioners, Hospice & Palliative Nurses Association (HPNA), ANCC, Leading Age, Gerontological Society of America (GSA), American Society on Aging (ASA), and American Association of Directors of Nursing Services (AADNS). A poster, "Nurses Improving Care for Healthsystem Elders (NICHE) Program: Expanding into Long-Term Care," was presented at AMDA—The Society for Post-Acute and Long-Term Care Medicine Annual Conference in 2017 with an updated poster presentation in the 2018 Annual Conference. A NICHE site readiness checklist was developed for prospective NICHE members to determine if they are ready to implement NICHE in their organization.

To raise awareness among the NICHE member hospitals and others regarding entry into the LTC market, specific sessions for LTC were developed for the 2017 and 2018 NICHE Annual Conference program. Recent LTC-focused sessions included (a) a luncheon for NICHE-LTC members and prospective member hospitals and LTC facilities interested in the NICHE-LTC program to network; (b) NICHE-LTC member presentations; and (c) review of LTC resources during the NICHE coordinator business meeting.

NICHE RECOGNITION

The NICHE-LTC program, over time, will follow the same overall NICHE member recognition levels. Members submit evaluation data at the end of the first year of membership capturing the extent to which the NICHE program model, in terms of their change project and educational staff development, is implemented on the participating units. In turn, the annual evaluation data are used to assign a NICHE recognition level to participating sites ranging from "member" to "senior-friendly" to "exemplar."

CHAPTER SUMMARY

With an expected increase in the number of older adults who will need LTC services and supports and a decrease in the number of healthcare professionals qualified to provide these services, the relevance of NICHE for the LTC setting is clear. The NICHE-LTC program seeks to improve care of older adults in LTC settings by providing education on how best to address transition of care issues, prevent avoidable hospital readmissions, assess and manage older adults with dementia, and communicate and collaborate with interprofessional team members.

The NICHE-LTC program accomplishes this goal via two different initiatives: an 8-week Leadership Training Program for nurse managers and clinical leaders, and clinical training for RNs, LPNs, and CNAs. Resources provided by this program include online courses, group conference calls, webinars, instructional videos, books, coaching, mentoring, person and caregiver resources, follow-up evaluation, and LTC-specific national conference sessions.

ACKNOWLEDGMENT

Thank you to The John A. Hartford Foundation for supporting NICHE Long-Term Care.

REFERENCES

Boltz, M., Capezuti, E., Fulmer, T., & Zwicker, D. (Eds.). (2016). *Evidence-based geriatric nursing protocols for best practice* (5th ed.). New York, NY: Springer Publishing.

Capezuti, E., Boltz, M., Cline, D., Dickson, V. V., Rosenberg, M.-C., Wagner, L., . . . Nigolian, C. (2012). Nurses Improving Care for Healthsystem Elders: A model for optimising the geriatric nursing practice environment. *Journal of Clinical Nursing, 21*, 3117–3125. doi:10.1111/j.1365-2702.2012.04259.x

Cramer, M. E., High, R., Culross, B., Conley, D. M., Nayar, P., Nguyen, A. T., & Ojha, D. (2014). Retooling the RN workforce in long-term care: Nursing certification as a pathway to quality improvement. *Geriatric Nursing, 35*(3), 182–187. doi:10.1016/j.gerinurse.2014.01.001

Deschodt, M., Zúñiga, F., & Wellens, N. (2017), Challenges in research and practice in residential long-term care. *Journal of Nursing Scholarship, 49*(1), 3–5. doi: 10.1111/jnu.12270

Harris-Kojetin, L., Sengupta, M., Park-Lee, E., Valverde, R., Caffrey, C., Rome, V., & Lendon, J. (2016). *Long-term care providers and services users in the United States: Data from the national study of long-term care providers, 2013–2014. Vital and Health Statistics, 3*(38). Hyattsville, MD: National Center for Health Statistics.

Murray, L. M., & Laditka S. B. (2010). Care transitions by older adults from nursing homes to hospitals: Implications for long-term care practice, geriatric education, and research. *Journal of the American Medical Directors Association, 11*(4), 231–238. doi:10.1016/j.jamda.2009.09.007

Sullivan-Marx, E. M., & Gray-Miceli, D. (Eds.). (2008). *Leadership and management skills for long-term care.* New York, NY: Springer Publishing.

Health System Interventions

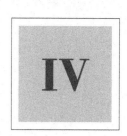

Program Expansion in the Age of Digital Learning and Engagement

Barbara Bricoli

Nothing demonstrated the success of Nurses Improving Care for Healthsystem Elders (NICHE) better than the annual conference where the work and innovations of hundreds of NICHE hospitals were showcased—building visibility for NICHE and engagement and loyalty from the NICHE hospitals. These NICHE advocates ensured new hospitals would seek designation which was critical to the long-term sustainability and growth of the NICHE program.
—Elizabeth Seka Gray, President, TSI Marketing Communications

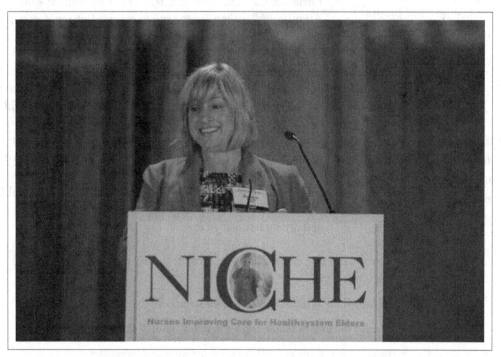

Barbara Bricoli.

CHAPTER OBJECTIVES

1. Describe development of the NICHE online learning modules and webinars
2. Describe benchmarking and recruitment of new NICHE sites
3. Discuss the process for encouraging hospital buy-in
4. Provide the rationale and process for NICHE benchmarking and evaluation

INTRODUCTION

Based on the geriatric resource nurse (GRN) model pioneered by Dr. Terry Fulmer, a geriatric nurse specialist at Boston's Beth Israel Hospital, and with funding from The John A. Hartford Foundation, NICHE evolved into a comprehensive hospital program based at New York University.

It was clear that for NICHE to scale, the team would need to tap into the burgeoning fields of digital learning, engagement, and cloud computing.

Nurses Improving Care for Healthsystem Elders (NICHE) aims to create better geriatric care environments for older adults in healthcare settings. Based on the geriatric resource nurse (GRN) model pioneered by Dr. Terry Fulmer, a geriatric nurse specialist at Boston's Beth Israel Hospital, and with funding from The John A. Hartford Foundation, NICHE evolved into a comprehensive hospital program based at New York University. In 2007, under the leadership of Dr. Elizabeth Capezuti, NICHE received a $5 million grant from The Atlantic Philanthropies to launch a period of rapid growth and expansion during which a sustainable business model was developed (see Chapter 2).

In 2007, with a solid base of 150 participating hospitals and prior to the launch of the new fee structure, an expanded NICHE operations team set out to develop a strong value proposition; a vast portfolio of tools and resources that would help hospitals build their geriatric capacity; a well-recognized designation for hospitals that would make them more competitive in the marketplace; a means for hospitals to measure their financial and clinical outcomes; and a cost-effective way to deliver all of the above. It was clear that for NICHE to scale, the team would need to tap into the burgeoning fields of digital learning, engagement, and cloud computing. In 2008, NICHE set out to develop and deploy technology to:

- *Convert existing content and new content to an online learning format*

- *House all the NICHE resources and curate other knowledge*

- *Market the program and build a pipeline of NICHE adopters*

- *Build a community of collaborative learners and advocates*

- *Support lean efficient business operations for a global customer base*

With a very lean operating budget, for NICHE to succeed the team would need to leverage technology to drive sales and support internal operations as well as deliver its goods and services to customers digitally.

ONLINE LEARNING

Developing and Launching Online Learning and a Learning Management System

At the time of NICHE expansion, a growing number of hospitals had begun to use learning management systems (LMSs) to deliver online learning and plan, implement, facilitate, and evaluate nurse education and learning. An LMS is a learning platform that can deliver content and administer, document, track, and report on the delivery of all methods of educational program delivery (Davis & Surajballi, 2014). Healthcare organizations were tapping into the flexibility and benefits provided by an LMS and e-learning, including the ability to centralize health information technology (IT) and nurse informatics educational content and resources; track learner activities; collect, aggregate, and store data on learners; and provide performance feedback to learners and educational providers (Sportsman, 2014).

It was vital that NICHE develop its own LMS and online courses to deliver content, foster collaboration, and align with healthcare organizational practices. One of the benefits of NICHE was the ability for hospitals to implement practices consistently across settings. NICHE promised a portfolio of content to help develop staff competency as well as deliver system-wide practice change initiatives. Furthermore, hospitals were looking for time- and cost-efficient educational programs. The economic downturn in 2008 caused hospitals to cut their travel and educational budgets for staff, limiting their ability to send people to in-person training and annual conferences offered by NICHE. These conditions accelerated NICHE's efforts to build online learning and collaboration. With staff shortages and a barrage of new regulations and reporting requirements, and the realization that hospital staff were ill prepared to care for the growing aging population, there was an increasing need for rapid delivery of content. E-learning offered a flexible and time-efficient way for healthcare organizations and nursing professional development practitioners to meet the challenges of educating staff who face a variety of challenges with varying schedules, diverse backgrounds, different work experiences, and unique learning requisites (White & Shellenbarger, 2017).

E-learning offered a flexible and time-efficient way for healthcare organizations and nursing professional development practitioners to meet the challenges of educating staff who face a variety of challenges with varying schedules, diverse backgrounds, different work experiences, and unique learning requisites

The development of NICHE online learning and resources happened iteratively. NICHE launched its first website in 2008. Shortly thereafter, a new core curriculum to build geriatric knowledge was made available. This curriculum was first offered as instructor-led presentations (nonpaying member sites were able to sign into the website and download the files and the accompanying instructor guides as a precursor to the anticipated online offerings that would be introduced in conjunction with the new membership fee structure). The original content was used by the first group of paying members, and NICHE requested and received feedback on the content. This content was then converted to e-learning modules using instructional design principles.

Next NICHE transformed the 2-day, face-to-face Leadership Training Program (LTP), the process by which new member hospitals assess their organizations' geriatric capacities and develop an implementation plan for NICHE, into a 6-week online blended learning program. Previously the LTP was a 2-day event held prior to the NICHE annual conference. The new online model utilized 30 hours of synchronous and asynchronous learning over 6 weeks. Participating hospitals would enroll their teams (a minimum of three staff from a hospital were required) and access online curriculum, videos, and assignments. Hospitals were assigned regional cohorts and assigned a NICHE mentor from their geographic regions. NICHE mentors, otherwise known as NICHE "faculty," were seasoned nurse leaders who had successfully implemented NICHE in their hospitals. NICHE faculty held periodic conference calls and webinars throughout the 6 weeks. This virtual, blended learning approach increased the depth and breadth of hospitals' implementation plans as it provided more time for participants to conduct thorough team-based analysis and assessment of their hospitals, engage with experts and peers for ongoing consultation and advice, and foster ongoing internal and external communication while they tested and piloted initiatives. The LTP also served as an indoctrination to the NICHE online program, setting hospitals up for successful implementation as they typically completed the LTP and then began enrolling their staff for training in the core curriculum, in particular the GRN program.

At the same time, the team set out to build an LMS to house all the resources. In fall 2009, a very basic platform was launched to host the first pilot LTP. While the LTP pilots were underway, the team was working with vendors to find the best long-term LMS solution. Always mindful of the fact that NICHE members would be using the NICHE LMS in addition to their internal hospital systems, NICHE sought to develop a platform that would be simple and compatible with their hospital systems. Over the years NICHE tried to provide solutions that would integrate the NICHE LMS with hospitals, but this proved problematic. NICHE launched its first fully functional LMS in 2010 and branded it as the NICHE Knowledge Center (KC; Bricoli, 2011). It was immediately successful. Nurse educators and other hospital staff were already becoming accustomed to the systems that their hospitals were providing and were hopeful that their hospital LMSs and the NICHE KC would reduce the amount of repetitive, face-to-face training, automate tracking, and simplify reporting.

Always mindful of the fact that NICHE members would be using the NICHE LMS in addition to their internal hospital systems, NICHE sought to develop a platform that would be simple and compatible with their hospital systems.

Webinars

Another digital learning tool introduced by NICHE was the webinar. Webinars were a great vehicle for quickly disseminating new information, engaging live audiences, and providing timely new information. The production times and costs were very low. NICHE would identify important topics and then identify subject matter experts to present on those topics. Topics were identified through the listserv (explained later) as well as by NICHE faculty and experts on relevant pressing issues (i.e., CMS "never events"[1]). Webinars were also an excellent way to enlist NICHE members to highlight their work and share their innovations, and a great way for NICHE to collaborate with other organizations on delivering content, such as the Oncology Nursing Society (ONS). Webinars were also complementary adjuncts to other resources. They provided real-life applications of innovations and best practices typically developed by member hospitals. NICHE developed a process in which individuals who presented their work at the annual NICHE conferences would be invited to present this work via a live webinar (presenters participated in a competitive process to present their work through podium and poster presentations at conferences). This content would inform the development of toolkits of resources around specific topics (webinars were just one component; there were also mini case studies, consumer resources, etc.).

By 2016, NICHE was delivering 22 webinars per year. Webinars were available to the general public for fees; fees for NICHE hospitals were included in membership. They were a great way to get nonmembers interested in becoming NICHE sites—a great introduction to NICHE resources.

The LMS housed the courses, webinars, LTP, and a large list of other clinical and organizational resources. It also housed discussion forums for collaboration between members and the NICHE team. A critical function of the LMS was inclusion of transcripts for learners and the ability for hospitals to track their staff and overall progress.

Benchmarking and Evaluation

An integral part of NICHE is a benchmarking service using several instruments essential for institutions to assess their strengths and weaknesses as they initiate the NICHE implementation process and to evaluate progress over time (Capezuti et al., 2013). These instruments included the NICHE Geriatric Institutional Assessment Profile (GIAP), a tool that helped hospitals measure their organizational cultures surrounding care of older adults (staff knowledge, attitudes, and perceptions of the care environment). With the launch of the business model, the GIAP went

---

[1]Never events are "serious and costly errors in provision of health care services that should never happen." (Centers for Medicare and Medicaid Services, www.cms.gov/newsroom/fact-sheets/eliminating-serious-preventable-and-costly-medical-errors-never-events)

from being a valuable tool that hospitals could purchase (or in many cases use for no cost) to a members-only tool that was bundled into the annual fee. Most hospitals chose to conduct the GIAP within 6 months of implementation of their NICHE programs (Capezuti et al., 2013) and were encouraged to repeat the GIAP periodically (every 1 or 2 years) to measure their progress.

The NICHE program evaluation is a 49-item self-evaluation tool that measures the depth (degree of application of evidence-based resources) and penetration (dissemination throughout the hospital) of programs. The original content was based on prior research that drew upon consumers, clinicians, and researchers to identify the components of geriatric programs. The instrument was developed by the NICHE research team, and content experts (clinicians, NICHE administrators) measured metrics aligned with the following dimensions: guiding principles, organizational structures, leadership, resources to build geriatric staff competence, interdisciplinary resources and processes, patient- and family-centered approaches, environment of care, and aging-sensitive practices (Boltz et al., 2013). Members reported high satisfaction with the content of the survey and its ability to monitor their progress; their compliance rate increased each year.

While the GIAP had been an integral part of NICHE since 1997, the first automated GIAP was introduced in 2007. In 2011, NICHE developed and launched a new version of the online benchmarking and evaluation platform to house the GIAP, the Annual Program Evaluation, and an annual institutional update that members completed. This new online system allowed NICHE coordinators to enroll their participants, complete surveys, view the progress of survey compliance, and generate reports. The system also supported internal data management for the internal NICHE team, both for research purposes as well as client relationship management, and utilization tracking. The ability for member hospitals to complete surveys online contributed to a large increase in surveys administered.

Getting Hospitals to Buy In

In 2009, when NICHE launched its online programs, hospitals were in the early stages of adopting e-learning, far behind many other industries. In many cases it was considered a new technology and not part of hospitals' strategic plans. One study from that period indicates that hospitals that were less bureaucratic and more innovative were more likely to adopt e-learning and the investigators posit that hospitals with innovative cultures have higher patient satisfaction rates and are more likely to be early adopters of new technologies (Hung, Chen, & Lee, 2009). These same attributes were often present in NICHE hospitals that were looking to provide better care for their older adult populations and were eager to adopt a program that utilized e-learning for successful implementation.

NICHE's introduction of online learning aligned with current trends and organizational goals. NICHE also determined that the introduction to the KC during the LTP was a way to indoctrinate new sites into the use of the system. NICHE was also able to articulate the cost efficiency of having staff utilize online courses. Even for those hospitals utilizing instructor-led courses, NICHE provided access to the core curriculum, specialty courses, and other in-service training for health system educators to use. They could download them from the KC and use them in their classroom setting.

In addition to the numerous resources available on the NICHE KC, the overall value proposition of NICHE was that everything was available and ready to use—saving hospitals invaluable time and dollars in developing their own content.

In addition to the numerous resources available on the NICHE KC, the overall value proposition of NICHE was that everything was available and ready to use—saving hospitals invaluable time and dollars in developing their own content. Furthermore, health systems were able to standardize their training practices across multiple settings. Additionally, the resources were utilized in other nonacute settings to improve care across the continuum (note that in 2015 NICHE began development of a program for nonacute care, which was launched in 2016).

In developing the LMS, NICHE knew that it had to have a hierarchical framework that allowed for each hospital to have the ability to track and monitor their staff's progress. Transcripts were built into the system. NICHE coordinators, individuals in the hospitals responsible for managing the NICHE programs, could view the progress of their staff and communicate with their peers at other hospitals and with the NICHE team all via the KC. Equally important was that through the New York University (NYU) College of Nursing, NICHE provided contact hours for continuing education (CE) credits to nurses and other healthcare providers. This was an important incentive for hospitals and increased the value of NICHE (Capezuti, Bricoli, & Boltz, 2013).

Success and Challenges

From 2010 to 2015, enrollment in the KC grew to 50,000. Hospitals enrolled their teams. Not all users were active, but this number demonstrates the level of hospitals' interest in providing access to their staffs. This number is also 63% higher than 2014 enrollments, indicating continued growth and retention. Other successes include the level of depth in the action plans produced by hospitals with the new LTP. The 6-week online program with ongoing mentorship and collaboration with peers resulted in hospitals producing more meaningful action plans. The benchmarking and evaluation program also expanded tremendously. By 2015, over 140,000 GIAPs were completed using the new system and the compliance rate on the annual program evaluation was 90%.

There were many challenges along the way. Online learning was a relatively new field. Despite continuous efforts to learn from other organizations of similar size (similar to NICHE), it was very difficult to find other success stories. In fact, NICHE served as a pioneer and leader in this field and was called upon to share its experience with other organizations. Another challenge was building the hierarchy in the LMS. The NICHE KC was designed to host several thousand users. When it grew to 50,000, the system did not have the capacity to handle it. Also, NICHE was looking for ways to embed its courses in hospitals' LMSs, as hospitals were requesting this. There were a few experiments in which NICHE licensed its course modules to hospitals to embed internally. This worked for those hospitals but it was not feasible for NICHE to manage this kind of licensing business with such a small staff. The benchmarking platform also began collapsing under the weight of such tremendous growth, In particular as NICHE expanded to other healthcare settings and created new surveys, the system was stretched to its limits and plans were underway to find a new solution as described in what follows.

COLLABORATION AND ENGAGEMENT

NICHE set out to build a learning community and brought together thousands of individuals working at member hospitals and healthcare organizations with researchers and faculty and content experts around the world. Online learning communities helped facilitate collaboration and knowledge sharing and helped members find solutions to problems. In addition, LMS options such as asynchronous discussion boards and group assignments (during the LTP) helped drive interprofessional collaboration and spark clinical innovation. Used in this way, the LMS platform was ideal for encouraging discussion among healthcare professionals who would not normally have the occasion to interact with one another (White & Shellenbarger, 2017).

Collaboration also took place in the creation of much of NICHE content. NICHE called upon its members to cocreate resources. Drawing upon their expertise and highlighting their best practices and innovations was an optimal way to share knowledge. Members viewed their contributions as an obligation to the organization—and while NICHE was not actually a membership association, they viewed it as such and took pride in ownership of the program. This collaboration was not only key to building brand loyalty, but also in creating meaningful resources, and positioned NICHE as a responsive organization. Overall, the majority of the digital content was member driven as NICHE was continuously engaged with its members, assessing the current climate, and responding to their needs. One successful mode of collaboration was the NICHE faculty and mentors program. NICHE invited experienced nurse leaders who had successfully implemented NICHE in their hospitals to be NICHE faculty and mentors. NICHE faculty worked with hospitals during the LTP and implementation process to provide mentorship and guidance (Capezuti et al., 2012). They also worked with the NICHE team to inform and update content. This collaboration was facilitated through online forums, communications, and courses.

Overall, the majority of the digital content was member driven as NICHE was continuously engaged with its members, assessing the current climate, and responding to their needs.

While NICHE recruited member hospitals to participate in research and other studies, it also supported members in developing their own quality improvement initiatives. To further this goal, NICHE launched an initiative with *BMJ* (formerly *British Medical Journals*) *Quality* to provide subscriptions to NICHE member organizations for access to a NICHE-specific portal on the *BMJ Quality* platform to develop quality improvement projects and receive mentorship and peer feedback from selected NICHE reviewers as well as the *BMJ Quality* reviewers. There would be a NICHE-specific portal where NICHE hospitals would collaborate among themselves and NICHE mentors would serve as reviewers. The NICHE portal would feature a digital NICHE journal. The *BMJ* would publish articles as well, provided they met the *BMJ* peer review process.

NICHE engaged members each year through an annual survey and reported the results at a virtual business meeting. Surveys guided agreement on the focus for the organization in upcoming years. In 2015, over 2,355 nurses and other healthcare providers from 225 NICHE member organizations completed the survey, an increase of 63% over the previous year's response. The survey results were reported at the virtual business meeting along with the current state of NICHE and goals for the future. The meeting also included Q&A and dialogue.

Prior to the expansion period, NICHE hosted a listserv where members would communicate with the NICHE team and one another. From this listserv, NICHE would gain understanding into members' needs. In 2010, NICHE transitioned the listserv to online forums embedded in the KC. The forums allowed NICHE to categorize topics, archive important information, and also align specific forums to courses such as the LTP and the GRN. The NICHE team and mentors communicated with hospitals during the designation process and the collaboration continued postdesignation for the life of members. Peer-to-peer collaboration was an important component of NICHE's success.

MARKETING

Although NICHE did employ traditional outbound communications such as journal print ads, conferences, and the occasional direct mail campaign, most of the marketing communications were inbound—or focused on attracting customers through relevant content. NICHE presented at relevant conferences, such as American Organiztion of Nurse Executives (AONE). Previous attempts to create relationships with organizations such as Voluntary Hospitals of America had proven unsuccessful. Customers would find NICHE through channels like search engines and social media. With a large database of members and potential members of over 50,000 email addresses, NICHE created tools, resources, and communications on a weekly and monthly basis with content specifically designed to bring the customer to NICHE.

NICHE News, a topic-based e-newsletter, e-blasts for new resources and webinar and conference registration, and the NICHE FAQ series, a Q&A for individual NICHE resources, gave NICHE the opportunity to reach out to its members and drive traffic back to the website. This practice of creating link-driven communications not only improved search engine optimization (SEO), increasing the quantity and quality of traffic to the website, one of the keys to moving NICHE up in Google rankings to the first page of search results, but brought members and potential members inbound to navigate throughout the NICHE website.

NICHE created a presence through multiple online social media platforms such as Facebook, Twitter, Pinterest, YouTube, and LinkedIn. Each platform served as a unique electronic solution for NICHE. Facebook gave NICHE members an opportunity to share accomplishments and post images and gave NICHE a platform to make announcements and bring new information to their attention—resources, events, opportunities, and healthcare news. NICHE created conference albums and posted all conference photos here so members could tag and repost. Twitter, another opportunity for NICHE to push notifications and bring industry news to members and potential members, also gave NICHE the opportunity to cover events live, create hashtags to drive conference traffic, and link to industry thought leaders. Even Pinterest gave NICHE an opportunity to connect directly with the "Sandwich Generation," collecting products, practices, organizations, and many other consumer interests like healthy recipes and senior friendly vacations, along with topics and keynotes from the NICHE conference.

The annual NICHE conference gave NICHE the opportunity to create interview videos, more than 80 in 2015; these were edited and released weekly on YouTube. In addition to creating new content for the NICHE website, members were able to link to the videos for their own organizations. The conference also brought two new platforms to NICHE, Cvent and CrowdCompass. Cvent enabled the automation of the registration process, integrated with online payment software, enhanced reporting, and simplified the CE process. The ability to link the individual to the sessions they attended generated a personalized survey and a unique personalized certificate with sessions and contact hours. CrowdCompass, the integrated mobile app for smartphones, tablets, and laptops by Cvent, made it easier for attendees to negotiate the conference, store and record information, and network with colleagues. Tied to the attendee's registration, the app gave each attendee his or her personalized agenda, access to the full conference schedule, keynote biographies, sponsors, site floor plans, area maps and attractions with descriptions, and full networking capabilities. Attendees could search, access, and bookmark information by day or speaker to come back to it after the conference.

The mobile app also gave NICHE the opportunity to crowdsource and hear in real time from their attendees with polling. Questions focused on the presentations and speakers as they were in the actual session and NICHE resources that could support the presentations. Results were calculated and pushed back to the attendees via the app as well. Cloning the event and apps for next year's conference saved time and money, giving the opportunity to open registration earlier, develop new features for the app, and send final evaluations for CEs the day after the conference concluded.

BUSINESS OPERATIONS

The NICHE expansion plan focused on North America and intended to penetrate states and Canadian provinces. It grew to include members in Australia, Singapore, and Bermuda. With the majority of the NICHE team based in New York, the most effective way to engage constituents was through digital and virtual engagement. Furthermore, some business operations would need to be up and running beyond East Coast business hours, as member sites needed to be serviced 7 days per week, 365 days per year. NICHE staff, consultants, and mentors were based in several states and regularly collaborated online. The NICHE team developed a combined virtual office that worked in conjunction with team members in the New York City office. This team in turn worked with hospitals around North America and the world.

In 2008, cloud computing was growing and NICHE leveraged this new technology to build its business. Starting with a robust web-based client relationship manager (CRM), NICHE developed a sales pipeline—a visual representation of sales prospects and where they were in the purchasing process. Pipelines also facilitated revenue forecasting and metrics for tracking the established targets for new hospitals.

The CRM also supported ongoing account management. Once a prospect became a designated hospital, the CRM served as an account in which all the activity was tracked—from membership due payments to webinars attended to the annual program evaluation data—the hospital's unique record contained all the activity related to their NICHE program. This robust database also facilitated marketing analytics and targeted marketing. Data from the CRM were integrated with the email marketing solution (Constant Contact) for marketing and communications. The CRM also integrated with the website. All leads from the website flowed to the CRM and alerted the sales team and the CRM populated the website with information about current membership so that anyone visiting the website would find the current NICHE hospitals.

Ongoing collaboration and file sharing was supported through Google Docs and Basecamp. In addition, the team regularly utilized platforms for screen sharing and web meetings for both internal and external meetings. Online accounting software enabled financial management to run seamlessly: NICHE was collecting several million dollars in members' dues throughout the year—invoices could be generated and emailed and funds received. Other digital solutions included event management systems and merchant accounts for online purchases. Cvent, the event management system, managed registration and scheduling for the annual conference. It also provided a survey system that allowed participants to complete surveys on sessions attended, track CE credits, and generate certificates. This system also allowed NICHE to capture large amounts of data on the conferences including individuals' attributes such as organizational roles, geographical locations, and educational levels. These data were also used to evaluate how participants reacted to the content and meeting experience, and what future content they were interested in.

Overall, NICHE invested a significant amount of time and money in collecting and managing data, both research and marketing related. Most business decisions were data driven.

CHAPTER SUMMARY

Technology played an undeniable role in the success of NICHE. When NICHE received a grant from The Atlantic Philanthropies to launch a period of expansion and build a sustainable business model, the team set out to leverage digital tools to build and enhance engagement of its members, deliver the developing content, and operate a lean business. Digital solutions for learning and engagement helped build greater loyalty and increase membership and brand awareness, propelling NICHE from 150 hospitals to over 700 highly engaged hospitals, nursing homes, and other postacute settings. With an iterative approach, NICHE was able to build and change business processes and the software that supports those processes, resulting in a successful transition to a sound and profitable business model as well as widespread dissemination of the NICHE program.

REFERENCES

Bricoli, B. (2011). NICHE resets knowledge center for greater access to tools, resources and information for the care of older adult patients. *Geriatric Nursing, 32*, 474. doi:10.1016/j.gerinurse.2011.09.010

Boltz, M., Capezuti, E., Shuluk, J., Brouwer, J., Carolan, D., Conway, S., . . . Galvin, J. E. (2013). Implementation of geriatric acute care best practices: Initial results of the NICHE SITE self-evaluation. *Nursing and Health Sciences, 15*(4), 518–524. doi:10.1111/nhs.12067

Capezuti, E., Boltz, M., Cline, D., Dickson, V. V., Rosenberg, M.-C., Wagner, L., . . . Nigolian, C. (2012). Nurses Improving Care for Healthsystem Elders: A model for optimizing the geriatric nursing practice environment. *Journal of Clinical Nursing, 21*(21-22), 3117–3125. doi:10.1111/j.1365-2702.2012.04259.x

Capezuti, E., Boltz, M., Shuluk, J., Denysyk, L., Brouwer, J. P., Roberts, M.-C., . . . Secic, M. (2013). Utilization of a benchmarking database to inform NICHE implementation. *Research in Gerontological Nursing, 6*(3), 198–208. doi:10.3928/19404921-20130607-01

Capezuti, E., Bricoli, B., & Boltz, M. P. (2013). Nurses Improving the Care of Healthsystem Elders: Creating a sustainable business model to improve care of hospitalized older adults. *Journal of the American Geriatrics Society, 61*, 1387–1393. doi:10.1111/jgs.12324

Davis, R., & Surajballi, V. (2014). Successful implementation and use of a learning management system. *Journal Continuing Education in Nursing, 45*(9), 379–381. doi:10.3928/00220124-20140825-12

Hung, S.-Y., Chen, C. C., & Lee, W.-J. (2009). Moving hospitals toward e-learning adoption: An empirical investigation. *Journal of Organizational Change Management, 22*(3), 239–256. doi:10.1108/09534810910951041

Sportsman, S. (2014). Learning management systems support RNs in mastering informatics. *Nursing Informatics & Technology: A blog for all levels of users.* Retrieved from http://community.advanceweb.com/blogs/nurses_18/archive/2014/11/17/learning-management-systems-support-rns-in-mastering-informatics.aspx

White, M., & Shellenbarger, T. (2017). Harnessing the power of learning management systems: An e-learning approach for professional development. *Journal for Nurses in Professional Development, 33*(3), 138–141. doi:10.1097/nnd.0000000000000348

The Business Proposition: Spreading and Scaling in the Age of Healthcare Reform

13

Barbara Bricoli and Judy Santamaria

Nurses are the appropriate professional group to discover and advance the knowledge necessary to provide care to the nation's elders. Therefore, I would strongly urge the Foundation's trustees and staff to continue to support this work.
—Trish Gibbons, DNSc, RN, former vice president for nursing at Beth Israel Deaconess Medical Center (BIDMC; 1995)

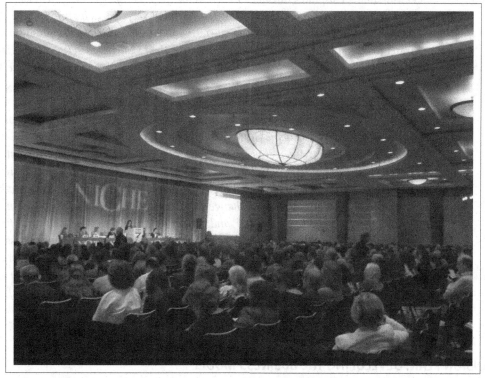

NICHE Conference 2013.

CHAPTER OBJECTIVES

1. Describe the factors important to development of the Nurses Improving Care for Healthsystem Elders (NICHE) business model
2. Discuss the roles of practicing nurses and nurse administrators in championing NICHE
3. Review the drivers that enhanced NICHE adoption
4. Discuss the influence of current healthcare initiatives on NICHE scaling and spreading

INTRODUCTION

The seeds of Nurses Improving Care for Healthsystem Elders (NICHE) were sown in 1981 when Dr. Terry Fulmer, a geriatric nurse specialist, initiated the Geriatric Resource Nurse (GRN) model at Boston's Beth Israel Hospital. Fulmer later adapted the GRN model within a geriatrician-led care team at Yale New Haven Hospital as part of The John A. Hartford Foundation's Hospital Outcomes Program for the Elderly. The early history of NICHE is well described in Chapter 2. By 2006, 157 hospitals were participating in NICHE, straining the existing infrastructure (Capezuti, Bricoli, & Boltz, 2013). The program had grown dramatically but did not have the funding nor the resources to service the existing sites. Additional funding was clearly needed to accelerate growth and expand capacity. An infusion of grant funding in 2007 allowed NICHE to launch a period of rapid growth and expansion during which a sustainable business model was developed.

As NICHE prepared to expand, there had been little success in the diffusion of similar models (Institute of Medicine [IOM], 2008) and the challenges associated with widespread adoption of models (Mezey et al., 2004) were not well documented nor understood (IOM, 2008). However, NICHE, a model driven by nurses, the most prevalent workforce in hospital settings, deployed a strategy that combined an approach to building evidence-based clinical protocols and organizational change practices with a robust delivery system to engage its audience, respond to their needs, and deliver services in an affordable and efficient way. By 2016, this focus on constituent (or customer) engagement and responsiveness layered on top of the successful nurse-driven model led to noticeably widespread adoption of NICHE by more than 700 hospitals and healthcare settings in North America and other countries.

This chapter describes the expansion of NICHE and the development of a business model for NICHE between the years 2007 and 2016.

THE EXPANSION PLAN: DEVELOPING THE BUSINESS MODEL

In 2006, the Atlantic Philanthropies Foundation, as part of a broad strategy to award nonprofits with capacity-building grants in the form of social venture capital, awarded a planning grant to Dr. Elizabeth Capezuti at New York University

Key to the plan was developing a strong value proposition so that hospitals would be willing to pay annual fees for the NICHE program, products, and services resulting in sustainable revenue streams that would fully support NICHE operations over time.

(NYU) to assess NICHE's capabilities, aspirations, and potential for growth. Facilitated by a business consultant, NICHE produced a 5-year business plan to build an internal infrastructure and programming to expand NICHE to hospitals nationally with the goal of having significant impact on the care older adults receive in hospitals. Key to the plan was developing a strong value proposition so that hospitals would be willing to pay annual fees for the NICHE program, products, and services resulting in sustainable revenue streams that would fully support NICHE operations over time. In 2007, the Atlantic Philanthropies Foundation awarded a $5 million grant to NYU to implement the business plan. This period of program expansion allowed NICHE to:

- Build organizational capacity and an internal infrastructure
- Develop a large portfolio of NICHE-specific resources
- Build a robust digital (online) platform to house and deliver education, resources, and peer collaboration
- Enhance the NICHE benchmarking service and program monitoring and evaluation
- Develop and launch targeted marketing strategies
- Grow NICHE to 500 hospitals (and other healthcare settings)
- Increase participation and activity of current NICHE sites
- Generate sufficient revenue to fund program operations (Capezuti et al., 2013)

Building Organizational Capacity

From 2007 to 2009, NICHE hired staff and consultants, reorganized operations, developed and updated new and existing resources, and created the infrastructure to launch the new business model. This built upon the existing relationships, educational content, and clinical tools that were developed during the prior decades within the NYU College of Nursing, specifically the *Try This:*® Geriatric Assessment Series and the geriatric nursing Clinical Practice Protocols developed by the NYU Hartford Institute for Geriatric Nursing. NICHE successfully transitioned from a grant-funded program to a growing organization with the ability to take on new sites, significant stability of participation (demonstrated by re-enrollment rates), and steady growth (demonstrated by new sites). Key features to the business model are highlighted in Box 13.1.

To increase participation and justify charging fees for the program, which had previously been available at a very low cost and required modest commitment,

> **BOX 13.1 Major Activities Conducted for Transition to a Fee-Based Model (2007–2009)**
>
> - Assigned a managing director and key staff, with 100% of their time dedicated to product development and constituent services
>
> - Established an online learning management system (LMS) to serve as a platform for the online Leadership Training Program (LTP) for new sites (replacing a 2-day in-person training) and to house and make accessible an extensive portfolio of tools and resources, called the Knowledge Center, to participating sites
>
> - Developed and launched a website
>
> - Expanded the annual conference and webinars
>
> - Implemented a recognition program and rigorous annual renewal process, including annual program evaluation and benchmarking
>
> - Invested significantly in and committed resources to sales outreach, follow-up, and services
>
> - Increased the formal engagement of active site leaders to help with the mentoring of new sites
>
> - Developed several revenue streams for services, resulting in sustainable operations

NICHE worked to create a strong value proposition to articulate to existing and potential adopters. The NICHE leadership began putting together a dedicated team to cultivate relationships with potential participants and to continuously service and engage existing participants.

From the onset, NICHE modeled itself after a healthcare association: recruiting and engaging members who paid fees and received valuable resources and a strong peer-to-peer network. In contrast, however, NICHE members were required to participate in an introductory Leadership Training Program (LTP), meet certain requirements, and, importantly, have commitment from institutional leadership. Individual members were not permitted because NICHE believed that healthcare organizations needed to make an organizational commitment to achieve systemic change.

Expanding the Product Portfolio

From 2008 to 2009, NICHE updated the existing resources and developed new clinical, educational, and organizational tools to increase geriatric knowledge and support organizational change. These early tools included the first versions of the GRN and Geriatric Patient Care Associate (GPCA) curriculum, and an updated version of the *NICHE Planning and Implementation Guide* to provide direction to sites during the implementation phase. Next followed a major overhaul of the LTP, the process by which new member hospitals assess their organizations' geriatric capacities and develop an implementation plan for NICHE.

The economic downturn of 2008 saw many hospitals limiting travel budgets for staff, and NICHE found that fewer hospitals were able to send nurses to the in-person LTP and conference. At the same time, the emerging practice of online learning was slowly being adopted by health systems around the United States (Hung, Chen, & Lee, 2009). These conditions accelerated the launch of on-line learning, starting with the transition of the LTP from a 2-day, in-person event held prior to the NICHE annual conference to an online model facilitated by NICHE faculty and mentors that utilized 30 hours of synchronous and asynchronous learning over 6 weeks. NICHE deployed a collaborative approach through engagement of experienced nurses who had successfully implemented NICHE in their hospitals as NICHE faculty and mentors to hospitals during the LTP and implementation process (Capezuti et al., 2012). These faculty mentors also served as champions or "brand ambassadors" for NICHE, presenting at conferences and webinars and in some cases publishing articles about their NICHE programs.

NICHE deployed a collaborative APPROACH through engagement of experienced nurses who had successfully implemented NICHE in their hospitals as NICHE faculty and mentors to hospitals during the LTP and implementation process.

The first online LTP was piloted in the fall of 2009 and was followed by the launch of the NICHE Knowledge Center (KC), an online learning management system (LMS) to facilitate online collaboration and house all NICHE content and transcripts for learners (staff at member hospitals; Bricoli, 2011). At the same time, NICHE worked to improve its benchmarking service, the Geriatric Institutional Assessment Profile (GIAP), a survey of staff knowledge, attitudes, and the geriatric care environment (Abraham et al., 1999; Boltz et al., 2008), by developing an online system to replace the paper-based system. The majority of NICHE content was for members only, as the cost to develop and maintain content was very expensive and NICHE resources added to the value of becoming a NICHE site. However, some content, including that from the Hartford Institute for Geriatric Nursing website, consultgeri.org, was still available as "open source," which helped introduce NICHE to nonmembers and demonstrated the value and quality of the resources. By 2010, when NICHE was ready to launch the fee-based model, a core set of tools and resources and a new web-based LTP created a strong value proposition. By 2015, the NICHE portfolio was extensive, having been created in large part by faculty, consultants, and members. NICHE also leveraged the resources of NYU and the Hartford Institute for Geriatric Nursing and collaborated with other organizations such as specialty associations and its own member hospitals to coproduce resources.

Moving From a Free to a Fee-Based Program

In 2009, with the positioning of an agile team, an extensive product portfolio, and a solid base of participants, NICHE prepared to launch the new fee-based program. Significant preparation and planning went into transitioning existing participants from a nonfee to a fee-based program requiring annual renewal. One year prior to the fee transition, a campaign was launched to educate participants and gain acceptance of the new fee model. This included several town hall–style conference calls. Concurrently, new sites that were interested in NICHE were indoctrinated early on in the sales cycle to anticipate a fee-based program. A significant challenge was to retain existing participants who were not used to the fee structure. While the campaign was in progress, planned releases of the new resources above, as well as the strengthening of the benefits of "designation," were introduced. NICHE provided tools for sites to gain stakeholder support: a webinar on "making the case for NICHE," a PowerPoint template for them to customize when presenting to decision makers, and customized cost–benefit analysis upon request.

All of this tied into an aggressive marketing and communications strategy to promote the benefits of NICHE to hospitals. Targeted marketing materials were developed for different audiences: the C-suite, educators, unit managers, physicians, marketing departments (and later patient experience leaders). One key decision to keep the price of NICHE for the first year just below $10,000 (and below $5,000 for subsequent years) allowed for quicker and more streamlined approval, often by a director-level champion. The price also bundled all NICHE services, including the GIAP. For the first 5 years, the $10,000 first-year fee did not cover the costs to acquire and service the customer, the hospital. As the program scaled, NICHE realized small operating margins, thus making it possible for NICHE to become "profitable" by year 6 of the expansion plan. All operating margins were reinvested in the ongoing development of the program and technological infrastructure, with a small amount held in reserve to support operations should the need arise.

THE VALUE PROPOSITION: FROM THE BEDSIDE NURSE TO THE C-SUITE

There were several drivers that contributed to the widespread adoption of NICHE. As the NICHE expansion plan launched, there was a growing sense of urgency in the United States related to how to care for the rapidly aging population, and health systems were increasingly aware of a gap in knowledge and expertise to care for this population. Older adults make up 13% of the population yet account for 37% of hospital discharges and 43% of hospital days (Hall, DeFrances, Williams, Golosinskiy, & Schwartzman, 2010) and are at greater risk to experience complications and adverse events during hospitalization (Kim, Capezuti, Kovner, Zhao, & Boockvar, 2010). During the early years of NICHE program expansion, hospital leaders were reluctant to invest in geriatric programs (population based) as they placed a priority on service lines, such as orthopedics, that generated revenue and were historically profitable. As hospitals began to focus on value-based care and population health, they began to see the value of investing in geriatric programs. Rapidly changing healthcare policies that advanced the imperative to lower costs, improve outcomes, and enhance patient experiences served as critical drivers for the adoption of NICHE. With

Rapidly changing healthcare policies that advanced the imperative to lower costs, improve outcomes, and enhance patient experiences served as critical drivers for the adoption of NICHE.

the advent of accountable care organizations (ACOs) and health system consoli-dations to drive efficiencies, NICHE was seen as a viable way to standardize care across service lines and settings. Yet even before the aforementioned policy shifts, nurses who were on the frontlines of delivering care to the older adult population were the earliest champions of NICHE, as they had a genuine concern and desire to improve care for older adults, recognized serious gaps in geriatric knowledge, and were seeking ways to build geriatric expertise in their hospital settings.

Bedside Nurse Champions

Nurses, the most prevalent workforce profession in hospitals, became increas-ingly aware that caring for an increasingly aging population required specialized knowledge and skills. Prior to the launch of the NICHE business model, nurses working on the units were most often the ones to identify and champion the program. In order to get the budget and time required for implementation, they needed to make the case for NICHE to the members of the hospital administration. The NICHE program emphasized the nurse's role and responsibility in decision making around the care of older adults (Capezuti et al., 2013; Fulmer, 2001). Par-ticipating in an LTP gave staff nurses and advanced practice nurses (APNs) the requisite skills to develop a comprehensive, geriatric program that would have a positive and measureable impact on nursing practice and patient care outcomes (Bub, Boltz, Malsch, & Fletcher, 2015). The NICHE program also aligned with the principles espoused by the ANCC Magnet program, including nurse competence, autonomy, and interdisciplinary collaboration, as these principles were core com-ponents of the NICHE GRN model (Nickoley, 2010).

Benefits to unit managers were apparent as NICHE clinical practice guidelines filled a training gap in responding to the special nursing needs of the older patient, and educational directors appreciated the fact that training curricula were "pack-aged" and ready to use. Those who participated in the LTP became leaders to their peers in caring for this population and often led quality improvement projects to measure the outcomes of NICHE programming. GRNs served as resources to other staff on the units. Additionally, many hospitals used NICHE participation, and de-velopment as a GRN, as advancement criteria in their clinical ladder programs.

Gaining the Attention of the C-Suite

In providing evidence-based best practices and educational tools that focused on strengthening care for the geriatric patient, NICHE served as an important resource for hospitals seeking to provide better care to older adults. NICHE, as it had in the very beginning, captured the attention of hospital chief nursing officers (CNOs) and other hospital leaders concerned about both clinical and financial results. It was viewed as a cost-efficient and effective way to use the existing resources, and build geriatric service lines and expertise. In particular, hospitals that were focused on Magnet designation and valued nurses' role in decision making saw NICHE as aligned with Magnet goals. NICHE also provided tools to demonstrate how NICHE guiding principles aligned with Joint Commission standards. CNOs leading health systems sought to standardize practice across multiple sites. NICHE's LTP program and tools, courses, and resources offered a framework for standardization.

NICHE leadership importantly created a value estimate document illustrating a cost comparison between the resources available through the bundled NICHE program payment and the costs to purchase these resources individually (Figure 13.1). Over the years, several NICHE hospitals developed their own cost

Value Estimate: **Cost and Benefits**

Save Your Hospital up to $**122,925** in the First Year **With NICHE**

Without NICHE

	With NICHE	Without NICHE
Leadership Training Program		
6 week online program for team of 3, includes 30 CEs	$0	$4,950
Annual Fee		
Licensing, membership fee, access to all below	$0	$5,500
Education and Training		
Online & Instructor Led Courses	$55,500	$0*
(100 users, 4 online courses, 37 CEs per user @ $15 per CE)		
Webinars up to 100 Users	$49,500	$0*
(25 users, 20 webinars, includes 1 CE per user @ $99 per webinar)		
Webinars additional CEs	$12,000	$0*
(50 users, 20 webinars, 1 CE per user @ $12 per CE)		
Project Management Tools		
Organizational Strategies, Clinical Improvement Models, Implementation Tools	$2500	$0
Consultation & Review		
Developing Action Plan, Sustaining NICHE Program, GIAP Review	$10,000	$0
Evaluation		
Geriatric Institutional Assessment Profile (GIAP), Unit Level Measures	$3,800	$0
Conference		
4 Day Conference, includes 20 or more CEs	$800	$725
Collaboration. Support. Peer Advice.	Priceless	Priceless
Total	**$134,100**	**$11,175**

FIGURE 13.1 *NICHE value estimate 2016.*

savings calculators related to their NICHE program, which included the cost savings related to reduced falls, pressure ulcers, and other conditions they deemed avoidable due to their NICHE programs. However, with the value estimate, NICHE is now able to demonstrate very simple costs related to staff training, project management tools, consultation, and benchmarking and evaluation tools, all included in the bundled NICHE fee. Purchased alone, these resources could cost over $100,000, whereas the NICHE program, including conference attendance, costs under $12,000.

NICHE was not simply a provider of continuing education courses but rather an organization-wide program to change culture, attitudes, and practice around caring for older adults.

An extensive marketing and communication strategy was developed, due largely to the support of the Atlantic Philanthropies grant, to engage healthcare providers and institutions more broadly. One-on-one conversations were often required to help the CNO and hospital leadership understand the benefits of NICHE, as it was important to communicate that NICHE was not simply a provider of continuing education courses but rather an organization-wide program to change culture, attitudes, and practice around caring for older adults.

SCALING AND SPREADING IN THE AGE OF HEALTHCARE REFORM

Over the last decade, there have been key policies and sweeping reforms driving transformation in the healthcare industry. From Centers for Medicare & Medicaid Services (CMS) "never events" to 30-day hospital readmission penalties, healthcare providers and payers have been seeking ways to reduce costs, improve quality, and achieve better population health. NICHE was able to align with the priorities of health systems.

CMS Never Events

In 2007, in an effort to reduce hospital-acquired conditions (HAC), CMS announced they would no longer reimburse hospitals for the increased costs related to treating what they considered preventable conditions that should never happen or "never events." NICHE had already been very much focused on providing resources to help hospitals reduce several of these conditions: catheter-associated urinary tract infections (CAUTIs), falls, and pressure ulcers. (Fulmer SPICES is a framework for assessing older adults that focuses on six common "marker conditions": sleep problems, problems with eating and feeding, incontinence, confusion, evidence of falls, and skin breakdown, and was developed well before never events and served as an intermediate interface with this CMS concept) One of the earliest marketing campaigns focused on "never events" and it was very successful in aligning NICHE with hospitals' priorities.

Institute of Medicine and the Triple Aim

In 2008, the IOM Committee on the Future Health Care Workforce for Older Americans released its report, *Retooling for an Aging America: Building the Health Care Workforce*, and made several recommendations to address the looming crisis in caring for the aging population. Dr. Fulmer was a member of that committee and was able to embed NICHE concepts into those deliberations. It was concluded that as the population of older adults grew to comprise approximately 20% of the U.S. population, they would face a healthcare workforce that was too small and untrained to meet their health needs. NICHE aligned with IOM's recommendations including the need to boost recruitment and retention of geriatric specialists and healthcare aides (IOM, 2008).

This focus on quality of care was further accelerated when the Institute for Healthcare Improvement (IHI, n.d.) produced the Triple Aim, a framework for optimizing health system performance by simultaneously focusing on the health of a population, the experience of care for individuals within that population, and the per capita cost of providing that care (IHI, n.d.). NICHE, with its focus on person- and family-centered care, tools to support avoiding costs related to HACs, and adaptability to all settings across the healthcare continuum, provided its constituents with a framework to meet the goals of the Triple Aim.

Value-Based Care

In 2010, the Patient Protection and Affordable Care Act (ACA) was signed into law and introduced major reforms, including several that impacted the way providers are reimbursed. The ACA imperative to reduce costs, improve quality, and address the needs of individuals across the healthcare continuum has greatly influenced how care is delivered. With the passage of the ACA, CMS introduced an array of value-based care models, such as the Medicare Shared Savings Program (MSSP) and the ACO model to support the goals of the Triple Aim and the ACA. Once again, the NICHE framework provided health systems that were sharing risk and participating in bundled payments with a mechanism to prepare for value-based payments and implement standardized practices across settings.

Consolidation and Integrated Health Systems

Due to the major reforms just mentioned and other industry trends to introduce more efficient operational and financial systems, the past decade has seen the hospital industry experience extensive consolidation through mergers and the formation of health systems. Hospital mergers more than doubled in 2012 from prior years (Gaynor & Town, 2012). With hospitals working to secure their market positions, improve operational and financial efficiencies, and manage population health, NICHE began to negotiate system-wide contracts. Several systems (e.g., Medstar and Riverside Health) adopted the program on a system level, providing program management through a centralized NICHE coordinator. NICHE offered discounts when more than one hospital in a system joined, and that further created the desire on the part of system CNOs to standardize programming across sites. One of the earliest systems to adopt NICHE was Trinity Health in 2011. In the case of Trinity, local hospitals were not mandated to adopt NICHE; it was voluntary. According to Gay Landstrom, former CNO of Trinity Health, "We have found NICHE learnings, assessments and processes to be completely in line with what we should be doing for all patients—taking accountability and coordinating their care" (Landstrom & Gray, 2012, para. 7). Other health systems, such as Medstar, required and financially supported NICHE adoption in all hospitals, and later other settings, such as home care.

System contracts could be challenging to negotiate and in fact sometimes impeded the adoption of NICHE by individual hospitals that were ready to join but held back as they waited for Group Purchasing Organizations (GPOs) or health system procurement offices to finalize contracts. In other cases, the process was seamless and multiple hospitals within a system were invoiced in the same manner as individual hospitals. In all cases, NICHE and CNOs recognized the value of system-wide participation and worked to make this happen.

SUCCESS BY THE NUMBERS

Several key performance indicators highlight the success of NICHE: rate of new participants enrolling annually, retention of existing members, level of penetration within member organizations, and the attendance at the annual conference.

Membership Enrollment and Retention

In 2011, the first full year of the newly updated program, NICHE recruited 64 new hospitals. By 2015, NICHE had recruited 94 new hospitals, a 30% increase. Existing hospitals (41 in 2015) also enrolled in the LTP to "refresh" their programs. Participation in the LTP represented a major commitment by a hospital, as it was mandatory for a minimum of three staff members from a hospital to participate and required 38 contact hours. From 2009 through 2015, NICHE maintained a membership retention rate between 95% and 97%. Member hospitals clearly found value in the program, as there was an annual budgetary commitment as well as an annual self-evaluation survey to assess a site's progress and implementation level. By 2016, there were over 700 NICHE sites (Figure 13.2).

Member hospitals clearly found value in the program, as there was an annual budgetary commitment as well as an annual self-evaluation survey to assess a site's progress and implementation level.

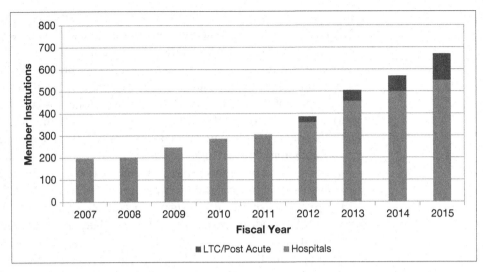

FIGURE 13.2 *NICHE membership growth from 2008 to 2015.*

Knowledge Center Enrollment

Once a hospital successfully completed the LTP and was designated as a NICHE member, it was provided full access to the NICHE KC. At this time, hospitals began implementation of their NICHE program by training staff, usually starting with GRNs. Enrollment in the KC indicates the depth and level of participation of hospitals. NICHE member organizations enrolled their staff in the KC and were able to manage and track their teams. NICHE did not auto-enroll staff; rather the hospital was required to request enrollment for all individuals. Several members enrolled hundreds of staff with the intention of having all staff complete, at minimum, the interdisciplinary "Introduction to Gerontology" course, which provided basic knowledge on providing geriatric-sensitive care across the hospital, while others enrolled fewer staff but focused on recruiting nurses to the GRN role and the GRN course. Still other hospitals enrolled only a few staff but downloaded the courses and training materials available to use for instructor-led sessions and in-service training. Regardless of where and how the training was delivered, hospitals completed an annual program evaluation and reported valuable information such as the number of GRNs trained and the number of units within the hospital that had implemented NICHE. By December 2015, there were over 50,000 enrolled users in the KC, a 63% increase over the same period in 2014.

Annual Conference Attendance

Commitment to NICHE was also demonstrated through the growth of the annual conference, which grew from 180 attendees in 2007 to 830 in 2015 (Figure 13.3). NICHE members received discounts on conference registration. The conference

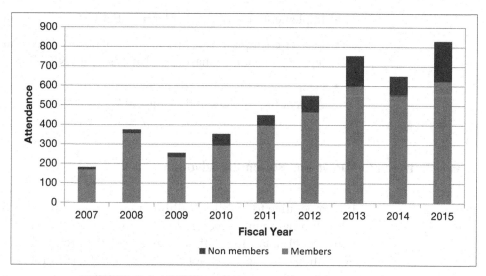

FIGURE 13.3 *NICHE conference attendance from 2007 to 2015.*

enjoyed a full roster of members and nonmembers who participated in a competitive process to present their work through podium and poster presentations. NICHE members served on conference committees, helping to shape the program and the selection of presentations.

NICHE offered member sites a promotional program by which they could spread the word about their NICHE program in their communities, including a media kit to announce membership, logos for adding to their website, and banners to hang in their hospitals. This full marketing and membership engagement program fostered loyalty to the NICHE program and bolstered membership retention rates.

CHALLENGES AND LIMITATIONS TO THE BUSINESS MODEL

Competing Initiatives

An obstacle to growing the NICHE program has always been the many important competing initiatives facing hospitals throughout the budget year. In particular, during the first few years of the NICHE program expansion, many hospitals were upgrading or implementing electronic health record (EHR) systems, an initiative that involved all nursing staff and significant management time and budget. Few CNOs were willing to start NICHE at the same time as the EHR rollout. Other competing initiatives involved:

- Changes in nursing leadership, as few new CNOs and interim CNOs wanted to start a new staff-wide project

- Budgetary constraints, which occasionally limited any new budget line items

- Implementation of another large initiative (e.g., a new oncology program)

- Loss of champions (e.g., unit nurse managers or educational directors who left the hospital) so that conversations about NICHE were put on hold

- General periods of turmoil in the healthcare market (e.g., the inception of the ACA or big changes in the political landscape)

Balance Between Top-Down and Bottom-Up Advocacy

It is imperative to have leadership buy-in for a program such as NICHE because NICHE programming required full-time equivalent (FTE) time for a coordinator, educational hours for staff, and resources for program planning and outcomes evaluation. Having the CNO champion the NICHE program was the surest way to foster success. However, buy-in of frontline staff is equally important. Since NICHE was designed to bring exemplary nursing practices to the bedside nurse, it was critical that the staff understood the benefits of the program and wanted to do it. Ideally, a hospital would allocate some FTE time to NICHE program coordination, though some hospitals did not do this and a successful program ensued simply because a staff member believed in the program and successfully championed it to peers.

And while NICHE is a nurse-driven program, it requires the efforts of an interdisciplinary team and a commitment from all levels of the organization. For this reason, a crucial component of the program is developing an interdisciplinary steering committee to guide the rollout of the program. (Fulmer used this approach early on at the Yale NICHE Program with excellent success.) This committee often included representatives from other disciplines (medicine, pharmacy, social work, rehab therapy) as well as from finance, patient satisfaction, and quality assurance.

NICHE EXPANSION BEYOND THE HOSPITAL

Demand for a Skilled Nursing Facility Program

While NICHE grew intentionally as a program for acute care hospitals, the goal had been to expand it to other settings. By 2011, many member hospitals began adapting NICHE hospital resources for use in skilled nursing facilities (SNFs) and other nonacute care settings (i.e., home health, short-term rehab, long-term care [LTC]). NICHE hospitals advocated for these SNFs to join because SNFs were owned by their systems, or were sites to which they frequently referred patients. NICHE formalized a pilot program for a new level of membership called affiliate (later associate) members. Affiliate members paid a small fee to use the resources and report back to NICHE on how to best adapt them for nonacute settings. Even before the 30-day readmission penalties and value-based care were introduced by CMS, hospitals wanted to ensure that once a patient left the hospital, he or she continued to receive the same evidence-based geriatric nursing care he or she had received in the hospital. Independent SNFs sought out NICHE because they recognized a lack of geriatric expertise in their organizations and wanted to be more attractive partners to referring hospitals. Whether part of a hospital system or independent, SNFs and other nonacute settings were facing many of the same pressures regarding quality outcomes and costs as are hospitals.

Funding for Expansion

In 2016, NICHE received a grant from The John A. Hartford Foundation to expand and adapt its well-known acute care designation program to LTC settings. The NICHE-LTC program began providing clinical, organizational, and quality improvement content pertinent to LTC settings. Other nonacute settings were also able to benefit from NICHE, including hospice, home care, and short-term rehabilitation. An LTP was developed to meet the needs of LTC. NICHE developed program materials on a range of topics specific to LTC. SNFs present specific challenges for the implementation of NICHE. For example, limited funds are available for education and new programs, chronic attrition and understaffing makes time commitments to learning and program development difficult, and a lack of access to updated technology can make web-based programs difficult to navigate. Please refer to Chapter 11 in this book for more information related to NICHE-LTC.

CHAPTER SUMMARY

The NICHE program, with its comprehensive portfolio of organizational, clinical, and educational resources as well as its collaborative approach to building leadership capabilities, has and continues to help hundreds of hospitals promote system-level change (Capezuti et al., 2013). A 2012 review of a grant-funded project testing the implementation of multiple geriatric care models in a small group of hospitals concluded that NICHE, "with its emphasis on developing geriatric-appropriate nursing practices throughout a hospital environment, was seen as a model on which organizations could build a foundation to improve a hospital's culture of quality and safety of inpatient care for older adults" (Leff et al., 2012, p. 1210).

With a substantial investment from the Atlantic Philanthropies Foundation in 2007, NICHE has been able to accomplish the rare transition from a primarily academic program to a sustainable business operation enabling it to expand to hundreds of hospitals and healthcare organizations in the United States and several more in Canada, Singapore, Australia, and Bermuda. In bringing together an agile, adaptable, and service-driven team, NICHE was able to develop and disseminate an evidence-based model, engage the adopters for continuous feedback and monitoring, foster collaboration among adopters and faculty, and consistently respond to constituents' needs. The opportunity for the future is to continue the spread and scale of the program in an economically strong model, with the future opportunity of private/public partnerships for accelerated change.

REFERENCES

Abraham, I. L., Bottrell, M. M., Dash, K. R., Fulmer, T. T., Mezey, M. D., O'Donnell, L., & Vince-Whitman, C. (1999). Profiling care and benchmarking best practice in care of hospitalized elderly: The Geriatric Institutional Assessment Profile. *The Nursing Clinics of North America, 34*(1), 237–255.

Boltz, M., Capezuti, E., Bowar-Ferres, S., Norman, R., Secic, M., Kim, H., . . . Fulmer, T. (2008). Changes in the geriatric care environment associated with NICHE (Nurses Improving Care for HealthSystem Elders). *Geriatric Nursing, 29*(3),176–185. doi:10.1016/j.gerinurse.2008.02.002

Bricoli, B. (2011). NICHE resets knowledge center for greater access to tools, resources and information for the care of older adult patients. *Geriatric Nursing, 32,* 474. doi:10.1016/j.gerinurse.2011.09.010

Bub, L., Boltz, M., Malsch, A., & Fletcher, K. (2015). The NICHE program to prepare the workforce to address the needs of older patients. In M. L. Malone, E. Capezuti, & R. Palmer (Eds.), *Geriatrics models of care: Bringing 'best practice' to an aging America* (pp. 57–70). New York, NY: Springer Nature.

Capezuti, E., Boltz, M., Cline, D., Dickson, V. V., Rosenberg, M.-C., Wagner, L., . . . Nigolian, C. (2012). Nurses Improving Care for Healthsystem Elders: A model for optimizing the geriatric nursing practice environment. *Journal of Clinical Nursing, 21*(21–22), 3117–3125. doi:10.1111/j.1365-2702.2012.04259.x

Capezuti, E. A., Bricoli, B., & Boltz, M. P. (2013). Nurses Improving the Care of Healthsystem Elders: Creating a sustainable business model to improve care of hospitalized older adults. *Journal of the American Geriatrics Society, 61,* 1387–1393. doi:10.1111/jgs.12324

Fulmer, T. (2001). The geriatric resource nurse: A model of caring for older patients. *American Journal of Nursing, 101*(5), 62. doi:10.1097/00000446-200105000-00023

Gaynor, M., & Town, R. (2012). The impact of hospital consolidation: Update. *Robert Wood Johnson Foundation.* Retrieved from http://www.rwjf.org/content/dam/farm/reports/issue_briefs/2012/rwjf73261

Hall, M. J., DeFrances, C. J., Williams, S. N., Golosinskiy, A., & Schwartzman, A. (2010). National hospital discharge survey: 2007 summary. *National Health Stat Report, 29,* 1–20.

Hung, S. Y,, Chen, C.C., & Lee, W.-J. (2009). Moving hospitals toward e-learning adoption: An empirical investigation. *Journal of Organizational Change Management, 22*(3), 239–256. doi:10.1108/09534810910951041

Institute for Healthcare Improvement. (n.d.) The IHI triple aim initiative. Retrieved from http://www.ihi.org/Engage/Initiatives/TripleAim/Pages/default.aspx

Institute of Medicine. (2008). *Retooling for an aging America: Building the health care workforce.* Washington, DC: National Academies Press.

Kim, H., Capezuti, E., Kovner, C., Zhao, Z., & Boockvar, K. (2010). Prevalence and predictors of adverse events in older surgical patients: Impact of the present on admission indicator. *Gerontologist, 50*, 810–820. doi:10.1093/geront/gnq045

Landstrom, G., & Gray, D. (2012). Trinity Health put sharper focus on geriatric care. *Health Progress, 93*(5), 34–39. Retrieved from https://www.chausa.org/publications/health-progress/article/september-october-2012/trinity-health-puts-sharper-focus-on-geriatric-care

Leff, B., Spragens, L. H., Morano, B., Powell, J., Bickert, T. Bond, C., . . . Siu, A. L. (2012). Rapid reengineering of acute medical care for Medicare beneficiaries: The Medicare Innovations Collaborative. *Health Affairs, 31*(6), 1204–1215. doi:10.1377/hlthaff.2011.1187

Mezey, M., Kobayashi, M., Grossman, S., Firpo, A., Fulmer, T., & Mitty, E. (2004). Nurses Improving Care to Healthsystem Elders (NICHE): Implementation of best practice models. *Journal of Nursing Administration, 34*, 451–457. doi:10.1097/00005110-200410000-00005

Nickoley, S. (2010). Aligning NICHE and magnet initiatives. In M. Boltz, J. Taylor, E. Capezuti, & T. Fulmer (Eds.), *NICHE planning and implementation guide* (pp. 58–61). New York, NY: Hartford Institute for Geriatric Nursing.

Large-Scale Evidence-Based Change: An Integrated Delivery System Approach to NICHE

14

Maureen P. McCausland

*Nurses will no longer accept the mere performance of tasks as their practice
goals or outcomes. Nor will they remain in systems that promote fragmented,
uncoordinated care leading to dissatisfaction for everyone—the patient, nurse, and
hospital. Instead, nurses seek opportunities to provide comprehensive, professional
care through a system that allows for continuity of patient care as well as the
opportunity for them to maximize their knowledge and skill.*

— Joyce Clifford, PhD, RN, FAAN

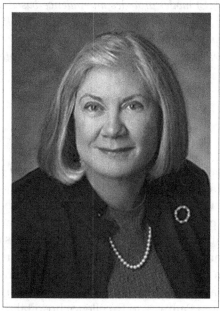

Maureen P. McCausland.

CHAPTER OBJECTIVES

1. Describe the experiences of a fully integrated health system with the NICHE program
2. Explain the elements used to select NICHE as a Signature Program aimed at creating systemness in the integrated health system
3. Describe the structure used to implement NICHE to achieve large-scale change in an integrated health system
4. Describe the challenges and mitigation strategies used to implement NICHE

INTRODUCTION

Leading nursing practice of large numbers of professional nurses and assistive personnel as they care for patients, families, and communities is both a responsibility and privilege. Chief nursing officers (CNOs) are charged with shaping nursing practice in fiscally responsible ways that produce positive outcomes for patients, their families, and communities while also creating a rewarding practice environment for professional nurses. Elders constitute a significant percentage of patients in healthcare settings and as such require specialized nursing care. The Nurses Improving Care for Healthsystem Elders (NICHE) model provides an evidence-based approach to organizing and delivering care to elders and their families while simultaneously providing opportunities for role expansion, professional development, and interprofessional collaboration. This chapter describes the experiences of a fully integrated health system with the NICHE program.

MEDSTAR HEALTH SYSTEM

MedStar Health is one of the largest integrated health systems in the Maryland and District of Columbia area. Care is delivered throughout the distributed care delivery network of 10 hospitals, a large visiting nurse association, and a total of 300 sites of care. The hospitals include nine acute care hospitals as well as an acute rehabilitation hospital. MedStar Health has an academic medical center and a large urban teaching hospital as well as seven community hospitals. MedStar Georgetown University Hospital and MedStar Franklin Square Medical Center are recognized as Magnet Hospitals while MedStar Washington Hospital Center is designated as a Pathway to Excellence hospital.

The 8,700 nurses practicing at MedStar are governed through a system-level collaborative governance model and CNO Council. Nurses from all areas of the care continuum from home to hospital to postacute and ambulatory sites are part of this governance system.

ORGANIZATIONAL ASSESSMENT OF THE NURSING ENVIRONMENT

When assuming the role of CNO, initial assessments guide priority setting with key stakeholders. Upon entering our major regional integrated delivery system in late 2010 as the first senior vice president and CNO, it was apparent that stakeholders from patients and families to the Board of Directors to clinical nurses and other clinicians understood that changes in nursing practice were necessary to assist the organization in meeting its goals of providing excellent patient care while becoming a satisfying and engaging practice environment for nurses.

"Systemness" is "a term that leaders use to define looking and acting more like a single integrated organization rather than a collection of independently functioning pieces" (McCausland, 2012, p. 307). MedStar Nursing was early in the systemness journey as evidenced by variability in nursing standards and practice. Historically, the hospital nursing services looked at specific nursing quality indicators such as patient falls and hospital-acquired pressure ulcers individually and interventions were similarly developed. Nurse-sensitive patient outcomes varied as well. Nursing programs of care had not yet been identified at the system level. These findings were true for geriatric patients and their families as well. As reported by Mack in a case study in Vignette C, in 2010 there was a targeted focus on improving the care of older adults through NICHE at only one MedStar hospital, the MedStar Washington Hospital Center.

MedStar Nursing was early in the systemness journey as evidenced by variability in nursing standards and practice.

THE INTEGRATED HEALTH SYSTEM APPROACH

Creation of the MedStar Health nursing professional practice model, a commitment to evidence-based nursing practice and leadership, and establishment of a system-level collaborative governance model became the foundation upon which MedStar Health Nursing Signature Programs were built. These Signature Programs are evidence based, fiscally responsible, and congruent with the system's strategic and operational priorities. NICHE was one of the two initial Signature Programs implemented across the system.

NICHE was chosen for adoption for four reasons. First, successful nursing programs are congruent with organizational priorities. The nation "has a distinctly older age profile than it did 16 years ago" according to U.S. Census Bureau population estimates released in June 2017 (U.S. Census Bureau, 2017). U.S. residents aged 65 and older grew to 15.2% of the population (N = 49.2 million) in 2016 compared to 12.4% (N = 35 million) in 2000. Mirroring the national demographics, elders comprise a significant patient population in the MedStar-distributed care delivery network. Patients aged 65 and older hover between 35% and 38% of patients receiving both inpatient and observation care in our hospitals. Older adults typically are 19% to 20% of patients receiving care in our emergency services. Focusing directly on improving nurses' care of older adults is congruent with MedStar Health 2020 and our vision, goals, and strategies and the MedStar Nursing strategic goal to "deliver exemplary evidence-based patient and family focused care across the continuum that is safe, reliable and fiscally responsible" (MedStar Health Nursing, 2013, p. 2).

Second, NICHE exemplifies an evidence-based approach to both executive nursing practice *and* clinical practice (Mezey et al., 2004). The MedStar Nursing Service chose the Iowa Model of Evidence-Based Practice to Promote Quality Care (Titler et al., 2001) upon the recommendation of the MedStar Nursing Research Council and endorsement from system-level nursing council members, the MedStar Nursing Leadership team, and the MedStar CNO Council. Review and selection of evidence-based programs demonstrates that nursing leaders follow the same approach they expect clinical nurses to use. The triggers for focusing on the nursing care of older adults were both problem focused and knowledge focused. The clinical trigger was performance on nursing-sensitive outcomes such as patient falls and hospital-acquired pressure ulcers. These variables were considered separately, for example. A holistic approach to care of older adults was missing. The knowledge-focused triggers were variability of nursing standards and care processes across the hospitals and the determination that the latest gerontological nursing science was not always available to MedStar professional nurses and curricula for professional development programs did not systematically include a focus on older adults as a specific patient population.

A holistic approach to care of older adults was missing.

Third, NICHE provides opportunities for clinical nurses and unlicensed patient care associates to develop expertise in caring for geriatric patients. It supports opportunities for role expansion of clinical nurses through the geriatric resource nurse (GRN) role, professional development using the curricula and strategies available from NICHE, and interprofessional collaboration as hospitals move through the levels of NICHE designation. The GRN role contributes to the nursing strategic goal of recruiting, engaging, and retaining appropriate numbers of professional nurses and patient care associates to support MedStar 2020.

Fourth, NICHE is a strong example of a fiscally responsible approach to patient- and family-centered care and professional nursing practice. The associated fees provide access to the latest scientific findings, recommendations based on expert judgment, and professional development content online and in person at the annual national meeting. Networking with colleagues from other NICHE organizations fosters the sharing of best practices. Educational content for both registered nurses and other associates from the same source helps to ensure that the messages are congruent.

LARGE-SCALE CHANGE

Implementing programs such as NICHE across an integrated delivery system in the fast-paced, uncertain, and complex healthcare environment requires new leadership approaches. While the MedStar NICHE program was implemented prior to the publication *Team of Teams: New Rules of Engagement for a Complex World* (McChrystal, 2015), the lessons from this work and the companion publication, *One Mission: How Leaders Build a Team of Teams* (Fussell, 2017), offer important strategies and tactics for nurse executives and leaders.

Historically, nursing professional practice models (Clifford & Horvath, 1990; Koloroutis, 2004) were characterized by a nursing practice system with a focus on accountability, continuity, and collaboration. The organizational structures in those organizations supported decentralized decision making and expected coherence to organizational values. The healthcare environment was challenging but the pace of change and of patient care was slower than in today's world.

Today, the pace of change has accelerated, the environment is more complex, and patient care and therapeutic interventions are more complex as well. The core capabilities of trust, common purpose, shared consciousness, and empowered execution (McChrystal, 2015, p. 245) now inform the MedStar Nursing approach to structure and processes at both the system level and the entity level.

System-Level Structure and Processes

The MedStar Health NICHE program is led at the system level by a Clinical Practice Program Specialist with clinical specialist preparation and certification. Her leadership activities are discussed in Vignette C in this book, "MedStar Health: Accelerating and Sustaining NICHE Implementation Through Systemness." Her role includes a combination of external and internal activities. Externally she coordinates with the national NICHE program office, presents scholarly work from NICHE, and hosts a significant number of MedStar professional nurses at the Annual NICHE Conference.

Her internal role and responsibilities include leading the development, implementation, and evaluation of the NICHE program. The system NICHE Steering Committee develops annual goals that are congruent with the MedStar Annual Operating Plan and MedStar Annual Nursing Goals. NICHE goals are tied to each of the balanced scorecard domains: Best Place to Work, Highest Quality and Safety, Best Patient Experience, Market Leader, and Financial Strength. She provides oversight of educational programs and data collection as appropriate, for example the Geriatric Institutional Assessment Profile (GIAP). She coordinates with the entity NICHE coordinators and fosters their sharing though a combination of monthly coordinating calls and entity site visits. She communicates and collaborates widely with a large group of stakeholders ranging from the MedStar Board of Directors and Patient Family Advisory Councils for Quality and Safety (PFACQS) to leaders of the local entities. She is actively involved in bringing an interprofessional perspective to NICHE and the care of older adults across the system. For example, she is socializing the idea of a geriatric emergency program. The NICHE Knowledge Center is a web-based resource for MedStar clinicians. MedStar Nursing also hosts an annual conference for the GRNs that brings national leaders directly to clinical nurses and nurse leaders.

The NICHE coordinator plays a major role in helping to cultivate the shared consciousness about the NICHE program components, evidence-based practices, and program outcomes essential for empowered execution at the local entity.

Entity-Level Structure and Processes

The entity structure and processes mirror those of the system level. All hospitals have NICHE coordinators, NICHE steering committees, and annual goals. Collaboration with their stakeholders, including their Board of Directors and communities, is a priority. Most entity NICHE programs work with their local PFACQS to gain input and support for their work. Building on the shared consciousness and sharing of best practices from across the system, local teams are empowered to add additional activities important to their patients, families, and communities. This empowered execution is celebrated locally and at the system level. The GRN role continues to be a critically important component of the NICHE program at all of our hospitals.

CHALLENGES AND MITIGATION STRATEGIES

NICHE was one of the first two evidence-based Signature Programs implemented across the MedStar Nursing Service. Gaining initial support from formal and informal nursing leaders as well as from clinical nurses was critical to our success. Communicating with and listening to those stakeholders helped to establish buy-in aimed at improving the nursing care we provide to older adults. It is the type of care that "we would want for our parents and family members." This is the common purpose of NICHE.

The early NICHE work was challenging as competing priorities and lack of widespread geriatric nursing expertise resulted in many questions and concerns that NICHE was "another flavor of the month" management strategy.

The early NICHE work was challenging as competing priorities and lack of widespread geriatric nursing expertise resulted in many questions and concerns that NICHE was "another flavor of the month" management strategy. The dedication of specific resources from corporate nursing demonstrated the real commitment to the program. Gradually, a base of support emerged throughout the system. As the program has matured, clinical nurses have been supported to attend the annual meetings, to present their work, and to attend our annual MedStar conference.

Entity NICHE coordinators do change roles and move on to other positions both within MedStar and in other healthcare systems. Providing ongoing orientation to new coordinators and support to all is critical to maintaining the program. The national NICHE education materials and courses are valuable resources.

Members of the MedStar Health CNO Council also change. Insuring their orientation to NICHE if they have not led a NICHE organization in the past is important. Their understanding and active support for the program is obviously necessary for success.

OUTCOMES

"Between 2010 and 2013, the NICHE journey to exemplary and sensitive geriatric care began at each MedStar hospital by select nurse leaders who completed the NICHE Leadership Training Program" (Mack, 2017). MedStar hospitals progressed through the levels of NICHE implementation. Today, every hospital has NICHE recognition. As a system, MedStar Health has achieved seven Senior Friendly and three Exemplar level NICHE implementation levels (see Vignette C).

MedStar hospitals progressed through the levels of NICHE implementation. Today, every hospital has NICHE recognition.

MedStar Health NICHE structure, process, and outcome measures (Donabedian, 1966) are delineated in the previously referenced Vignette C by Karen Mack. The NICHE program is an internal exemplar of successfully implementing large-scale change. The progress MedStar nurses have made in the care of older adult hospital patients is significant. It truly is "the care we wish for our parents and family members."

CHAPTER SUMMARY

MedStar Health is an example of an integrated health system that has successfully implemented NICHE as one of its Signature Programs. MedStar chose NICHE for four reasons:

- *NICHE's focus on improving nursing care of older adults, who compose 35% to 38% of MedStar's patients*

- *NICHE's evidence-based approach to both executive nursing practice and clinical practice*

- *Opportunity for nurses and unlicensed patient care associates to develop expertise in caring for geriatric patients*

- *NICHE's fiscally responsible approach to patient- and family-centered care and professional nursing practice*

The MedStar Health NICHE program is led at the system level by a certified clinical practice program specialist and at the entity or hospital level by NICHE coordinators and steering committees. Challenges faced during implementation included competing priorities, skepticism over change, lack of widespread geriatric nursing expertise, and turnover in council members and coordinators. Today, however, NICHE has been effectively implemented in all 10 hospitals of MedStar Health.

REFERENCES

Clifford, J. C., & Horvath, K. (Eds.). (1990). *Advancing professional nursing practice: Innovations at Boston's Beth Israel hospital.* New York, NY: Springer Publishing.

Donabedian, A. (1966). Evaluating the quality of medical care. *The Millbank Quarterly, 44,* 166–203. doi:10.1111/j.1468-0009.2005.00397.x

Fussell, C. (2017). *One mission: How leaders build a team of teams.* New York, NY: Portfolio/Penguin.

Koloroutis, M. (Ed.). (2004). *Relationship based care: A model for transforming practice.* Minneapolis, MN: Creative Health Care Management.

Mack, K. (2017). *MedStar health "Nurses Improving Care for Healthsystem Elders (NICHE): Fiscal year 2017 annual report.* Clinton, MD: MedStar Southern Maryland Hospital Center. Retrieved from https://ct1.medstarhealth.org/content/uploads/sites/17/2016/03/MSMHC_2018_Nursing_Annual_Report_low.pdf

McCausland, M. P. (2012). Opportunities and strategies in contemporary health system executive leadership. *Nursing Administration Quarterly, 36*(4), 306–313. doi:10.1097/NAQ.0b013e3182669300

McChrystal, S. (2015). *Team of teams: New rules of engagement for a complex world.* New York, NY: Portfolio/Penguin.

MedStar Health Nursing. (2013). *MedStar health nursing strategic plan: Fiscal years 2013–2017.* Columbia, MD: Author. Retrieved from https://ct1.medstarhealth.org/content/uploads/sites/114/2015/03/AtaGlance-0315.pdf

Mezey, M., Kobayashi, M., Grossman, S., Firpo, A., Fulmer, T., & Mitty, E. (2004). Nurses improving care to health system elders (NICHE): Implementation of best practice models. *Journal of Nursing Administration, 34*(10), 451–457. Retrieved from https://journals.lww.com/jonajournal/Abstract/2004/10000/Nurses_Improving_Care_to_Health_System_Elders.5.aspx

Titler, M. G., Kleiber, C., Steelman, V., Rakel, B., Budreau, G., Everett, L.Q., . . . Goode, C. (2001). The Iowa model of evidence-based practice to promote quality care. *Critical Care Nursing Clinics of North America, 13*(4), 497–509. doi:10.1016/S0899-5885(18)30017-0

U.S. Census Bureau. (2017). *The nations' older population is still growing.* Retrieved from https://www.census.gov/newsroom/press-releases/2017/cb17-100.html

External Forces that Align with NICHE

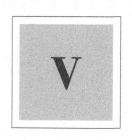

External Regulations and NICHE

15

Kimberly Glassman

*I think healthcare is more about love than about most other things. If there isn't
at the core of this two human beings who have agreed to be in a relationship
where one is trying to help relieve the suffering of another, which is love,
you can't get to the right answer here.*

—Donald Berwick, MD, MPP, FRCP

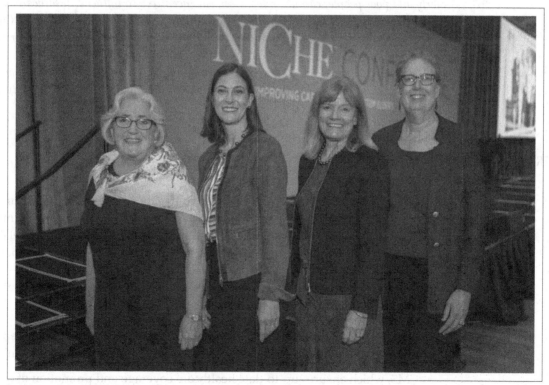

From left: Catherine O'Neill D'Amico, Mattia Gilmartin, Terry Fulmer, Eileen Sullivan-Marx.

INTRODUCTION

Contemporary hospitals and other healthcare delivery settings operate within a complex constellation of legal, financial, and other rules and regulations designed to ensure quality and safe patient care practices, as well as working environments that protect healthcare workers. The organizations involved in creating, monitoring, and enforcing these rules and regulations have varying degrees of authority and power to compel healthcare organizations to comply with their requirements. Governmental agencies, such as the Centers for Medicare & Medicaid Services (CMS), which is fiscally responsible for care of eligible elderly and poor people, can use reimbursement incentives to influence healthcare organizational practices. Nongovernmental organizations (NGOs), such as The Joint Commission (TJC), possess significant authority to influence healthcare practices as a result of its reputation and demonstrated outcomes of its policies, programs, and services. This chapter explores some of the major governmental and NGOs that impact on care of the elderly, particularly in hospitals, and examines how the NICHE program fits into the larger picture.

FEDERAL GOVERNMENT ORGANIZATIONS

The most prominent federal entity involved in healthcare is the U.S. Department of Health and Human Services (DHHS). The Secretary of Health and Human Services is a member of the President's cabinet and oversees all health-related policies (DHHS trategic Plan FY 2018–2022, available at www.hhs.gov/about/strategic-plan/index.html).

DHHS is responsible for ensuring the health and well-being of the nation and includes operating divisions such as the:

- Administration on Aging (AoA), which promotes the dignity and independence of older people and helps society prepare for an aging population

- CMS, which ensures up-to-date healthcare coverage and promotion of quality care for medically vulnerable populations. CMS maintains a user-friendly searchable database that allows consumers to examine the performance of hospitals (known as Hospital Compare) on important healthcare outcomes, including patient satisfaction

- Agency for Healthcare Research and Quality (AHRQ), which supports, conducts, and disseminates research that improves access to care and the outcomes, quality, cost, and utilization of healthcare services

Hospitals and other healthcare delivery settings are also bound by the rules and regulations of their state departments of health, which vary considerably across the 50 states and territories. Regulation is believed to protect the public, and provides a threshold of standards for basic care delivery (Frieden, 2013).

NONGOVERNMENTAL AND NONPROFIT ORGANIZATIONS

The United States has a long history of nongovernmental organizations (NGOs) and nonprofit (or not-for-profit) organizations dedicated to providing services, advocacy, and resources to address specific issues. NGOs are defined as follows:

> [A]ny nonprofit, voluntary citizens' group which is organized on a local, national or international level. Task-oriented and driven by people with a common interest, NGOs perform a variety of service and humanitarian functions, bring citizen concerns to Governments, advocate and monitor policies and encourage political participation through provision of information. Some are organized around specific issues, such as human rights, environment or health (www.ngo.org/ngoinfo/define.html).

In current parlance, the NGO label is typically given to organizations operating on an international level.

Nonprofit organizations dedicate themselves to social activities that are not-for-profit and nongovernmental. To a great extent, the term "nonprofit organization" refers to the financial structure of an organization and does not necessarily mean that the organization is not profitable. On the contrary, many nonprofits are fiscally successful but use their profits to benefit the organization rather than shareholders or other stakeholders. There are literally thousands of nonprofit organizations dedicated to healthcare issues in the United States from large national organizations like the American Cancer Society and the Alzheimer's Association to local advocacy groups that promote care in specific geographical locations or for specific populations. The rest of this chapter will discuss the key governmental agencies and nonprofit organizations that have relevance to care of the elderly and the NICHE program.

BACKGROUND: HOSPITAL REGULATIONS

The healthcare landscape is increasingly complex. Health organizations must be attentive in meeting and addressing rules and regulations from both governmental and nongovernmental agencies. Aside from the federal- and state-level

Hospitals and healthcare systems, including community-based agencies, all deal with a plethora of regulations and anticipate annual regulatory visits from governmental and NGOs.

agencies, such as CMS and state health departments (DOH), there are many nongovernmental, nonprofit agencies that provide services and programs that help hospitals meet and exceed federal requirements. While large hospital-focused organizations such as TJC and American Hospital Association may come to mind, specialty organizations, such as the American Nurses Credentialing Center (ANCC), the accreditation arm of the American Nurses Association that oversees the Magnet Recognition Program, are also important. Hospitals and healthcare systems, including community-based agencies, all deal with a plethora of regulations and anticipate annual regulatory visits from governmental and NGOs.

Governmental organizations (CMS, state health departments, city health departments) provide regulatory oversight addressing adherence to public health laws and regulations. They may conduct regular on-site surveys of hospitals and healthcare organizations, or they may arrive unannounced to address a complaint from a patient or the public. During those visits, the governmental regulatory agency may review adherence to other standards, in addition to the allegation they are investigating.

TJC, founded in 1951, is an independent, not-for-profit organization that accredits and certifies nearly 21,000 healthcare organizations and programs in the United States. TJC accreditation and certification is recognized nationwide as a symbol of quality that reflects an organization's commitment to meeting certain performance standards. Its stated mission is to continuously improve healthcare for the public, in collaboration with other stakeholders, by evaluating healthcare organizations and inspiring them to excel in providing safe and effective care of the highest quality and value.

A more recent player in hospital accreditation, Det Norske Veritas Healthcare, Inc. (DNVHC), was approved in 2008 by CMS to deem hospitals in compliance with the CMS Conditions of Participation for hospitals, a role similar to TJC. Believing that the current accreditation programs in the United States had little impact on business practices that are responsible for creating quality and controlling costs, DNVHC was formed and proposed an accreditation model that focused on "improvement" and "sustainability." DNV, which means "the Norwegian truth," originated in Norway and its mission is dedicated to safeguarding life, property, and the environment (Fennel, 2014).

NGOs (like TJC and DNVHC) offer the public an added level of scrutiny against a different set of standards. As hospital and other healthcare organization accrediting bodies, TJC and DNVHC generally survey healthcare organizations using their own standards and measures that allow hospitals to assess their outcomes and performance. TJC surveys hospitals every 3 years; DNVHC surveys annually, but on different standards each year.

Both focus on creating a culture where organizations develop an obsession with quality and safety, such that there are regular review practices in place from members of the healthcare organization in a self-appraisal. TJC and most other accrediting bodies require organizations to self-appraise, and enter the results into a database. Those data may be used by TJC on their site visits.

HOW GOVERNMENTAL AGENCIES AND NONGOVERNMENTAL AGENCIES WORK TOGETHER

The relationship between CMS and accrediting bodies such as TJC is complex. Hospitals must meet eligibility standards established by the federal government in order to receive reimbursement from the federally funded programs Medicare and/or Medicaid. CMS has been designated as the organization responsible for certification of hospitals, deeming them certified and meeting established standards.

TJC sets its standards and establishes elements of performance based on the CMS standards. CMS has approved TJC as having standards and a survey process that meets or exceeds the established federal requirements. TJC is one of several organizations approved by CMS to certify hospitals. If a hospital is certified by TJC, it is deemed eligible to receive Medicare and/or Medicaid reimbursement. Hospitals must be a member and pay a fee to TJC to be included in their survey process.

By complying with the standards set by the organizations, there is greater consistency of care, better processes for patient and staff safety, and thus higher quality of care.

In short, CMS requires hospitals to demonstrate their ability to meet federal requirements for participating in healthcare delivery in order to receive federal reimbursement and TJC accreditation is one method that provides evidence of meeting this requirement (TJC, 2018). It is important to note that CMS does conduct random validation surveys of hospitals that are certified by TJC. CMS may also conduct complaint-based investigations and surveys. In the final analysis, the goal of these programs, then, is to ensure quality care and patient safety. By complying with the standards set by the organizations, there is greater consistency of care, better processes for patient and staff safety, and thus higher quality of care.

TJC accredits approximately 4,023 general, pediatric, long-term acute, psychiatric, rehabilitation, and specialty hospitals, and 366 critical access hospitals, through a separate accreditation program. Approximately 77% of the nation's hospitals are currently accredited by TJC, and approximately 88% of hospitals that are accredited in the United States are accredited by TJC (TJC, 2016). TJC also offers certification on a wide range of clinical specialties such as comprehensive stroke care and palliative care (TJC, n.d.).

WHERE DOES NICHE FIT?

The NICHE program serves as a "specialty" designation that recognizes nurses' excellence in caring for older adults. Hospitals may have more than one specialty designation that reflects excellence in a wide range of patient care and provider measures. For example, Baby Friendly USA is an accrediting body that sets standards for breastfeeding and other baby-related issues in a hospital setting. NICHE requires rigorous self-assessment, described elsewhere in this publication, and provides hospitals and health systems with increasing levels of geriatric nursing expertise through education and training. As the number of certified hospital-based geriatric nurses increases, older adults are assured higher quality of care delivered by knowledgeable and expert nurses (Biel, Grief, Patry, Ponto, & Shirey, 2014).

There are anecdotal but important correlations between NICHE organizations and successful regulatory surveys (NICHE Advisory Board meeting, 2015; Wurt, personal communication). The rigor in the educational program and ongoing development of nursing practice provides hospitals with a level of nursing expertise that can and does improve patient outcomes. NICHE hospitals may be able to demonstrate superior outcomes for prevention of falls, hospital-acquired pressure injury, and hospital-associated infections in older adults, thus improving the hospitals' publically reported measures in the nurse-sensitive domains.

NICHE hospitals may be able to demonstrate superior outcomes for prevention of falls, hospital-acquired pressure injury, and hospital-associated infections in older adults, thus improving the hospitals' publically reported measures in the nurse-sensitive domains.

NICHE alone does not improve patient outcomes. Because NICHE is an educational curriculum designed to increase nursing knowledge and competency in the care of hospitalized elders, the implementation of the program is key. Geriatric resource nurses (GRNs) must be developed and nurtured to lead practice in the organization. Empowering the GRNs to review unit-level data across the organization and develop targeted interventions for improvement in underperforming areas is one way to ensure that their expert knowledge impacts the hospital. The investment for NICHE can be communicated through improved patient outcomes demonstrated by evidence-based and standardized practice for the care of older adults.

NICHE AND MAGNET RECOGNITION

Magnet recognition for hospitals remains the gold standard for nursing practice and the impact nurses have on patient outcomes and improving care.

Magnet recognition for hospitals remains the gold standard for nursing practice and the impact nurses have on patient outcomes and improving care. Approximately 500 hospitals across the world have obtained ANCC Magnet recognition (ANCC 2017); this is a credential of organizational recognition of nursing excellence.

The original Magnet research study, conducted in 1983, identified 14 characteristics of organizations best able to recruit and retain nurses during the nursing shortages of the 1970s and 1980s (McClure, Poulin, Sovie, & Wandelt, 1983). These characteristics remain known as the ANCC Forces of Magnetism, which provide the conceptual framework for the Magnet appraisal process.

The Forces of Magnetism are attributes or outcomes that exemplify nursing excellence. The full expression of the Forces of Magnetism is required to achieve Magnet designation and embodies a professional environment guided by a strong and visionary nursing leader who advocates and supports excellence in nursing practice. The 14 forces are noted below, and align with the American Nurses Association's *Nursing Administration: Scope and Standards of Practice* (2016):

- **Force 1: Quality of Nursing Leadership.** Knowledgeable, strong, risk-taking nurse leaders follow a well-articulated, strategic, and visionary philosophy in the day-to-day operations of nursing services. Nursing leaders, at all organizational levels, convey a strong sense of advocacy and support for the staff and for the patient. The results of quality leadership are evident in nursing practice at the patient's side.

- **Force 2: Organizational Structure.** Organizational structures are generally flat, rather than tall, and decentralized decision making prevails. The organizational structure is dynamic and responsive to change. Strong nursing representation is evident in the organizational committee structure. Executive-level nursing leaders serve at the executive level of the organization. The Chief Nursing Officer (CNO) typically reports directly to the Chief Executive Officer. The organization has a functioning and productive system of shared decision making.

- **Force 3: Management Style.** Healthcare organization and nursing leaders create an environment supporting participation. Feedback is encouraged, valued, and incorporated from the staff at all levels. Nurses serving in leadership positions are visible, accessible, and committed to effective communication.

- **Force 4: Personnel Policies and Programs.** Salaries and benefits are competitive. Creative and flexible staffing models that support a safe and healthy work environment are used. Personnel policies are created with direct care nurse involvement. Significant opportunities for professional growth exist in administrative and clinical tracks. Personnel policies and programs support professional nursing practice, work/life balance, and the delivery of quality care.

- **Force 5: Professional Models of Care.** There are models of care that give nurses responsibility and authority for the provision of direct patient care. Nurses are accountable for their own practice as well as the coordination of care. The models of care (i.e., primary nursing, case management, family-centered, district, and holistic) provide for the continuity of care across the continuum. The models take into consideration patients' unique needs and provide skilled nurses and adequate resources to accomplish desired outcomes.

- **Force 6: Quality of Care.** Quality is the systematic driving force for nursing and the organization. Nurses serving in leadership positions are responsible for providing an environment that positively influences patient outcomes. There is a pervasive perception among nurses that they provide high quality care to patients.

- **Force 7: Quality Improvement.** The organization possesses structures and processes for the measurement of quality and programs for improving the quality of care and services within the organization.

- **Force 8: Consultation and Resources.** The healthcare organization provides adequate resources, support, and opportunities for the utilization of experts, particularly advanced practice nurses. The organization promotes involvement of nurses in professional organizations and among peers in the community.

- **Force 9: Autonomy.** Autonomous nursing care is the ability of a nurse to assess and provide nursing actions as appropriate for patient care based on competence, professional expertise, and knowledge. The nurse is expected to practice autonomously, consistent with professional standards. Independent judgment is expected within the context of interdisciplinary and multidisciplinary approaches to patient/resident/client care.

- **Force 10: Community and the Healthcare Organization.** Relationships are established within and among all types of healthcare organizations and other community organizations, to develop strong partnerships that support improved client outcomes and the health of the communities they serve.

- **Force 11: Nurses as Teachers.** Professional nurses are involved in educational activities within the organization and community. Students from a variety of academic programs are welcomed and supported in the organization; contractual arrangements are mutually beneficial. There is a development and mentoring program for staff preceptors for all levels of students (including students, new graduates, experienced nurses, etc.). In all positions, staff serve as faculty and preceptors for students from a variety of academic programs. There is a patient education program that meets the diverse needs of patients in all of the care settings of the organization.

- **Force 12: Image of Nursing.** The services provided by nurses are characterized as essential by other members of the healthcare team. Nurses are viewed as integral to the healthcare organization's ability to provide patient care. Nursing effectively influences system-wide processes.

- **Force 13: Interdisciplinary Relationships.** Collaborative working relationships within and among the disciplines are valued. Mutual respect is based on the premise that all members of the healthcare team make essential and meaningful contributions in the achievement of clinical outcomes. Conflict management strategies are in place and are used effectively, when indicated.

- **Force 14: Professional Development.** The healthcare organization values and supports the personal and professional growth and development of staff. In addition to quality orientation and in-service education addressed earlier in Force 11, Nurses as Teachers, emphasis is placed on career development services. Programs that promote formal education, professional certification, and career development are evident. Competency-based clinical and leadership/management development is promoted and adequate human and fiscal resources for all professional development programs are provided (ANCC, 2017).

The Magnet Model has evolved to incorporate the Forces of Magnetism into five components: Transformational Leadership (TL), Structural Empowerment (SE), Exemplary Professional Practice (EP), and New Knowledge, Innovation, and Improvements (NK), all supported by Empirical Outcomes (EO) that reflect achievements in each of the domains (ANCC, 2013).

Transformational Leadership

The CNO in a Magnet-recognized organization is a knowledgeable, transformational leader who develops a strong vision and well-articulated philosophy, a professional practice model (PPM), and strategic and quality plans in leading nursing services. The transformational CNO communicates expectations, develops leaders, and evolves the organization to meet current and anticipated needs and strategic priorities. Nursing leaders at all levels of the organization demonstrate advocacy and support on behalf of staff and patients (ANCC, 2017, p. 19).

Empirical Outcomes

Professional nursing makes an essential contribution to patient, nursing workforce, organizational, and consumer outcomes. The empirical measurement of quality outcomes related to nursing leadership and clinical practice in Magnet-recognized organizations is imperative (ANCC, 2017, p. 15).

Structural Empowerment

Magnet structural environments are generally flat, flexible, and decentralized. Nurses throughout the organization are involved in shared governance, decision-making structures, and processes that establish standards of practice and address opportunities for improvement (ANCC, 2017, p. 25).

Exemplary Professional Practice

A PPM is the overarching, conceptual framework for nurses, nursing care, and interprofessional patient care. It is a schematic description of a system, theory, or phenomenon that depicts how nurses practice, collaborate, communicate, and develop professionally to provide the highest quality of care for those served by the organization (e.g., patients, families, communities). The PPM illustrates the alignment and integration of nursing practice with the mission, vision, values, and philosophy that nursing has adopted. At the organizational level, nurse executives ensure that care is patient and family centered. Magnet-recognized organizations take the lead in research efforts to create and test models that promote the professional practice of nurses (ANCC, 2017, p. 39).

New Knowledge, Innovations, and Improvements

Magnet-recognized organizations conscientiously integrate evidence-based practice and research into clinical and operational processes. Nurses are educated about evidence-based practice and research, enabling them to appropriately explore the safest and best practices for their patients and practice environment and to generate new knowledge. Published research is systematically evaluated and used. Nurses serve on the board that reviews proposals for research and knowledge gained through research is disseminated to the community of nurses (ANCC, 2017, p. 59).

NICHE can provide significant evidence of meeting the Magnet standards.

NICHE can provide significant evidence of meeting the Magnet standards. Participating in the NICHE program demonstrates TL, as nurse leaders advocate for applying for NICHE, and there is the financial investment of the application fee and time for nurses to learn to support the NICHE journey. NICHE takes a village, and all disciplines must be involved in providing expert care to older adults, but nursing taking the lead is strong evidence for this TL element. SE reflects the educational foundation NICHE provides to nurses and other disciplines to gain the knowledge of caring for hospitalized elders. The learning modules and sitting for the ANCC geriatric certification examination are strong evidence for this element. There are many exemplars that can be used for EP. NICHE embeds a culture of outcomes in the organization, and NICHE hospitals must review their data on their older patient populations (Nurses Improving Care for Healthsystem Elders, n.d.). Showing improvements in hospital-acquired pressure injury reduction, management of delirium, and falls prevention among the older adult population are common exemplars for this element (EP). NICHE also can be used for NK. The NICHE program in and of itself is an innovation. Some hospitals use NICHE as a platform for small studies and rigorous quality improvement initiatives that provide learning opportunities for clinical nurses to present at national meetings, including the annual Magnet conference and the NICHE conference.

Magnet and NICHE have many synergies that provide hospitals with a framework to display and test their excellence in the care of older adults. The achievement of Magnet recognition can be supported by implementation of the NICHE program, and the NICHE journey from progressive to exemplar is evidence of engagement in professional practice that reflects all of the Magnet elements.

The NICHE program provides hospitals and health systems with a strong, evidence-based curriculum to support the knowledge and professional development of geriatric nurses. This knowledge, in turn, empowers and enables nurses to deliver expert care to hospitalized older adults. Expert nursing care of older adults produces improved patient outcomes. These outcomes are rewarded by regulatory agencies—both governmental and NGOs—but most importantly, excellent patient outcomes benefit the patients and their families. NICHE has the potential to ensure that the care provided to older adults is of the highest quality.

CHAPTER SUMMARY

Hospitals and other healthcare delivery settings are regulated by federal governmental agencies, such as DHHS (including CMS), state departments of health, and nongovernmental and nonprofit organizations, such as TJC. Several organizations, including TJC, are approved by CMS to certify hospitals. If a hospital is certified by TJC, it is eligible to receive reimbursement from Medicare and Medicaid. By helping improve health outcomes for older adults, NICHE can help hospitals and other member organizations to meet federal, state, and nongovernmental regulations and standards and achieve Magnet recognition. Attributes that exemplify nursing excellence and help a hospital achieve Magnet designation are known as the Forces of Magnetism. These 14 attributes are grouped together in five categories:

- *Transformational leadership*

- *Empirical outcomes*

- *Structural empowerment*

- *Exemplary professional practice*

- *New knowledge, innovations, and improvements*

REFERENCES

American Nurses Association. (2016). *Nursing administration: Scope and standards of practice* (2nd ed.). Silver Spring, MD: Author. Retrieved from https://www.nursingworld.org/nurses-books/nursing-administration-scope-and-standards-of-practice-2nd-edition

American Nurses Credentialing Center. (2013). *2014 Magnet application manual.* Silver Spring, MD: Author.

American Nurses Credentialing Center. (2017). *2019 Magnet application manual.* Silver Spring, MD: Author.

Biel, M., Grief, L., Patry, L. A., Ponto, J., & Shirey, M. (2014). *The relationship between nursing certification and patient outcomes: A review of the literature.* Birmingham, AL: American

Board of Nursing Specialties. Retrieved from http://www.nursingcertification.org/resources/documents/research/certification-and-patient-outcomes-research-article-synthesis.pdf

Fennel, V. (2014). Understanding Det Norske Veritas Healthcare's National Integrated Accreditation for Healthcare Organizations program. *Becker's Clinician Leadership & Infection Control*. Retrieved from https://www.beckershospitalreview.com/quality/understanding-det-norske-veritas-healthcare-s-national-integrated-accreditation-for-healthcare-organizations-program.html

Frieden, T. R. (2013). Government's role in protecting health and safety. *New England Journal of Medicine, 368*(20), 1857–1859. doi:10.1056/NEJMp1303819

The Joint Commission. (n.d.). What is certification? Retrieved from https://www.jointcommission.org/certification/certification_main.aspx

The Joint Commission. (2016). Facts about the Joint Commission. Retrieved from https://www.jointcommission.org/facts_about_the_joint_commission

The Joint Commission. (2018). Facts about federal deemed status and state recognition. Retrieved from https://www.jointcommission.org/facts_about_federal_deemed_status_and_state_recognition

McClure, M. L., Poulin, M. A., Sovie, M. D., & Wandelt, M. A. (1983). *Magnet hospitals: Attraction and retention of professional nurses.* Kansas City, MO: American Nurses Association.

Nurses Improving Care for Healthsystem Elders. (n.d.). *Leadership training program overview.* Retrieved from https://nicheprogram.org/sites/niche/files/inline-files/LTP_timeline.pdf

Consumers in an Age-Friendly Era: NICHE as a Vehicle for Change

16

Susan C. Reinhard

While the Nurses Improving Care for Healthsystem Elders (NICHE) program provides the resources and tools to support the highest level of evidence-based nursing practice for our older adults, it is so much more than that—It is a transformative program that transcends barriers, dispels negative assumptions, and provides nurses with the skills, expertise, confidence, and passion for providing holistic, complex, evidence-based-care.

—Fran Cartright, PhD, MS, BS, AAS, Senior Director of Nursing, Oncology Services and Medicine, New York University Langone Medical Center

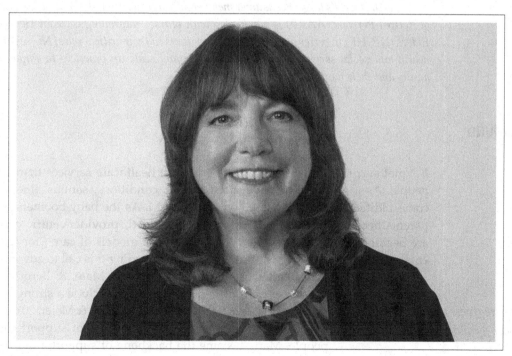

Susan C. Reinhard.

> ### CHAPTER OBJECTIVES
>
> 1. Discuss the growing urgency of placing consumers and family caregivers at the center of care
> 2. Highlight the historical path toward an impactful partnership between NICHE and the American Association of Retired Persons (AARP), the world's largest consumer membership organization
> 3. Encourage nurses and their colleagues to lead the way toward excellence in supporting family caregivers

INTRODUCTION

Older adults and those who help support them are taking center stage in today's healthcare transformation discussions. Older people are major consumers of health and long-term services and supports (LTSS) across many different settings. And, their family caregivers are increasingly recognized as essential members of the care circle (James & Hughes, 2016). This is particularly true as new payment systems for healthcare incentivize efficient return of the patient to home settings, which often necessitates family caregivers to provide complex care (Reinhard, 2018).

As the world's largest consumer membership organization, the American Association of Retired Persons (AARP) is partnering with Nurses Improving Care for Healthsystem Elders (NICHE) to better support family caregivers in their critical roles. Nurses and other health and social service colleagues can create and scale up practices to empower older adults and their families.

BACKGROUND

It is not surprising that older adults use more healthcare services than younger people. As a group, they have more chronic conditions, serious illnesses, and comorbidities (National Council on Aging, n.d.). As the baby boomers of aging parents become firsthand witnesses to fragmented, provider-centric care, they are beginning to demand more consumer-centric models of care—for their parents and for themselves. Healthcare leaders are heeding this call to advance more age-friendly health systems (Fulmer, Mate, & Berman, 2017), and these transformed systems must include a strong focus on family caregivers (Sladoba, Fail, Norman, & Meier, 2018).

Family caregivers are the first line of support for older people.

Family caregivers are the first line of support for older people. Many become the backbone of support, often for long periods of time. They include relatives, neighbors, and friends who help with daily living needs resulting from a limitation in physical, mental, or cognitive functioning (Schulz & Eden, 2016).

There are about 40 million family caregivers in the United States, more than 34 million of whom care for an adult aged 50 years or more. They are a diverse group in age, gender, income, education, and ethnicity (National Alliance for Caregiving, 2015). While it is true that most are women, men are catching up. Forty percent of family caregivers are men. And young people are stepping in as well. One in four caregivers is a millennial. Most (60%) of family caregivers are employed, while collectively they are also providing $470 billion in free care (Reinhard, Feinberg, Choula, & Houser, 2015). They should be considered an invaluable resource, particularly because their pool is shrinking. While there were seven potential family caregivers for each adult aged 80 or older in 2010, there will be only three in 2050 (Redfoot, Feinberg, & Houser, 2013).

The role of family caregivers is becoming more complex as they are expected to perform tasks that would make new nursing students tremble (Reinhard, 2001).

About half of family caregivers are performing medical/nursing tasks, such as the administration of multiple medications, injections, wound care, tube feedings, colostomy care, and other technically sophisticated interventions

As identified in the groundbreaking *Home Alone* report, about half of family caregivers are performing medical/nursing tasks, such as the administration of multiple medications, injections, wound care, tube feedings, colostomy care, and other technically sophisticated interventions (Reinhard, Levine, & Samis, 2012). They do not consistently receive instruction on how to perform these tasks, and express concern that they may be making a mistake or hurting the person for whom they care.

Supported through funding from the John A. Hartford Foundation, this *Home Alone* research led to national recognition of the serious gap between what family caregivers are expected to do and the instruction and support they receive to do it. The purpose of this chapter is to describe the search for solutions to this gap, including a review of state policy, resource development and coalition building, and a discussion of how the collaboration with NICHE substantially enhances past and future AARP efforts on behalf of consumers.

POLICY DEVELOPMENT

The *Home Alone* research quickly led to advocacy for policy changes at the state level (Reinhard & Ryan, 2017). AARP developed model legislation, the Caregiver Advise, Record, Enable (CARE) Act, to require hospitals to ask anyone admitted to a hospital if they have someone who helps provide care (a family caregiver), and if so, whether they want that person(s) to be included in the medical record. If the patient wishes, this routine admission procedure opens up the inclusion of the family caregiver into the care team. If the caregiver is going to be helping the patient with care tasks after discharge, instruction must be offered and the date of discharge identified as soon as possible. NICHE conducted outreach to its sites encouraging them to support the CARE Act (see example in Appendix 16.1). As of January 2018, 39 states and territories have enacted the CARE Act, and more

The goal of the CARE Act National Scan is to uncover facilitators and barriers to implementing this family caregiver-focused intervention, and uncover promising practices to quickly spread innovation.

are on the way. A national scan on implementation began in late 2016, 2 years after the first two states pioneered this legislation. The goal of the CARE Act National Scan is to uncover facilitators and barriers to implementing this family caregiver-focused intervention, and uncover promising practices to quickly spread innovation. Nursing leaders are bringing attention to this transformative policy (Mason, 2017).

RESOURCE DEVELOPMENT

One innovation is the development of instructional videos to teach family caregivers how to perform specific medical/nursing tasks. After convening a diverse group of family caregiver advocacy organizations, researchers, providers, and philanthropists interested in exploring how we might fill the gap between expectations and support for family caregivers providing complex care in December 2014, it was evident that we need better understanding of caregivers' learning needs and ways to meet them.

Qualitative research provided direction. Focus group findings informed a list of "dos and don'ts" for developing videos as one teaching tool (Levine & Reinhard, 2016). Family caregivers wanted to see themselves in the videos, to be clearly seen as a partner in care. Existing patient teaching videos did not include a family caregiver. Rather, they often show a patient performing a task on themselves, or show a clinician performing a task. Family caregivers also wanted the tone to reflect that family members are usually anxious about the caregiving roles and do not think learning the task will be easy. They do not want the person who is giving the instruction to be overly enthusiastic or cheerful. Family caregivers from multicultural communities expressed a desire to see themselves and the nuances specific to their cultures reflected. This included the opportunity to have the videos done "in language."

This foundational research informed the development of a "No Longer Alone" series of videos, with tip sheets and published, peer-reviewed articles on the evidence underlying the instructions (Harvath, Lindauer, & Sexson, 2017; Lindauer, Sexson, & Harvath, 2017a, 2017b; Reinhard & Young, 2017; Sexson, Lindauer, & Harvath, 2017a, 2017b). The first pilot videos were released at the NICHE Annual Conference in 2016, with much input and feedback gathered for subsequent videos. Currently, there are series on medication administration, mobility, and wound care that can be found at www.aarp.org/nolongeralone. There are currently 23 videos, including seven in Spanish, with more planned for 2018 and beyond. The goal is to create best practice models for providers, manufacturers, faculty, and others to use as they develop their own teaching tools. They are getting the attention of thought leaders (Graham, 2017) as we conduct consumer evaluation of the first set and create plans for broad dissemination.

COALITION BUILDING

To bring together a multi-stakeholder group that will help create practical solutions for better supporting family caregivers providing complex care, the AARP Public Policy Institute launched the Home Alone Alliance[SM] (Appendix 16.2). Home Alone Alliance[SM] members provide expertise for resource development, the CARE Act National Scan, and additional research, including follow-on research to the *Home Alone* report. NICHE was among the first to join this coalition, helping to open doors in hospitals that participate in the CARE Act National Scan. NICHE may also include Home Alone Alliance[SM] instructional resources (e.g., videos) in its work with member hospitals. And, these videos can be included in NICHE teaching modules for nurses and other health professionals to practice communication with family caregivers.

HOW NICHE IS SUPPORTING A CONSUMER- AND FAMILY-FOCUSED MODEL OF CARE

The author of this chapter was first introduced to NICHE two decades ago. The first introduction came through NICHE presentations to advisory boards, publications, and national nurse leader organizations. In 2007, this author joined AARP, a consumer membership organization with nearly 40 million members, to lead its Public Policy Institute. In 2009, AARP received funding from the John A. Hartford Foundation and the Valeria Langeloth Foundation to support a pilot study to explore simple ways that nurses could reach out to family caregivers. AARP invited NICHE to collaborate on this effort, and the pilot study was conducted at five NICHE sites. This was the first time AARP had focused on how health and social service professionals could better support family caregivers. The NICHE leaders from these hospitals helped design and implement a tool to ask family caregivers two broad questions: What questions do you have regarding care today? What questions do you have about care at home? Structured tools can be helpful in establishing an expectation of practical communication and respect (Reinhard, Capezuti, Bricoli, & Choula, 2017). Ideally, the nurse and other colleagues would ask the family caregiver a question that few say they are ever asked by anyone: "How are YOU doing?"

Having supported the CARE Act, NICHE leaders provided AARP access to its 2017 NICHE Conference participants in a 2017 breakfast meeting. Approximately 100 nurses and nurse leaders attended and provided insight into how to best conduct the CARE Act National Scan, and trends they have noticed among family caregivers performing complex medical/nursing tasks. Participants repeatedly emphasized the importance of including a broad range of health professionals in National CARE Act Scan interviews, including nurses at all levels (from bedside to executive leadership), allied health professionals (e.g., physical therapy), pharmacists, and case/care managers. They also recommended including health information technology, electronic health records, and admissions/registrar staff.

A few participants even suggested looking beyond the four walls of a hospital at people such as emergency medical services (EMS) professionals.

Additionally, participants identified potential barriers to supporting family caregivers. These included caregiver willingness to learn, comprehension of instruction, and health literacy. They also identified potentially promising practices in their own settings, such as integrating pharmacy staff on hospital floors and staff education related to supporting family caregivers. Local presentations in New Jersey NICHE hospitals and additional national conferences in 2017 enriched that guidance.

FUTURE DIRECTIONS

The opportunity to engage with nurses and their other NICHE colleagues during annual meetings is a key strategy to continue the highly successful partnership between AARP and NICHE.

The opportunity to engage with nurses and their other NICHE colleagues during annual meetings is a key strategy to continue the highly successful partnership between AARP and NICHE. A preconference at the 2018 NICHE Conference will highlight early findings from the CARE Act National Scan site visits and solicit promising practices for teaching family caregivers how to confidently care for those who need their help. Creativity and scaling are essential to really transform our healthcare systems into patient- and family-centered care models.

CHAPTER SUMMARY

We need clear and supportive communications among health and social service professionals, patients, and family caregivers to promote the highest quality outcomes for patients and families (Reinhard & Choula, 2012). Engagement of family caregivers has been linked to substantial reductions in patient readmissions (Rodakowski et al., 2017). We need this kind of support across health systems, and NICHE leaders are in key positions to make this happen. Organizations that advocate for consumers urge professionals to speak up for those who need them most.

REFERENCES

Fulmer, T., Mate, K., & Berman, A. (2018). The age-friendly health system imperative. *Journal of the American Geriatrics Society, 66*(1), 22–24. doi:10.1111/jgs.15076

Graham, J. (2017). Video help is on way for family caregivers who must draw blood or give injections. *Kaiser Health News.* Retrieved from https://khn.org/news/video-help-is-on-way-for-family-caregivers-who-must-draw-blood-or-give-injections

Harvath, T. A., Lindauer, A., & Sexson, K. (2017, May). Managing complex medication regimens. *American Journal of Nursing, 117*(Suppl. 1 5), S3–S6. doi:10.1097/01.NAJ.0000516386.89892.f3

James, E., & Hughes, M. (2016). Embracing the role of family caregivers in the U.S. health system. *Health Affairs*. Retrieved from https://www.healthaffairs.org/do/10.1377/hblog20160908.056387/full

Levine, C., & Reinhard, S. (2016). *"It all falls on me": Family caregiver perspectives on medication management, wound care, and video instruction*. Washington, DC: AARP Public Policy Institute. Retrieved from https://www.aarp.org/content/dam/aarp/ppi/2016-08/AARP1078_FamilyCaregiver_SpotlightSep6v5.pdf

Lindauer, A., Sexson, K., & Harvath, T. A. (2017a). Medication management for people with dementia. *American Journal of Nursing, 117*(Suppl. 1 5), S17–S21. doi:10.1097/01.NAJ.0000516389.35634.84

Lindauer, A., Sexson, K., & Harvath, T. A. (2017b). Teaching caregivers to administer eye drops, transdermal patches, and suppositories. *American Journal of Nursing, 117*(Suppl. 1 5), S11–S16. doi:10.1097/01.NAJ.0000516388.97515.ca

Mason, D. (2017). Supporting family caregivers, one state at a time: The CARE act. *news@JAMA*. Retrieved from https://newsatjama.jama.com/2017/12/13/jama-forum-supporting-family-caregivers-one-state-at-a-time-the-care-act

National Alliance for Caregiving. (2015). Caregiving in the United States 2015. *AARP Public Policy Institute*. Retrieved from http://www.aarp.org/ppi/info-2015/caregiving-in-the-united-states-2015.html

National Council on Aging. (n.d.). Healthy aging facts. Retrieved from https://www.ncoa.org/news/resources-for-reporters/get-the-facts/healthy-aging-facts

Redfoot, D., Feinberg, F., & Houser, A. (2013). The aging of the baby boom and the growing care gap: A look at future declines in the availability of family caregivers. *AARP Public Policy Institute*. Retrieved from http://www.aarp.org/home-family/caregiving/info-08-2013/the-aging-of-the-baby-boom-and-the-growing-care-gap-AARP-ppi-ltc.html

Reinhard, S. (2001). Nursing's role in family caregiver support. In K. J. Doka & J. D. Davidson (Eds.), *Caregiving and loss: Family needs, professional responses* (pp. 181–190). Washington, DC: Hospice Foundation of America.

Reinhard, S. (2018). The family context. In T. Fulmer & B. Chernof (Eds.), *Handbook for geriatric assessment* (5th ed., pp. 81–88). Burlington, MA: Jones & Bartlett.

Reinhard, S., Capezuti, E., Bricoli, B., & Choula, R. (2017). Feasibility of a family-centered hospital intervention. *Journal of Gerontological Nursing, 43*(6), 9–16. doi:10.3928/00989134-20160516-01

Reinhard, S., & Choula, R. (2012). *Meeting the needs of diverse family caregivers*. Washington, DC: AARP Public Policy Institute. Retrieved from https://www.aarp.org/content/dam/aarp/research/public_policy_institute/ltc/2012/meeting-needs-diverse-family-caregivers-insight-AARP-ppi-ltc.pdf

Reinhard, S., Feinberg, L. F., Choula, R., & Houser, A. (2015). Valuing the invaluable 2015 update: Undeniable progress, but big gaps remain. *AARP Public Policy Institute*. Retrieved from http://www.aarp.org/ppi/info-2015/valuing-the-invaluable-2015-update.html

Reinhard, S., Levine, C., & Samis, S. (2012). *Home alone: Family caregivers providing complex chronic care*. Retrieved from https://www.aarp.org/content/dam/aarp/research/public_policy_institute/health/home-alone-family-caregivers-providing-complex-chronic-care-rev-AARP-ppi-health.pdf

Reinhard, S., & Ryan, E. (2017). *From* Home Alone *to the CARE act: Collaboration for family caregivers*. Washington, DC: AARP Public Policy Institute. Retrieved from https://www.aarp.org/content/dam/aarp/ppi/2017/08/from-home-alone-to-the-care-act.pdf

Reinhard, S., & Young, H. (2017). Nurses supporting family caregivers. *American Journal of Nursing, 117*(Suppl. 1 5), S2. doi:10.1097/01.NAJ.0000516385.05140.b0

Rodakowski, J., Rocco, P., Ortiz, M., Folb, B., Schulz, R., Morton, S., … James, A. E. (2017). Caregiver integration during discharge planning for older adults to reduce resource use: A metaanalysis. *Journal of the American Geriatrics Society, 65*(8), 1748–1755. doi:10.1111/jgs.14873

Schulz, R., & Eden, J. (Eds.). (2016). *Families caring for an aging America*. Washington, DC: National Academies Press.

Sexson, K., Lindauer, A., & Harvath, T. A. (2017a). Administration of subcutaneous injections. *American Journal of Nursing, 117*(Suppl. 1 5), S7–S10. doi:10.1097/01.NAJ.0000516387.89892.ba

Sexson, K., Lindauer, A., & Harvath, T. A. (2017b). Discharge planning and teaching. *American Journal of Nursing, 117*(Suppl. 1 5), S22–S24. doi:10.1097/01.NAJ.0000516390.43257.c8

Sladoba, J., Fail, R., Norman, G., & Meier, D. (2018). A study of family caregiver burden and the imperative of practice change to address family caregivers' unmet needs. *Health Affairs*. Retrieved from https://www.healthaffairs.org/do/10.1377/hblog20180105.914873/full

Appendix 16.1

Outreach Letters to NICHE Site

Dear Colleague,

NICHE and the AARP Public Policy Institute have worked together over the past 4 years, through pilots and the development of a toolkit, to show how nursing professionals and hospitals can support family caregivers of older adult patients. As you are aware, one of the main factors that a NICHE designation demonstrates is a hospital's commitment to "enhancing the patient and family experience." Results from our work show that supporting family caregivers as they seek to provide support to their loved one improves not only the caregiver experience but the patient experience in the hospital as well. We plan to continue our work with the AARP Public Policy Institute in the development of best practice ideas in the area of caregiver training and support.

In an effort to transform foundational research into action, AARP has developed model caregiving legislation titled the CARE Act. Currently, 10 AARP state offices are working with stakeholders on legislation or regulation that calls for greater support of family caregivers as they strive to give the best possible care to their loved ones leaving the hospital setting. The legislation's provisions are simple but profound:

- Provide each patient the opportunity to identify a family caregiver who will be documented in the patient's record.

- Ensure that the family caregiver is notified by hospital personnel, in a reasonable amount of time, prior to a patient's discharge or transfer to another licensed facility.

- Provide the caregiver with an opportunity to play a role in developing a plan of care and give the caregiver an opportunity to learn about and receive a live demonstration of the care they are expected to provide to the family member once back home.

AARP values conversations with stakeholders such as you. NICHE leaders, in particular, are familiar with best practices associated with supporting both the patient and the family caregiver. While NICHE does not take a position on the legislation, we would like to offer you the opportunity to become involved in the discussion and help shape the conversation in this important area.

If you would like to discuss further, please contact Patrick Willard (phone number redacted) at the AARP National Office or Dave McNally (phone number redacted) at your AARP state office.

We thank you for your continued commitment to improving the care and lives of your older adult patients and their families.

Thank you,
Barbara Bricoli, MPA
Managing Director

Appendix 16.2

The Home Alone Alliance^{SM}

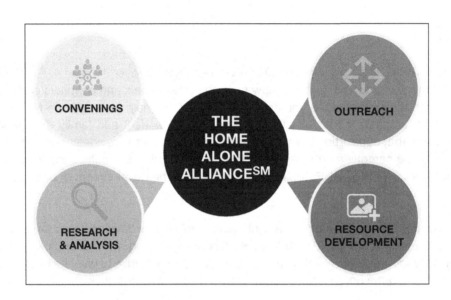

HOME ALONE ALLIANCE^{SM} FOUNDING PARTNERS

- AARP
- The Betty Irene Moore School of Nursing at University of California Davis
- Family Caregiver Alliance
- United Hospital Fund

HOME ALONE ALLIANCE^{SM} ADDITIONAL MEMBERS

- American Journal of Nursing
- The John A. Hartford Foundation
- Atlas of Caregiving
- Center to Advance Palliative Care
- Coalition to Transform Advanced Care

- Easterseals
- Home Instead Senior Care
- National Alliance for Caregiving
- National League for Nursing
- New York University Rory Meyers College of Nursing
  - Hartford Institute for Geriatric Nursing
  - NICHE
- Rosalyn Carter Institute for Caregiving
- U.S. Department of Veterans Affairs

Quality Geriatric Care in an International Context: The Case of South Korea

17

Hongsoo Kim

Our international colleagues have done so much to further the work of NICHE globally. Every culture in the world is experiencing demographic changes that impact care of older adults. We are so fortunate to learn from them along this journey.
—Terry Fulmer, President, The John A. Hartford Foundation

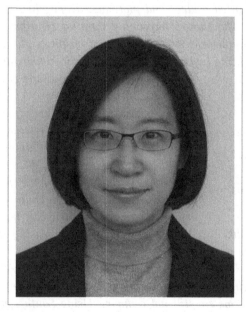

Hongsoo Kim.

CHAPTER OBJECTIVES

1. Explain the need for quality geriatric care in an international context using the case of South Korea, which has the most rapidly aging population in the world
2. Provide examples of efforts to improve geriatric care in the acute care setting in South Korea
3. Discuss the implications of the NICHE program in advancing geriatric care practice in South Korea
4. Suggest factors to be considered in cross-national learning of innovative geriatric practices

INTRODUCTION TO QUALITY GERIATRIC CARE IN AN INTERNATIONAL CONTEXT

Quality geriatric care is a key facet of high-performing healthcare organizations, but it is not always easy to provide. Older people often have complex conditions that require healthcare organizations to fundamentally shift away from their usual approaches to business. Such changes are possible only with system-wide innovations led by visionary, committed leaders and motivated teams, including frontline staff, with proper resources. The Nurses Improving Care for Healthsystem Elders (NICHE) is a U.S. program implemented in hundreds of hospitals and other settings that has been reported as being instrumental in effectively supporting nurse-led, system-wide efforts to improve geriatric care (Boltz et al., 2008; Capezuti, Briccoli, & Boltz, 2013).

The need for quality geriatric care is not unique to older people in the United States but rather is common for most developed countries with aging populations.

The need for quality geriatric care is not unique to older people in the United States but rather is common for most developed countries with aging populations (World Health Organization [WHO], 2015). The need is likely to be more intense and urgent in East Asian countries, where the speed of population aging is much faster than in the Western countries but the workforce and delivery of specialized geriatric care has been less developed in general (World Bank, 2016); the good news is the increasing awareness of the need for quality geriatric care.

The Republic of Korea (South Korea) is an East Asian country with one of the most rapidly aging populations (World Bank, 2016), yet innovations to build senior-friendly health systems are still not common. Using South Korea as a case study, this chapter begins by presenting the complex care needs of older Koreans and the various efforts led by governments, academics, and hospitals to improve the quality of geriatric care in the country, including innovative geriatric care programs at two academic medical centers. A discussion of what Korean acute care organizations can learn from NICHE, a nurse-led, evidence-based, system-wide approach to improving geriatric care follows. Finally, factors to be considered for successful cross-national learning from innovative geriatric care models and practice are suggested.

CARE NEEDS OF AGING POPULATIONS AND IMPACTS ON HEALTH SYSTEMS

South Korea (hereafter Korea) constitutes the southern part of the Korean peninsula, with a land border in the north shared with the Democratic People's Republic of Korea (North Korea). Korea's maritime borders are shared with China to the west and Japan to the east. The total population of Korea is 51.25 million, about one sixth the population of the United States (323.1 million; World Bank, 2016). The GDP per capita of South Korea was 27,538.8 USD, compared with the United States's 57,638.2 USD, in 2016 (1 USD = 1,000 KRW; World Bank, 2017).

Korea has had a national health insurance (NHI) program with universal health coverage for over four decades (Na & Kwon, 2015). The National Health Insurance Services under the Ministry of Health and Welfare is the single insurer, and all Koreans are beneficiaries of the NHI from birth to death regardless of income level. South Korea also introduced public long-term care insurance (LTCI) programs in 2008 (Kim & Cheng, 2018); all Korean citizens aged 65 years or older or people under the age of 65 with senile conditions are eligible when they have certain levels of limitations in daily activities, based on the nationally standardized care need assessment system.

People aged 65 or older were about 13.8% of the total population in South Korea in 2015, and the proportion will be almost double in 2030 (24.5%) and triple in 2060 (41.0%; Statistics Korea, 2016). Thanks to rapid economic growth and the achievement of universal health coverage, the life expectancy of South Koreans has reached 82.16 years (vs. 78.7 years for Americans; World Bank, 2016). The average life span of South Korean women born in 2030 is expected to reach 90, the longest among 35 industrialized countries in a recent study published in *The Lancet* (Kontis et al., 2017).

Living longer does not guarantee healthy longevity, however, similar to other developed countries. The average healthy life expectancy, defined as the expected life span without illness, is estimated at 73.2 years, about 9 years shorter than the overall life expectancy (WHO, 2015). In addition, about 9 out of 10 (89.2%) older Koreans have at least one chronic condition diagnosed by a physician, and 7 out of 10 (69.7%) have multiple chronic conditions (the average number of chronic conditions per person has been reported as 2.6; Chung et al., 2014). The top three reasons for death of older Koreans were all chronic conditions—cancer, cardiovascular diseases, and cerebrovascular diseases (Statistics Korea, 2017). A high suicide rate among older people (58.6 per 100,000 people; Statistics Korea, 2016) also warns of an urgent need for quality geriatric mental health services.

The increasing life span and complex care needs of its citizens, along with the high prevalence of chronic conditions, have resulted in a rapid increase in healthcare utilization and expenditure in Korea.

The increasing life span and complex care needs of its citizens, along with the high prevalence of chronic conditions, have resulted in a rapid increase in healthcare utilization and expenditure in Korea. This is related to Korea's health system, which is characterized by good access to healthcare, weak primary care, and limited gatekeeping for hospitalizations (Kim & Cheng, in press). Older people, composing about 13.8% of the total population, spent approximately 38.0% of the total NHI expenditure in 2016 (Statistics Korea, 2017). The average medical cost per person aged 65 years and over was almost three times higher than the average cost in the overall population. The high utilization of healthcare is partially attributed to a policy to promote good access to care for older people: the copayment for a physician consultation for a light condition in a primary care clinic is about 1.5 USD (1 USD = 1,000 KRW) under the NHI. The number of physician consultations per year in South Korea is 16.0, number one among OECD countries (OECD average = 6.9, U.S. = 4.0; Organization for Economic Cooperation and Development, 2017).

RECENT EFFORTS TO IMPROVE QUALITY OF GERIATRIC CARE

Good access to healthcare contributes to the increased longevity of South Koreans, but the sustainability of the national health system will be threatened if the healthcare utilization of older people continues to increase rapidly. Expansion of service and cost coverage of the NHI is still the main health policy agenda in South Korea (Na & Kwon, 2015), but there seems to be room to improve the effectiveness and quality of care for older adults as a strategy for system sustainability, though this has been less explored and reported in the literature.

A large number of geriatric studies on a wide range of issues including healthy aging and geriatric syndromes of individual older persons have been actively conducted and published in international as well as domestic journals in Korea (Kim, Park, Jang, & Kwon, 2011; Park & Kim, 2016; Park, Kim, Ryu, & Cho, 2016). A government-funded, multidisciplinary national cohort study on frailty has been recently launched (Won et al., 2016). International and also Asian conferences on frailty and sarcopenia were held in Korea in 2013 and 2016, respectively. Systems to produce nationally representative longitudinal surveys and national statistics on the health and well-being of older people are also well established; key longitudinal surveys include the Korean Longitudinal Study of Aging (KLoSA; Jang, 2016) and the Survey of Living Conditions and Welfare Needs of Korean Older Persons (Chung et al., 2014). Yet only a few system-wide initiatives led by healthcare and long-term care (LTC) organizations exist so far. Two good examples of geriatric care programs at academic medical centers in Korea are selected, and their key characteristics are described in what follows.

SEOUL NATIONAL UNIVERSITY BUNDANG HOSPITAL'S MULTIDISCIPLINARY GERIATRIC MEDICINE CENTER

Since the healthcare utilization of older people has increased, and their needs are complex, several academic medical centers have introduced geriatric-specialist centers or clinics called "geriatric medicine clinics," "healthy aging clinics," or "geriatric medicine centers"; a common characteristic of these programs is the so-called "one-stop service" characterized by coordinated care across various medical specialties. This approach is possible because most acute care hospitals have hospitalists of various specialties in South Korea, unlike in the United States. The Geriatric Medicine Center (GMC) at Seoul National University Bundang Hospital (SNUBH; hereafter SNUBH-GMC) is known as the first program of this kind.

SNUBH-GMC was established in 2003 as an independent, geriatrics-specialized, multidisciplinary medical service center including four specialties: geriatric internal medicine, endocrinology internal medicine, rehabilitation medicine, and mental health medicine.

SNUBH is a 1,326-bed teaching hospital located in Suwon, a city near Seoul, the capital city. SNUBH-GMC was established in 2003 as an independent, geriatrics-specialized, multidisciplinary medical service center including four specialties: geriatric internal medicine, endocrinology internal medicine, rehabilitation medicine, and mental health medicine (www.snubh.org/dh/gc). As the foundation of multidisciplinary collaboration, a comprehensive geriatric assessment (CGA) is conducted to identify physical, mental, social, and nutritional needs. Table 17.1 includes the contents of a CGA of SNUBH-GMC. CGA cases consistently increased from 300 cases in 2004 to 2,000 cases in 2017.

Based on the CGA, multidisciplinary case conferences and rounding for inpatients are conducted twice per week. The team consists of pharmacists, nutritionists, geriatrics internal physicians, and rehabilitation physicians. CGA data are also actively used for frailty studies, especially developing prediction models for treatment outcomes to improve clinical practice. For older patients in the pre-operation stage, the extent of frailty based on the CGA can inform clinicians' predictions of the risks of length of stay, death, complications, and/or discharge to LTC institutions (Choi et al., 2015, 2017; Kim et al., 2014).

Medication management is another key area of success that the multidisciplinary geriatrics team, including pharmacists certified in geriatric pharmacy, has achieved at SNUBH-GMC. The team recently reported a meaningful decrease in polypharmacy in terms of the number of drugs prescribed, from 10.5 at admission to 6.5 at discharge per person on average, which saved a medication expenditure

TABLE 17.1 Contents of Comprehensive Geriatric Assessment at SNUBH-GMC

Medical	Problem list
	Comorbid conditions and disease severity
	Medication review
	Nutritional status
Functional	Basic ADLs
	IADLs
	Activity/exercise status
	Gait and balance/grip strength
Psychological	Mental status (cognitive) testing
	Mood/depression testing
Social	Informal support needs and assets
	Care resource eligibility/financial assessment

ADLs, activities of daily living; IADLs, instrumental activities of daily living; SNUBH-GMC, Geriatric Medicine Center at Seoul National University Bundang Hospital.

of about 460 USD per person (1 USD = 1,000 KRW) through a CGA-based safe medication-use program applied to 300 older inpatients between July 2016 and June 2017 (Jung, 2017).

Geriatric nurse practitioners (GNPs) perform key roles in operating programs at SNUBH-GMC. GNPs conduct CGAs and, in collaboration with other professionals on the team, develop care plans for older people visiting outpatient clinics. GNPs also coordinate care for hospitalized older adults from admission to discharge. GNPs conduct CGAs at admission and coordinate the development of discharge plans by communicating and sharing information with clinicians and administrators from various departments in SNUBH and also with postacute or LTC institutions. Counseling and educating family caregivers is another important role of GNPs at SNUBH-GMC. They also develop and share educational materials for staff at hospitals and collaborating partner organizations (e.g., LTC hospitals, nursing homes; H. J. Yoo, RN, APN, personal communication, January 8, 2018).

KONKUK UNIVERSITY MEDICAL CENTER'S SENIOR-FRIENDLY HOSPITAL INITIATIVE

Recently, the concept of a senior-friendly hospital (SFH) has attracted attention from the geriatrics and gerontology community in Korea. Konkuk University Medical Center (KUMC) is the first acute care hospital to introduce a system-wide effort to promote senior-friendly services (Kim et al., in press). As an 870-bed academic medical center located in Seoul, KUMC identified the special needs of older patients, envisioned transforming KUMC into a leading SFH, and in 2016 launched an initiative to meet their vision (Lee, 2016). The goal of KUMC's SFH initiative was to provide seniors with safe and special services, for which the hospital aimed to improve under the leadership of a SFH taskforce three areas: care process, communication and services, and physical environment (Lee, 2016).

Konkuk University Medical Center (KUMC) is the first acute care hospital to introduce a system-wide effort to promote senior-friendly services.

First, for the care process improvement, the hospital developed a senior-friendly care process based mainly on Taiwan's Framework for Age-Friendly Hospitals (Chiou & Chen, 2009) and the 48/6 Model of Care, an integrated care initiative for hospitalized seniors in British Columbia, Canada (British Columbia Provincial Seniors Hospital Care Working Group, 2012). The 48/6 Model of Care is characterized by provision of a CGA within 48 hours of admission and managing six key functional areas: cognition, mobility, medication management, nutrition, pain, and incontinence. KUMC's senior-friendly care process was refined through extensive literature review on SFHs, workgroup discussions, input from various members of KUMC and experts, and also pilot tests (Kim et al., in press).

The finalized care process begins with a screening and evaluation in 10 domains within 24 hours of admission, based on which a treatment plan and a discharge plan are also developed (Table 17.2). For this screening, the 10-item Geriatric Screening

TABLE 17.2 Ten Domains of Geriatric Care Assessment and Management in KUMC's SFH Initiative

DOMAIN	PRINCIPLE OF MANAGEMENT
Cognition impairment	Support the optimal level of cognitive function through effective treatment strategies promoting the functional independence of all patients, including those with dementia
Depression	Prevent situations that can cause or exacerbate depression
Delirium	Prevent situations that can cause or exacerbate delirium
Polypharmacy	Reduce the risk of drug interactions Review medicines to prevent and resolve potential side effects
Functional decline	Maintain the patient's functional ability
Dysphagia	Provide safe meals and prevent pneumonia caused by dysphagia
Malnutrition	Provide proper nutrition Identify and avoid hospital procedures that can cause nutritional imbalances
Urinary incontinence	Maintain urinary function through urinary management and healthy lifestyle practices Use urinary catheters only when medically necessary
Fecal incontinence	Maintain normal bowel function
Pain	Assess and manage acute and chronic pain Identify common causes of acute and chronic pain

KUMC, Konkuk University Medical Center; SFH, senior-friendly hospital.

for Care-10 (GSC-10) was developed (Lee et al., 2017). During the hospital stay, an individualized treatment program is provided by a multidisciplinary team with shared information. At discharge and/or transition, the relevant care plan and education are provided to older patients and their family members. Information on the patient's care needs at discharge is shared with community-based providers and also informal caregivers to promote continuity of care (Kim et al., in press).

Second, along with care process improvement, senior-friendly communication and service are provided, including an escort service for older people and their families when navigating the hospital and fast-track service for administrative and test processes in order to decrease wait time. Third, the hospital conducted modifications of the physical environment to promote safety and convenience (e.g., introducing safety belts, sidebars for fall prevention, chairs for seniors to rest in; Lee, 2016).

In implementing the SFH initiatives, nurses in each unit conduct screenings in 10 domains using the GSC-10 and also screen for safety risks causing pressure ulcers and falls. When older patients are at risk for any geriatric issues, research nurses conduct more detailed assessments for the triggered issues and consult with relevant specialists, if necessary. At discharge, nurses conduct screening of older patients using the GSC-10 again and provide discharge care, including education about medications, what to do in an emergency, which symptoms to report, contact info, and so on. The SFH taskforce also developed and disseminates guidelines for preventive care for pressure ulcers, fall, pain, dysphagia, functional decline, cognitive issues, and incontinence, which staff nurses can use in their practice (Y. Kim, RN, PhD, personal communication, January 7, 2018).

IMPLICATIONS OF NICHE FOR ADVANCING GERIATRIC CARE IN KOREA

NICHE has been mainly a hospital-based program, but it recently expanded to other settings including the LTC setting (Santamaria, 2016). NICHE aims to implement best practices for hospitalized older adults (Boltz et al., 2008; Kim et al., 2007). NICHE designates nurses as the change agents, not for nursing practice only, but for system-wide efforts to improve quality of geriatric care. NICHE is a nurse-led program in which nurses play a crucial role in developing and running programs for clinical improvement, coordinating efforts of interdisciplinary teams, and mobilizing human and capital resources. The geriatric resource nurse (GRN) model is a signature care model widely adopted by NICHE member organizations (Capezuti, Briccoli, & Boltz, 2013; Fulmer et al., 2002). As an education and clinical intervention model, the GRN model involves geriatric advanced practice nurses training staff nurses in a unit to be clinical resources on common geriatric syndromes for other nurses and interdisciplinary teams (Capezuti et al., 2012). NICHE provides a system of services, resources, and networks to empower nurses to facilitate and support a positive geriatric care environment in collaboration with other professions across departments in their institutions. NICHE's success is also because it took an approach to providing necessary support to stimulate changes in practice that can be tailored to an individual organization's goals, needs, and capacities, rather than taking a prescriptive approach (Hendrix, Matters, West, Stewart, & McConnell, 2011).

NICHE is also known for its evidence-based emphasis. Its Geriatric Institutional Assessment Protocol (GIAP) survey can provide an opportunity for a healthcare organization to assess its readiness and capacity to provide quality geriatric care, according to the staff's perceptions (Kim, Capezuti, Boltz, & Fairchild, 2009). Second, a benchmarking service using the national GIAP database provides information on an institution's strengths and weaknesses, compared to its relevant counterparts, in the four domains of the GIAP survey: aging-sensitive care delivery, resource availability, institutional values regarding older adults and staff, and capacity for collaboration (Capezuti, Boltz, Shuluk, et al., 2013). Third, NICHE's evidence-based protocols and best practice models for common geriatric syndromes are powerful resources for nursing practices. In addition, the technical and practical assistance and support for program implementation through an annual NICHE conference, webinars, and a listserv of member organizations are useful (Hendrix et al., 2011). More details about the NICHE program can be learned from other chapters in this book.

What are the lessons and implications of NICHE for the advance of geriatric care programs in acute care hospitals in Korea? An obvious one is that NICHE takes a system-wide approach to improving quality of geriatric care with the endorsement and support of hospital leadership and administrators/managers, with the engagement of direct care staff at the bedside, and with clinical leaders. KUMC's SFH initiative, previously described, took a similar path: the initiative obtained the hospital president's support and a multidisciplinary team from diverse professions was selected for the SFH taskforce. A senior-friendly care process and administrative services, as well as physical environmental modifications, were implemented across the institution with input from direct care staff and leadership groups. KUMC has reported in a preliminary survey the positive experiences of older patients (Lee, 2016), and more rigorous evaluation of the SFH initiative is underway. Except KUMC, few hospitals in Korea are known for making system-wide efforts to improve geriatric care. Awareness of the importance and benefits of quality geriatric care should be increased. Demonstrating a business case for innovative geriatric care programs would be valuable for making hospitals commit to, and invest in, caring for older adults as their core business. Relevant health policies should also be in place that give hospitals incentives to make an effort to improve quality of care and reduce low-value care.

Second, NICHE is a nurse-driven program to improve care for older patients. It suggests Korean hospitals should consider giving nurses more active roles as change agents in system-wide efforts to improve geriatric care. Nurses are the largest group of the hospital workforce, and many of them work closely with patients at bedside in both Korea and the United States. NICHE demonstrates the huge potential of empowering and increasing the competency of direct nursing care staff, nurse clinical leaders, and clinical educators in improving quality of geriatric care. The GRN model, in which a staff nurse is trained as an educator and consultant for geriatric care in a unit (Capezuti et al., 2012), also seems applicable for Korean acute care hospitals. Nursing leaders and hospital administrators in Korea should examine the benefits of a nurse-led approach in improving geriatric care and also assess the feasibility and usability of such approaches as well as any modifications that may be necessary for successful implementation in Korea's clinical context.

Several key features of NICHE give insights for the direction of efforts to advance geriatric care programs in acute care hospitals in Korea.

Third, several key features of NICHE give insights for the direction of efforts to advance geriatric care programs in acute care hospitals in Korea. It is critical to secure the support of senior hospital leadership and the chief nursing officer for SFH initiatives or system-wide programs to improve geriatric care quality. Assessing institutional readiness for senior-friendly care (e.g., NICHE's GIAP survey) at the beginning of SFH initiatives would be informative. Rich educational programs, evidence-based resources for best practice, an online knowledge center, and webinars are strong foundations for increasing the competency of nurses in leading innovative geriatric care quality programs.

CHAPTER SUMMARY

As population aging is a shared concern, cross-national learning about innovative geriatric models that work in practice in one country is informative and gives new insights for other countries in advancing their own practice. On the other hand, different practice environments, health systems and policies, and cultural contexts should also be carefully considered in assessing what we can learn from each other and how the lessons can be translated into each country's context, in light of its respective needs.

This chapter presented two leading geriatric care programs at acute care settings in Korea and also discussed the lessons learned from NICHE for advancing geriatric care programs in Korea. The full NICHE program is not likely to be easily replicated in other countries, including Korea, as the success of NICHE is rooted in the achievements of the U.S. geriatric nursing community as a whole in advancing geriatric nursing science and the profession in academia and practice. The valuing of geriatric nursing care in the United States is also well demonstrated by the consistent financial support of the NICHE headquarters at New York University College of Nursing (NYUCN), from The John A. Harford Foundation, and numerous other sources over the past two decades (Capezuti, Boltz, et al., 2013). Yet the important roles and potential of nurses in chronic care management and coordination of complex care for older adults have been reported and discussed in academia and among policy makers in various countries (Institute of Medicine, 2011; Kang & Kim, 2014; McGilton et al., 2016; Yoo & Kim, 2016). For those countries, including Korea, NICHE can give new insights into how to promote geriatric nursing care in our own countries. As a part of such efforts, several features of NICHE discussed in this chapter can be adopted, tailored, and tested for each country's needs and contexts in order to educate and empower clinical nurses to contribute to system-wide improvements in geriatric care in collaboration with other professions.

ACKNOWLEDGMENTS

I appreciate Professor Kwang-il Kim and Ms. Hyun Jung Yoo at SNUBH and Professor Jongmin Lee and Dr. Yoon-Sook Kim at KUMC for their generous support in providing information on the geriatric care programs at their institutions.

REFERENCES

Boltz, M., Capezuti, E., Bowar-Ferres, S., Norman, R., Secic, M., Kim, H., . . . Fulmer, T. (2008). Changes in the geriatric care environment associated with NICHE (Nurses Improving Care for HealthSystem Elders). *Geriatric Nursing, 29*(3), 176–185. doi:10.1016/j.gerinurse.2008.02.002

British Columbia Provincial Seniors Hospital Care Working Group. (2012). Hospital care for seniors: 48/6 Approach. Retrieved from https://bcpsqc.ca/wp-content/uploads/2018/05/Key-Messages-for-48_6-24Sept2012-1.pdff

Capezuti, E., Boltz, M., Cline, D., Dickson, V. V., Rosenberg, M.-C., Wagner, L., . . . Nigo-lian, C. (2012). Nurses Improving Care for Healthsystem Elders: A model for optimis-ing the geriatric nursing practice environment. *Journal of Clinical Nursing, 21*(21–22), 3117–3125. doi:10.1111/j.1365-2702.2012.04259.x

Capezuti, E., Boltz, M., Shuluk, J., Denysyk, L., Brouwer, J. P., Roberts, M.-C., . . . Secic, M. (2013). Utilization of a benchmarking database to inform NICHE implementation. *Research in Gerontological Nursing, 6*(3), 198–208. doi:10.3928/19404921-20130607-01

Capezuti, E. A., Briccoli, B., & Boltz, M. P. (2013). Nurses Improving the Care of Healthsys-tem Elders: Creating a sustainable business model to improve care of hospitalized older adults. *Journal of the American Geriatrics Society, 61*(8), 1387–1393. doi:10.1111/jgs.12324

Chiou, S.-T., & Chen, L.-K. (2009). Towards age-friendly hospitals and health services. *Archives of Gerontology and Geriatrics, 49* (Suppl. 2), S3–S6. doi:10.1016/S0167-4943(09)70004-4

Choi, J.-Y., Cho, K.-J., Kim, S.-W., Yoon, S.-J., Kang, M.-G., Kim, K.-I., . . . Kim, C.-H. (2017). Prediction of mortality and postoperative complications using the hip-multidimen-sional frailty score in elderly patients with hip fracture. *Scientific Reports, 7,* 42966. doi:10.1038/srep42966

Choi, J.-Y., Yoon, S.-J., Kim, S.-W., Jung, H.-W., Kim, K.-I., Kang, E., . . . Kim, C.-H. (2015). Pre-diction of postoperative complications using multidimensional frailty score in older female cancer patients with American Society of Anesthesiologists physical status class 1 or 2. *Journal of the American College of Surgeons, 221*(3), 652–660.e2. doi:10.1016/j.jamcollsurg.2015.06.011

Chung, K., Oh, Y., Kang, E., Kim, J., Sunwoo, D., Oh, M., . . . Lee, K. (2014). *The survey of living conditions and welfare needs of Korean older persons.* Seoul, South Korea: Institute for Health and Social Affairs & Korea Ministry of Health and Welfare. Retrieved from https://wish.welfare.seoul.kr/upload/data/_20150409150150361.pdf

Fulmer, T., Mezey, M., Bottrell, M., Abraham, I., Sazant, J., Grossman, S., & Grisham, E. (2002). Nurses Improving Care for Healthsystem Elders (NICHE): Using outcomes and benchmarks for evidenced-based practice. *Geriatric Nursing, 23*(3), 121–127. doi:10.1067/mgn.2002.125423

Hendrix, C. C., Matters, L., West, Y., Stewart, B., & McConnell, E. S. (2011). The Duke-NICHE program: An academic-practice collaboration to enhance geriatric nursing care. *Nursing Outlook, 59*(3), 149–157. doi:10.1016/j.outlook.2011.02.007

Institute of Medicine. (2011). *The future of nursing: Leading change, advancing health.* Washington, DC: National Academies Press.

Jang, S.-N. (2016). Korean Longitudinal Study of Ageing (KLoSA): Overview of research design and contents. In N. A. Pachana (Ed.), *Encyclopedia of geropsychology* (pp. 1–9). Singapore: Springer.

Jung, Y.-S. (2017). Comprehensive review of prescribed medications for older adults can reduce drug cost. *Medicine Magazine.* Retrieved from http://www.bosa.co.kr/news/articleView.html?idxno=2073601

Kang, S. B., & Kim, H. (2014). The relationship between home-visit nursing services and health care utilization among nursing service recommended beneficiaries of the public long-term care insurance. *Korean Academy of Health Policy and Management, 24*(3), 283–290. doi: 10.4332/KJHPA.2014.24.3.283

Kim, H. (in press). Ten years of public long-term care insurance in South Korea: An overview and future policy agenda. In T. Hu (Ed.), *Health care reforms and health policy research in Asia.* Singapore: World Scientific Publishing.

Kim, H., Capezuti, E., Boltz, M., & Fairchild, S. (2009). The nursing practice environment and nurse-perceived quality of geriatric care in hospitals. *Western Journal of Nursing Research, 31*(4), 480–495. doi:10.1177/0193945909331429

Kim, H., Capezuti, E., Boltz, M., Fairchild, S., Fulmer, T., & Mezey, M. (2007). Factor structure of the geriatric care environment scale. *Nursing Research, 56*(5), 339–347. doi:10.1097/01.NNR.0000289500.37661.aa

Kim, H., & Cheng, S-H. (2018). Assessing quality of primary diabetes care in South Korea and Taiwan using avoidable hospitalizations. *Health Policy, 122*(11), 1222–1231. doi: 10.1016/j.healthpol.2018.09.009

Kim, H., Park, S.-M., Jang, S.-N., & Kwon, S. (2011). Depressive symptoms, chronic medical illness, and health care utilization: Findings from the Korean Longitudinal Study of Ageing (KLoSA). *International Psychogeriatrics, 23*(8), 1285–1293. doi:10.1017/S1041610211000123

Kim, S.-W., Han, H.-S., Jung, H.-W., Kim, K.-I., Hwang, D. W., Kang, S.-B., & Kim, C.-H. (2014). Multidimensional frailty score for the prediction of postoperative mortality risk. *JAMA Surgery, 149*(7), 633–640. doi:10.1001/jamasurg.2014.241

Kim, Y. S., Lee, J., Moon, Y., Kim, H. J., Shin, J., Park, J-M., et al. (in press). Development of senior-specific, citizen-oriented healthcare service system in South Korea based on the Canadian 48/6 Model of Care.

Kontis, V., Bennett, J. E., Mathers, C. D., Li, G., Foreman, K., & Ezzati, M. (2017). Future life expectancy in 35 industrialised countries: Projections with a Bayesian model ensemble. *The Lancet, 389*(10076), 1323–1335. doi:10.1016/S0140-6736(16)32381-9

Lee, J. (2016). *Senior-friendly care process in the acute care hospital setting.* Paper presented at the 25th Aging Society Forum—Senior-friendly healthcare services: Current status and future agenda. Seoul, South Korea.

Lee, J., Kim, Y.-S., Choi, J., Moon, Y., Park, J.-M., Uhm, K. E., . . . Han, S.-H. (2017). Development of screening tool for the elderly based on 48/6 Model of Care: The Geriatric Screening for Care-10 (GSC-10). *Ponte Academic Journal, 73*(7), 234–244. doi:10.21506/j.ponte.2017.7.14

McGilton, K. S., Bowers, B. J., Heath, H., Shannon, K., Dellefield, M. E., Prentice, D., . . . Mueller, C. A. (2016). Recommendations from the International Consortium on Professional Nursing Practice in long-term care homes. *Journal of the American Medical Directors Association, 17*(2), 99–103. doi:10.1016/j.jamda.2015.11.001

Na, S., & Kwon, S. (2015). *Building systems for universal health coverage in South Korea*. Retrieved from http://documents.worldbank.org/curated/en/367221468186565282/pdf/98266-WP-Box385353B-PUBLIC-UHC-in-South-Korea.pdf

Organization for Economic Cooperation and Development. (2017). *Health at a glance 2017: OECD indicators*. Paris, France: OECD Publishing.

Park, J.-E., Kim, H., Ryu, Y., & Cho, S.-I. (2016). Factors associated with hypertension control by sex: A systematic review. *Health and Social Welfare Review, 36*(2), 581–613. doi:10.15709/hswr.2016.36.2.581

Park, Y., & Kim, H. (2016). Gender differences in healthy lifestyle clusters and their relationship with depressive symptoms among middle-aged and older adults in Korea. *Korean Journal of Health Education and Promotion, 33*(1), 1–12. doi:10.14367/kjhep.2016.33.1.1

Santamaria, J. (2016). The Nurses Improving Care for Healthsystem Elders (NICHE) long-term care designation program. *Geriatric Nursing, 37*(6), 507. doi:10.1016/j.gerinurse.2016.10.004

Statistics Korea. (2016). 2016 statistics on the aged. Retrieved from http://kostat.go.kr/portal/eng/pressReleases/1/index.board?bmode=read&aSeq=358082

Statistics Korea. (2017). 2017 statistics on the aged [press release]. Retrieved from http://kostat.go.kr/portal/eng/pressReleases/1/index.board?bmode=read&aSeq=363974

Won, C. W., Lee, Y., Choi, J., Kim, K. W., Park, Y., Park, H., . . . Jang, H. C. (2016). Starting construction of frailty cohort for elderly and intervention study. *Annals of Geriatric Medicine and Research, 20*(3), 114–117. doi:10.4235/agmr.2016.20.3.114

World Bank. (2016). Live longer and prosper: Aging in East Asia and Pacific. Retrieved from https://openknowledge.worldbank.org/handle/10986/23133

World Bank. (2017). World Bank open data. Retrieved from https://data.worldbank.org

World Health Organization. (2015). *World report on ageing and health*. Retrieved from http://apps.who.int/iris/bitstream/10665/186463/1/9789240694811_eng.pdf?ua=1

Yoo, A., & Kim, H. (2016). Factors associated with physical restraints use of older adults in nursing homes and long-term care hospitals. *Korean Journal of Health Economics and Policy, 22*(1), 39–58.

Evaluation — Are We Reaching Our Target?

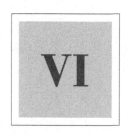

Program Evaluation, Dissemination, and Implementation Science: Concepts and Models to Evaluate NICHE Programs in Healthcare Organizations

18

Peri Rosenfeld

*Under the brilliant direction of Dr. Terry Fulmer, laid the foundation for repairing
a fragmented and unscientific approach to the care of older adults. These efforts
have led to an improved understanding of the unique needs of the elderly and the
availability of evidence-based practice interventions to support these needs.
The resulting impact is improved geriatric nursing care today, tomorrow,
and in the many years to come for older adults across settings.*

—Meredith Wallace Kazer, PhD, APRN, FAAN, Dean & Professor,
American Association of Colleges of Nursing-Wharton Executive Leadership Fellow,
Fairfield University, Marion Peckham Egan School of Nursing and Health Studies

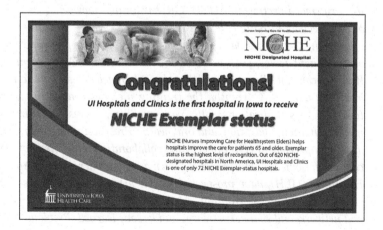

1. Describe trends in the development of translational research
2. Discuss dissemination and implementation science as it pertains to hospital program evaluation
3. Review concepts, frameworks, and models to increase the effective diffusion and integration of evidence-based practices
4. Provide examples of how implementation science pertains to the Nurses Improving Care for Healthsystem Elders (NICHE) program

INTRODUCTION

The NICHE program seeks to improve eldercare practices in healthcare organizations (or health systems) through nurse-specific educational and training programs, as well as consultation services and access to evidence-based resources. Most commonly, NICHE's geriatric resource nurse (GRN) model is adopted to train registered nurses (RNs) to serve as leaders of interdisciplinary teams and frontrunners of changes. As described in Chapters 8 and 9, GRN training focuses on enhancing the ability of RNs to recognize geriatric syndromes and conditions and promoting interprofessional collaboration to address challenges in patient care and influence organizational responses to emerging geriatric issues.

A significant component of the GRN skill set involves knowledge of nurse sensitive indicators (NSIs), which are measures and indicators that reflect the structure, processes, and outcomes of nursing care (Montalvo, 2007) with particular focus on the elderly. With regard to clinical outcomes, NSIs often focus on adverse events associated with nursing practices, including medication errors, falls, pressure injuries, and iatrogenic infections such as central line-associated bloodstream infection (CLABSI) and catheter-associated urinary tract infection (CAUTI). GRN training, however, goes beyond NSIs to include other aspects of nursing care as it relates to the geriatric population. GRNs learn, among other things, evidence-based geriatric practices, the appropriate use and interpretation of assessment tools—such as SPICES, the Confusion Assessment Measure (CAM), the Braden Scale, and Beers—and other clinical knowledge specific to the care of older adults and their families. Currently, the training includes completing four online modules on topics such as medications, falls, pain, mobility, depression/delirium/dementia, incontinence, nutrition, hydration, and oral health. Prospective GRNs are encouraged to conduct quality improvement (QI) projects and collaboration with interprofessional members of the care team. Some NICHE programs, such as the one here at New York University Langone Health (NYULH), have prospective GRNs attend seminars on selected, timely topics to supplement the online training. At the annual NICHE national conference, GRNs meet and network, and share experiences and lessons learned. Previous chapters provide greater detail on GRN training and expectations.

Once trained, as the name implies, GRNs are expected to serve as geriatric experts and resources to RNs, patient care technicians, and other unit-based personnel. Many sit for the national American Nurses Credentialing Center (ANCC) Geriatric Nurse Certification. NICHE organizations that invest in expanding their numbers of GRNs create a workforce with enhanced geriatric knowledge that prepares them for a wide range of activities. The underlying premise is that after acquiring new knowledge and skill, GRNs will disseminate and implement their newly learned practices on their respective units and, together with GRNs in other units, collectively influence practice in their organizations. In other words, GRN training prepares them to disseminate and integrate geriatric evidence-based practices (EBPs) in their respective units and, with multiple GRNs, beyond.

In reality, if the ultimate goal is to create culture change in NICHE organizations, the training of GRNs to possess the appropriate knowledge and competence is the relatively easy part. Even when armed with EBPs and tools, changing practice is difficult. GRNs are expected, to some extent, to lead change—on their units and elsewhere—disseminating their heightened knowledge of geriatric nursing and implementing available EBPs. Measuring patient outcomes is important but understanding the effectiveness of program elements, such as fidelity (i.e., consistency to processes) and sustainability, is often neglected. In the practice arena, tying outcomes to specific nursing processes can be difficult particularly in light of weak or absent standards of care. Lack of attention to fidelity and standardization can lead to variations in outcomes and jeopardizes the likelihood of sustainability. The success of GRNs to disseminate and implement practice changes depends on many organizational factors that can facilitate or impede progress. Anticipating and examining these potential facilitators and barriers can help boost the success of any NICHE program.

This chapter outlines recent developments in a relatively new area within the field of program evaluation known broadly as "translational research," including dissemination and implementation science (D&I). D&I provides concepts, frameworks, and models to increase the likelihood of effective diffusion and integration of EBPs, as embodied in programs such as NICHE.

DISSEMINATION AND IMPLEMENTATION

The field of D&I science is related to traditional program evaluation research and focuses on assessing how well initiatives and programs meet their desired outcomes. While proponents of EBPs focus on evaluating the strength of available evidence for particular practices or settings, D&I posits that effective use of EBP and other innovative practices does not organically spread across institutions; they require a systematic approach to getting the word out and promoting standardized processes to implementing change. Each year, healthcare systems devote significant amounts of resources to conduct research and identify EBP to improve service delivery, patient outcomes, and other measures. However, relatively little is known about how best to ensure that these EBPs, as well as findings of studies and projects, are disseminated in a standardized manner and integrated into the delivery of care services.

Relatively little is known about how best to ensure that these EBPs, as well as findings of studies and projects, are disseminated in a standardized manner and integrated into the delivery of care services.

Dissemination science connotes the systematic study of processes and factors that lead to the widespread use of an evidence-based intervention by the target population. Its focus is to identify the best methods that enhance the uptake and utilization of the intervention (Schillinger, 2010). *Implementation science* seeks to understand the processes and factors that are associated with successful integration of evidence-based interventions within a particular setting. *Implementation* also assesses whether the core components of the original intervention were faithfully incorporated into the real-world setting (Schillinger, 2010). Similarly, implementation research can help identify barriers to, and enablers of, effective adoption of evidence-based innovations.

In short, D&I research provides frameworks to examine, understand, and overcome barriers to the adoption, adaptation, integration, scale-up, and sustainability of innovation and evidence-based interventions, tools, policies, and guidelines. Simply put, D&I asks: how are new scientific discoveries and advances translated and transferred to people and settings to improve healthcare outcomes (Brownson, Colditz, & Proctor, 2012; Luke, 2012; Meissner et al., 2013)? All too often innovations and efforts at EBP die on the vine due to the absence of a well-grounded dissemination plan and/or insufficient attention paid to implementation fidelity (Breitenstein, Fogg, et al., 2010; Breitenstein, Gross, et al., 2010).

> *Simply put, D&I asks: how are new scientific discoveries and advances translated and transferred to people and settings to improve healthcare outcomes.*

Many attempts to implement specific interventions that have been found to be effective in research studies fail to translate into meaningful patient care outcomes. It is important to examine not only summative outcomes but also formative outcomes to assess whether there was an effective implementation plan that is specific to the setting, prolongs sustainability, and promotes dissemination into other settings (Damschroder et al., 2009).

The NICHE program, particularly as implemented at individual healthcare institutions, is predicated on the notion that EBP and practice change hinge on GRN knowledge and expertise of geriatric nursing assessments and practices. With its emphasis on EBP tools and common curricula to increase geriatric nursing knowledge, NICHE programs frequently neglect formal program evaluation. NICHE organizations may benefit from the systematic approaches of D&I that examine factors associated with successful adoption of EBP and innovative ideas. Some of the concepts and models associated with D&I follow as they relate to the integration of NICHE programs in healthcare organizations.

> *NICHE organizations may benefit from the systematic approaches of D&I that examine factors associated with successful adoption of EBP and innovative ideas.*

There is widespread recognition that scientific research findings often languish for years before being translated into practice and that more effective methods of diffusion of EBPs and innovative ideas are necessary. This emphasis on translating research into practice stimulated wide-ranging ideas about effective methods to disseminate and implement innovation and EBP. The next section presents some of the early and current approaches in the field.

ROGERS'S DIFFUSION OF INNOVATIONS THEORY

"Diffusion of innovations" is a theory that seeks to explain how, why, and at what rate new ideas spread (Rogers, 2003). Typically seen through the lens of introducing technological changes, the diffusion of innovation theory has value to practice changes, as well. Rogers proposes that four main elements influence the spread of a new idea: (a) the innovation itself, (b) the communication channels, (c) time, and (d) the social system. Inherent in the theory, the speed with which innovations are adopted (or change is produced) is related to the nature of the innovation, the way it is communicated, and the environment in which it is introduced.

Dissemination of new ideas to large, diverse groups of individuals, such as RNs and other healthcare providers dispersed in large organizations, is not uniform. Some folks catch on faster than others; some resist change. Rogers identifies five types of responses to change (Figure 18.1): innovators, early adopters, early majority, late majority, and laggards. The theory posits that time to adoption is dependent on the types of individuals involved in the change. Innovators and early adopters are quickest to accept change, people in the late majority group are typically skeptical about innovation and change, and laggards may be averse to change altogether. An individual's likelihood of adopting innovation is often related to his or her position within the organization, proximity to opinion leaders, and level of education.

The dissemination and integration of new practices, as promoted by NICHE-trained RNs, encounters much of the same patterns found with other innovative ideas. A very small group of early innovators, such as Fulmer, Inoue, Mezey, and others, predicted the future needs of older adults and promoted innovations, such as NICHE (Capezuti et al., 2012; Capezuti, Briccoli, & Boltz, 2013; Capezuti, Bub, & Boltz, 2013; Mezey et al., 2004; Mezey, Boltz, Esterson, & Mitty, 2005; Wallace & Fulmer, 2003; Wallace & Shelkey, 2011). Early adopters, such as the pilot organizations like NYULH and others, recognized the value of the message of the

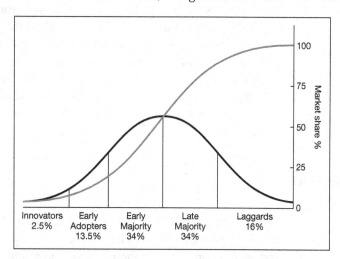

FIGURE 18.1 *Rogers's Diffusion of Innovations Theory: Five types of response to change.*
Source: Adapted from Rogers, E. M. (2003). Diffusion of innovations (5th ed.). New York, NY: Free Press.

innovators and developed programs at their institutions. With over 700 health system members, the national NICHE program is increasingly well known.

However, all NICHE member organizations are not alike and each has successfully adopted varying amounts of NICHE-recommended geriatric practices. A recent attempt to classify the range of geriatric nursing practice changes implemented by NICHE organizations (Boltz et al., 2013) resulted in four levels of NICHE implementation: (a) Early Implementation, (b) Progressive Implementation, (c) Senior Friendly Implementation, and (d) Exemplar Implementation. The progression reflects the varying rates of diffusion of innovation found in different organizations. Though no longer a formal feature of NICHE membership, the four levels correspond well with Rogers's framework.

All NICHE member organizations are not alike and each has successfully adopted varying amounts of NICHE-recommended geriatric practices.

FRAMEWORK FOR SPREAD

The gap between "best practice" and "common practice" hinges on the ability of healthcare organizations and providers to disseminate, spread, and adopt innovation (Massoud, Nielsen, Nolan, Schall & Sevin, 2006). Building on Rogers's diffusion of innovation, the Institute for Healthcare Improvement (IHI) launched a campaign to encourage organizations to proactively plan for spreading new ideas/change and to recognize potential hazards that can impact an organization's success in translating research in the form of EBPs into practice. According to the IHI, among the key issues to consider when developing a "plan for spread" are (a) support of leadership; (b) setup for spread (target population, pilot sites, etc.); (c) strengthening the social system (key messengers, what technology will be used); (d) developing a communication plan; and (e) developing a measurement and feedback system (IHI, 2004). IHI also outlines a range of practical tips for successful dissemination of new ideas called the "7 Spreadly Sins," which identifies barriers and potential minefields when spreading innovations as well as tips such as having realistic expectations and monitoring and refining plans based on feedback (IHI, 2015). This practical "how-to" approach allows organizations to determine their readiness for launching a dissemination/spread project and helps identify potential landmines that can derail their initiative (Nolan, Schall, Erb, & Nolan, 2005).

THE TIPPING POINT

Though not a scientific method, Gladwell's *The Tipping Point* (2000) discusses key factors that contribute to the likelihood that people will recognize and accept change and innovation. The tipping point is "the moment of critical mass, the threshold, the boiling point" when scales tip in the direction of acceptance (Gladwell, 2000).

Similar to Rogers, Gladwell identifies types of people and conditions that facilitate change and identifies types of individuals who enable change and support the efforts of change agents. Gladwell, like Rogers, recognizes that specific types of change agents, when working together, increase the probability of successful adoption of innovation and change. There are the "few" who get things started: *Connectors* are the people who know large numbers of people and who are in the habit of making introductions. *Mavens* are "information specialists," or "people we rely upon to connect us with new information." *Salesmen* are "persuaders"; they tend to have an indefinable trait that goes beyond what they say, which makes others want to agree with them. *Cheerleaders*, and other champions, spread the word and enthusiasm to larger groups of people. These individuals, with different skill sets, are similar to Rogers's innovators and early adopters who see opportunities for change and improvement.

In addition to recognizing types of change agents, there is the "Stickiness Factor" of the message you are trying to transmit. A "sticky" message is one that is memorable and important. Effective, visible programming and marketing are components of stickiness.

Robust NICHE programs typically have strong leaders promoting the program. These connectors, for example, the chief nursing officer and VPs and directors of nursing, are situated in positions that provide access to opinion leaders in the organization. Existing experts in geriatric care (nursing and interprofessional colleagues) may be the mavens that ensure that the science is right, and NICHE coordinators and GRNs may be the salesmen and cheerleaders, convincing others of the value of the desired change or innovation. It is difficult to determine the "stickiness" of the NICHE message in individual organizations. The NICHE brand may be increasingly visible among some healthcare organizations, but it is unknown how well it is understood among RNs and other providers at individual institutions. It may not be necessary to have all the potential change agents identified by Gladwell at your program, though the success of a NICHE program is likely associated with strong leadership, coordination, interprofessional collaboration, and a clear "sticky" message to disseminate.

The success of a NICHE program is likely associated with strong leadership, coordination, interprofessional collaboration, and a clear "sticky" message to disseminate.

MODELS OF TRANSLATIONAL SCIENCE AND DISSEMINATION AND IMPLEMENTATION SCIENCE

Over time, more scientific methodologies and models emerged to study and monitor dissemination and implementation efforts more systematically. Translating evidence-based knowledge and innovation into practice requires a multifaceted approach with attention to both dissemination and adoption patterns (Gonzales, Handley, Ackerman, & O'Sullivan, 2012). Many models currently exist to enable organizations and policy makers to study the progression of their effort to promote change (Aarons, Horowitz, Dlugosz, & Ehrhart, 2012; Brownson,

Dreisinger, Colditz, & Proctor, 2012; Meissner et al., 2013; Mitchell, Fisher, Hastings, Silverman, & Wallen, 2010). One such model is known as RE-AIM, which provides one approach for evaluating dissemination and implementation efforts (Gaglio, Shoup, & Glasgow, 2013; Glasgow, Vogt, & Boles, 1999). The acronym stands for *Reach*, *Effectiveness*, *Adoption*, *Implementation*, and *Maintenance* (Figure 18.2). *Reach* refers to the number and representativeness of the population. *Effectiveness* is the impact on outcomes. *Adoption* refers to the uptake by the organization and staff. *Implementation* refers to program consistency (fidelity) and *Maintenance* is the extent to which a program or policy becomes institutionalized or part of the routine organizational practices and policies. The vast majority of evaluations using RE-AIM do not examine all five components, nor did the developers of the model

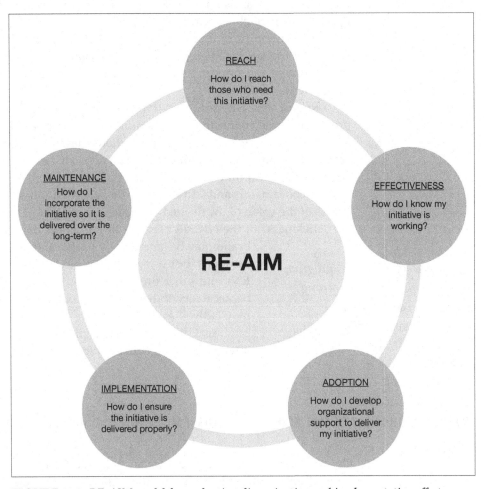

FIGURE 18.2 *RE-AIM model for evaluating dissemination and implementation efforts. RE-AIM, Reach, Effectiveness, Adoption, Implementation, and Maintenance.*
Source: Adapted from Ory, M. G., Altpeter, M., Belza, B., Helduser, J., Zhang, C., & Smith, M. L. (2015). Perceived utility of the RE-AIM framework for health promotion/disease prevention initiatives for older adults: A case study from the U.S. evidence-based disease prevention initiative. Frontiers in Public Health, 2. doi:10.3389/fpubh.2014.00143

intend for it to be comprehensive (Ory et al., 2015b). However, it is useful to consider the range of factors that are at play when evaluating a program designed to impact practice change, like NICHE. RE-AIM shares some of the practicality of IHI's *Framework for Spread* and illustrates that dissemination and implementation are cyclical processes that require consistent attention to feedback and sustainability (Dzewaltowski, Glasgow, Klesges, Estabrooks, & Brock, 2004).

As awareness about the field of translational science grows, new conceptual dissemination and implementation models are now available. Mitchell and colleagues grouped 47 conceptual models related to EBP, knowledge uptake and adoption, and translational science into four general categories related to each model's particular objective and focus: (a) Models on EBP, Research Utilization and Knowledge Transformation Processes; (b) Strategic/Organizational Change Models That Promote Uptake and Adoption of New Knowledge; (c) Models on Knowledge Exchange and Synthesis for Application and Inquiry; and (d) Designing and Interpreting Dissemination Research Models (Mitchell et al., 2010). Using these categories, nursing studies predominantly adopt the EBP/Research Utilization models including the Iowa Model of Evidence-Based Practice, Johns Hopkins Nursing Evidence-Based Practice Model and Guidelines, and Stetler's Model of Research Utilization (Mitchell et al., 2010). Rogers's diffusion of innovation is an example of models that promote uptake and adoption of new knowledge. Among the most popular models in the area of designing and interpreting dissemination research are RE-AIM and the Consolidated Framework for Implementation Research (CFIR).

As the field became more complex, the developers of CFIR conducted a meta-analysis of 18 different D&I theories to identify areas of overlap and inconsistencies in terminology and definitions (Damschroder et al., 2009). As a result of this meta-analysis, CFIR is something of a warehouse that provides clear identification of constructs and definitions to assist in evaluating processes and outcomes of implementing innovations in organizations, large and small. Studies that adopt CFIR standard definitions and common procedures can benefit from the experiences of other D&I researchers. As with RE-AIM, researchers and program evaluators select the CFIR components most relevant to the particular objectives of their initiatives and studies (www.cfirguide.org).

CHAPTER SUMMARY

The key takeaway from this review of recent developments in "translating evidence into practice" is the critical need to systematically plan for and monitor the pace and progress of efforts to disseminate and implement new ideas, EBPs, and innovations. Regrettably, many EBP and QI initiatives fail to make the sustained impact hoped for. The early work of Rogers emphasized that diffusion of new ideas and practices does not happen automatically; a variety of factors can facilitate the likelihood and pace of change. Rogers, Gladwell, and others isolated and identified the types of individuals and groups that could facilitate and accelerate the likelihood of translating and sustaining EBPs at the bedside to improve patient and organizational outcomes. Recent developments in D&I science provide more rigorous models for planning, executing, and sustaining change in healthcare settings.

Over the past few decades EBP and QI have become critical elements in nursing practice and RNs are encouraged to conduct unit-based projects to pilot initiatives that address patient and staff needs. GRNs and other NICHE-related professionals are expected to be at the helm of some of these initiatives. However, training GRNs alone will not necessarily lead to diffusion of ideas, produce a tipping point, or effectively translate science to bring about practice change. It is difficult to be a change agent in contemporary high-demand, fast-paced healthcare settings—even when all parties agree that the change is desirable. This chapter provides some of the concepts and resources from the fields of translational D&I science that underscore the importance of integrating program evaluation into any effort to change practice. NICHE organizations (especially those with significant GRN workforces) can utilize these approaches, concepts, and models to evaluate their programs and bring about the desired changes in care of health system elderly.

REFERENCES

Aarons, G., Horowitz, J., Dlugosz, L., & Ehrhart, M. (2012). The role of organizational processes in dissemination and implementation research. In R. Brownson, G. Colditz, & E. Proctor (Eds.), *Dissemination and implementation research in health: Translating science to practice* (pp. 128–153). New York, NY: Oxford University Press.

Boltz, M., Capezuti, E., Shuluk, J., Brouwer, J., Carolan, D., Conway, S., ... Galvin, J. E. (2013). Implementation of geriatric acute care best practices: Initial results of the NICHE SITE self-evaluation. *Nursing & Health Sciences, 15*(4), 518–524. doi:10.1111/nhs.12067

Breitenstein, S. M., Fogg, L., Garvey, C., Hill, C., Resnick, B., & Gross, D. (2010). Measuring implementation fidelity in a community-based parenting intervention. *Nursing Research, 59*(3), 158–165. doi:10.1097/NNR.0b013e3181dbb2e2

Breitenstein, S. M., Gross, D., Garvey, C. A., Hill, C., Fogg, L., & Resnick, B. (2010). Implementation fidelity in community-based interventions. *Research in Nursing & Health, 33*(2), 164–173. doi:10.1002/nur.20373

Brownson, R. C., Colditz, G. A., & Proctor, E. K. (Eds.). (2012). *Dissemination and implementation research in health: Translating science to practice.* New York, NY: Oxford University Press.

Brownson, R. C., Dreisinger, M., Colditz, G. A., & Proctor, E. K. (2012). The path forward in dissemination and implementation research. In R. C. Brownson, G. A. Colditz, & E. K. Proctor (Eds.), *Dissemination and implementation research in health: Translating science to practice* (pp. 498–508). New York, NY: Oxford University Press. doi:10.1093/acprof:oso/9780199751877.003.0024

Capezuti, E., Boltz, E., Cline, D., Dickson, V., Rosenberg, M., Wagner, L., ... Nigolian, C. (2012). Nurses Improving Care for Healthsystem Elders: A model for optimizing the geriatric nursing practice environment. *Journal of Clinical Nursing, 21,* 3117–3125. doi:10.1111/j.1365-2702.2012.04259.x

Capezuti, E., Briccoli, B., & Boltz, M. (2013). Nurses Improving the Care of Healthsystem Elders: Creating a sustainable business model to improve care of hospitalized older adults. *Journal of the American Geriatrics Society, 61*(8), 1387–1393. doi:10.1111/jgs.12324

Capezuti, E., Bub, L., & Boltz, M. (2013). *The NICHE guide: The geriatric resource nurse model. NICHE planning and implementation guide.* New York: New York University.

Damschroder, L. J., Aron, D. C., Keith, R. E., Kirsh, S. R., Alexander, J. A., & Lowery, J. C. (2009). Fostering implementation of health services research findings into practice: A consolidated framework for advancing implementation science. *Implementation Science, 4*(1), 50. doi:10.1186/1748-5908-4-50

Dzewaltowski, D. A., Glasgow, R. E., Klesges, L. M., Estabrooks, P. A., & Brock, E. (2004). RE-AIM: Evidence-based standards and a web resource to improve translation of research into practice. *Annals of Behavioral Medicine, 28*(2), 75–80. doi:10.1207/s15324796abm2802_1

Gaglio, B., Shoup, J. A., & Glasgow, R. E. (2013). The RE-AIM framework: A systematic review of use over time. *American Journal of Public Health, 103*(6), e38–e46. doi:10.2105/AJPH.2013.301299

Gladwell, M. (2000). *The tipping point: How little things can make a big difference.* New York, NY: Little, Brown and Company.

Glasgow, R. E., Vogt, T. M., & Boles, S. M. (1999). Evaluating the public health impact of health promotion interventions: The RE-AIM framework. *American Journal of Public Health, 89*(9), 1322–1327. doi: 10.2105/ajph.89.9.1322

Gonzales, R., Handley, M. A., Ackerman, S., & O'Sullivan, P. S. (2012). A framework for training health professionals in implementation and dissemination science. *Academic Medicine: Journal of the Association of American Medical Colleges, 87*(3), 271–278. doi:10.1097/ACM.0b013e3182449d33

Institute for Healthcare Improvement. (2004). *Spread planner.* Boston, MA: Author.

Institute for Healthcare Improvement. (2015). IHI "seven spreadly sins." Retrieved from http://www.ihi.org/resources/Pages/Tools/IHISevenSpreadlySins.aspx

Luke, D. (2012). Viewing dissemination and implementation research through a network lens. In R. Brownson, G. Colditz, & E. Proctor (Eds.), *Dissemination and implementation research in health: Translating science to practice* (pp. 154–174). New York, NY: Oxford University Press.

Massoud, M. R., Nielsen, G. A., Nolan, K., Schall, M. W., & Sevin, C. (2006). *A framework for spread: From local improvements to system-wide change.* IHI Innovation Series White Paper. Cambridge, MA: Institute for Healthcare Improvement.

Meissner, H. I., Glasgow, R. E., Vinson, C. A., Chambers, D., Brownson, R. C., Green, L. W., … Mittman, B. (2013). The U.S. training institute for dissemination and implementation research in health. *Implementation Science, 8*(1), 12. doi:10.1186/1748-5908-8-12

Mezey, M., Boltz, M., Esterson, J., & Mitty, E. (2005). Evolving models of geriatric nursing care. *Geriatric Nursing, 26*(1), 11–15. doi:10.1016/j.gerinurse.2004.11.012

Mezey, M., Kobayashi, M., Grossman, S., Firpo, A., Fulmer, T., & Mitty, E. (2004). Nurses Improving Care to Health System Elders (NICHE): Implementation of best practice models. *Journal of Nursing Administration*, *34*(10), 451–457. doi:10.1097/00005110-200410000-00005

Mitchell, S. A., Fisher, C. A., Hastings, C. E., Silverman, L. B., & Wallen, G. R. (2010). A thematic analysis of theoretical models for translational science in nursing: Mapping the field. *Nursing Outlook*, *58*(6), 287–300. doi:10.1016/j.outlook.2010.07.001

Montalvo, I. (2007). The National Database of Nursing Quality Indicators® (NDNQI®). *Online Journal of Issues in Nursing*, *12*(3). doi:10.3912/OJIN.Vol12No03Man02

Nolan, K., Schall, M. W., Erb, F., & Nolan, T. (2005). Using a framework for spread: The case of patient access in the Veterans Health Administration. *Joint Commission Journal on Quality and Patient Safety*, *31*(6), 339–347. doi:10.1016/s1553-7250(05)31045-2

Ory, M. G., Altpeter, M., Belza, B., Helduser, J., Zhang, C., & Smith, M. L. (2015a). Perceived utility of the RE-AIM framework for health promotion/disease prevention initiatives for older adults: A case study from the U.S. evidence-based disease prevention initiative. *Frontiers in Public Health*, *2*. doi:10.3389/fpubh.2014.00143

Ory, M. G., Altpeter, M., Belza, B., Helduser, J., Zhang, C., & Smith, M. L. (2015b). Perceptions about community applications of RE-AIM in the promotion of evidence-based programs for older adults. *Evaluation & the Health Professions*, *38*(1), 15–20. doi:10.1177/0163278714542335

Rogers, E. M. (2003). *Diffusion of innovations* (5th ed.). New York, NY: Free Press.

Schillinger, D. (2010). An introduction to effectiveness, dissemination and implementation research. Retrieved from http://accelerate.ucsf.edu/files/CE/edi_introguide.pdf

Wallace, M., & Fulmer, T. (2003). Fulmer SPICES: An overall assessment tool of older adults. *Alabama Nurse*, *30*(3), 26.

Wallace, M., & Shelkey, M. (2011). How to try this: Best practices in nursing care to older adults: Monitoring functional status in hospitalized older adults. See Katz Index of Independence in Activities of Daily Living (ADL) section. Retrieved from https://consultgeri.org/try-this/general-assessment/issue-2

Building and Sustaining a Robust NICHE Program

19

Amy Berman, Carrie Lehman, and Mattia Gilmartin

> *Striving to provide the highest quality of care for older adults is the very heart of what we do as geriatric nurses every day. Over the past 25 years, how many hip fractures have been prevented because of NICHE? How many hospital stays were shortened because of NICHE? How many nurses left their shift satisfied that they made a difference in the life of an older persoan because of NICHE? NICHE provides an opportunity for nurses to take a leadership role on the interprofessional team to implement evidence-based geriatric practice at the bedside.*
> —Ellen Flaherty, PhD, MSN, APRN, Director, Dartmouth Centers for Health & Aging & former President of the American Geriatrics Society

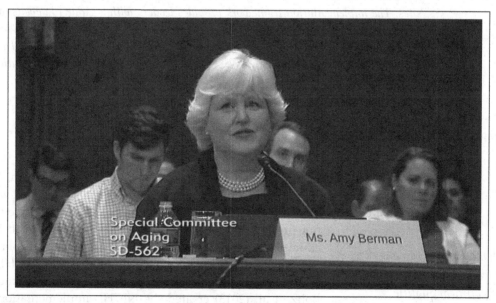

Amy Berman.

CHAPTER OBJECTIVES

1. Define "sustainability" within the context of large-scale clinical practice change initiatives
2. Describe the Nurses Improving Care for Healthsystem Elders (NICHE) program characteristics at the early, progressive, senior-friendly, and exemplar implementation levels
3. Articulate the role of community benefit in sustainability
4. Identify the role of development staff in support of sustainability

INTRODUCTION

NICHE was conceptualized as a nurse-led, interprofessional, system-wide approach to improving care for older adults by improving staff leadership, competence, and processes of care. Initially focused in the hospital setting, and later expanded to address the needs of older adults in long-term care settings such as nursing homes and assisted living facilities, the goal of the NICHE program is to develop person-centered care environments that maximize nurses' contributions to patient outcomes. The challenge with any quality improvement effort is the ability to achieve ongoing sustainability.

The challenge with any quality improvement effort is the ability to achieve ongoing sustainability.

The purpose of this chapter is twofold. First, we present the NICHE implementation framework that is used to guide the adoption and sustainability of the program at member sites. The implementation framework provides leaders with a guide to develop organizational systems and care processes that enable age-friendly healthcare. Second, we discuss NICHE program sustainability with a specific focus on the role of financial resources, including philanthropic support, as a strategy to support ongoing implementation efforts at member sites.

NICHE IMPLEMENTATION FRAMEWORK

Leaders can expect that the NICHE program will evolve in its depth, breadth, and complexity and that there are discernable characteristics associated with each stage of program development. Implementation of the NICHE practice model is not prescribed. Instead, leaders have the freedom to improve clinical services that align with the healthcare needs of the older adults whom they serve to gain full benefit of the NICHE model.

The implementation framework provides leaders with a blueprint to identify clinical quality improvement priorities, establish clinical governance structures, and develop expertise in geriatric nursing practice.

To guide program development activities at member sites, Boltz et al. (2013) created the NICHE implementation framework (see Appendix 19.1). The eight dimensions of the framework align with the NICHE principles of (a) evidence-based care at the bedside; (b) patient- and family-centered environments; (c) healthy and productive practice environments; and

(d) multidimensional quality measures. Designed as a self-evaluation tool, the implementation framework provides leaders with a blueprint to identify clinical quality improvement priorities, establish clinical governance structures, and develop expertise in geriatric nursing practice.

The eight components of the NICHE Implementation Framework are:

- **Guiding Principles**—This dimension focuses on the development and operationalization of the NICHE principles and values that are used to mobilize staff around a shared vision for high-quality, nurse-led care for older adults and their families.

- **Organizational Structures**—This dimension outlines criteria to create an effective interdisciplinary steering committee that is responsible for implementing the NICHE program in local settings.

- **Leadership**—This dimension specifies the roles of advanced practice nurses, nurse managers, geriatric resource nurses (GRNs), and frontline staff to align program goals and quality improvement initiatives on participating units. As NICHE programs mature, the leadership dimension specifies the requirements for regional and national leadership to share promising clinical innovations and best practices among the NICHE members.

- **Staff Competencies**—This dimension specifies the requirements for educating nursing staff and frontline personnel on concepts and principles of aging and care of older adults. Continuing professional education requirements and career advancement systems are also outlined in this dimension.

- **Interdisciplinary Resources and Processes**—This framework dimension outlines the development and use of an interdisciplinary care plan, care coordination, and transitions within and across nursing units and levels of care. The availability of educational, consultative, and material resources, including the use of evidence-based care models, is emphasized.

- **Patient- and Family-Centered Approaches**—This dimension outlines requirements for promoting consumerism through the development of family councils to gain feedback from older adults and their families to shape age-friendly programs and services. This dimension also emphasizes expanding nursing services outside the hospital walls to advance community outreach and population health programs.

- **Environment of Care**—This dimension focuses on changing the physical environment to enhance mobility, socialization, and participation in care activities during episodes of hospitalization, rehabilitation, and extended custodial care.

- **Quality**—This dimension assesses the extent to which evidence-based clinical guidelines, tailored to the needs of older adults, are used consistently on the NICHE nursing units. As the local programs mature, the role of the GRN and frontline staff to lead quality improvement projects is specified.

Implementation Levels

The implementation framework generates information to determine the scale, scope, and sustainability of the NICHE program along the trajectory of early, progressive, senior-friendly, and exemplar levels. The implementation framework is used by the NICHE faculty at New York University Rory Meyers College of Nursing to assess the extent to which the principles and practices of age-friendly care are operationalized on participating clinical nursing units. The NICHE implementation levels are characterized by the following attributes.

Early Implementation Level

In the beginning stages of program implementation, the emphasis is on establishing governance structures, identifying clinical quality improvement priorities, and establishing frontline clinical leadership by initiating the GRN and Geriatric Patient Care Associate/Certified Nursing Assistant (PCA/NA) roles on pilot units. Much of the emphasis in the early stage of program development is on establishing the guiding coalition to advance geriatric care that aligns with the organization's larger clinical quality improvement and population health priorities. Identifying leaders and assessing and educating frontline staff on geriatric nursing principles on participating units is emphasized.

Progressive Implementation Level

As sites mature, the hallmark of the progressive implementation stage includes establishing a comprehensive geriatric acute care model and implementing the GRN practice model on at least one nursing unit. In this stage, sites are using clinical practice guidelines and evaluating clinical outcomes on multiple nurse-sensitive quality indicators on the units using the GRN model.

Senior-Friendly Implementation Level

As the systems and structures to support the NICHE program are embedded within the organizational culture and processes, senior-friendly sites focus on establishing family- and community-oriented programs and take a more active regional leadership role to promote age-friendly care. Senior-friendly sites are characterized by active GRN and Geriatric Patient Care Associate/Certified Nursing Assistant (GPCA/GCNA) programs on multiple units that serve older adults and the widespread use of clinical practice guidelines to support nurse-sensitive quality outcomes.

Exemplar Implementation Level

Exemplar sites are characterized by the depth and breadth of specialized services catering to the older adults. Exemplar NICHE sites have institutionalized and sustained geriatric services throughout the organization. Exemplar sites also assume a national leadership role to advance geriatric nursing excellence by engaging in activities such as hosting regional conferences and sharing innovative nursing practices through publications, webinars, or presentations to the larger NICHE membership.

NICHE Member Recognition Program

To celebrate the commitment and important work that is vital to advancing geriatric nursing excellence, NICHE offers a membership recognition program. The ultimate goal of the NICHE recognition program is to support practice and organizational transformation efforts to achieve senior-friendly and exemplar program implementation levels.

The ultimate goal of the NICHE recognition program is to support practice and organizational transformation efforts to achieve senior-friendly and exemplar program implementation levels.

Members voluntarily complete a self-evaluation report that is used to assess the extent to which the NICHE program principles and practices set forth in the implementation model are embedded in the daily work practices on the designated nursing units. In turn, participating sites are awarded a recognition level and receive a certificate and marketing materials to publicize the NICHE program achievements to key stakeholders.

At the completion of the first year in the NICHE program, new members are invited to complete a survey and submit a practice portfolio to showcase the program structure and progress with implementing the action plan goals developed during the Leadership Training Program. Members receive feedback from the NICHE faculty to adjust ongoing implementation plans, identify barriers to change, and accelerate clinical practice improvement efforts. Existing members at the progressive, senior-friendly, and exemplar recognition levels initiate the review process and submit practice portfolios and surveys to validate the depth, breadth, and sustainability of the NICHE program and to move to the next recognition level. Long-Term Care program members complete a similar self-evaluation process at the end of the first year in NICHE to describe changes in clinical practice and the integration of the NICHE practice principles in daily practice.

SUSTAINING LARGE-SCALE PRACTICE IMPROVEMENT INITIATIVES

"Sustainability" is defined by the Merriam-Webster dictionary as the capacity to harvest or use a resource so that the resource is not depleted. In the context of organizational change and practice improvement, sustainability focuses on solidifying new work processes or performance improvements over an extended period of time (Buchanan et al., 2005).

Sustainability is a significant challenge for change initiatives in the healthcare sector (Buchanan Fitzgerald, & Ketley, 2007). The goal in any effort to improve care is to embed the innovation into operations, making this the default practice. This includes developing or adopting evidence-based care processes and embedding them into policies and procedures, the clinical record, and the quality dashboard.

Several factors associated with both the nature of the change and characteristics of the local context need to be taken into account when deciding to implement and sustain complex programs like NICHE. It is useful to take the following characteristics of innovations into consideration to understand the long-term sustainability of change initiatives.

- Experimentation—The adoption of innovation oftentimes involves a period of experimentation to meet the needs of the local setting.

  ○ *Example*: A GRN implementing hourly rounds may need to test two or three different report sheets to design a communication tool that both fits into the unit routines and is useful for the nursing staff to tailor the interventions encompassed in the hourly rounding program.

- Fit—In some instances, a change may not work as intended or it may have unintended consequences that need to be addressed. In these situations, a common course of action is to either redesign the change so it fits the context or abandon the change and search for a better solution.

  ○ *Example:* A group of GRNs were interested in implementing a medication education program that was successful at another NICHE hospital in the region. The original medication education program relied on one-on-one teaching and handouts with instructions for how to properly take common medications. Because the population characteristics in the two regions were different, the GRNs discovered that the medication handouts were not very effective in getting the key points across to the older adults and families in their area. Thus, the GRNs decided not to use the original handouts in their medication education program. Instead, they created index cards with shorter and simpler directions that included graphics that proved to be a better fit for the learning needs of the local community members.

- Developmental stage—Early stage changes may impede progress of larger, more substantial change that is required at a later stage of the change process. Well-established and mature work processes on local units may be abandoned or undone by larger organizational change initiatives.

  ○ *Example*: The GRNs on a large medical–surgical unit were early adopters of delirium screening and intervention at their hospital. The nurses developed a comprehensive protocol that included a delirium order set embedded in the electronic health record (EHR). When the hospital changed

EHR vendors as part of a larger organization-wide initiative to upgrade the information technology systems, the delirium order set was not included. The GRNs had to work through the approval processes to reestablish the delirium order set within the unit EHR, which took many months to accomplish.

Sustainability of Organizational Change

Observers have identified a number of factors that support or hinder the sustainability of large-scale change initiatives such as NICHE (Buchanan et al., 2005). Factors that influence sustainability of organizational change include:

- Cultural—Is the environment ready to accept the practice change? Do the new practices match the values and needs of the organization? Is there a sense of urgency that the status quo is not acceptable and change needs to happen? Are the performance expectations and incentives to imbed the new behaviors into daily practice clear?

- Financial—Is the change contributing to improvements on key performance measures? Are the perceived benefits greater than the perceived costs? Are there sufficient human and capital resources available to support the change initiative?

- Political—Does the change have the support of powerful stakeholders within and outside of the organization? Are the influential formal and informal leaders supportive of the change and any shifts in power or available resources that may occur with a particular change?

- Context—Is the change consistent with social norms, popular opinion, and the dynamics of local market competition? How might health policy and legislation enhance or hinder the adoption and sustainability of a change initiative? Does the public understand the need for the innovation or new work practices?

- Timing and sequence of implementation—Has enough attention been paid to managing the change process? Has enough time elapsed to assess the benefits, costs, or unrealized improvements of a particular change project?

The process of implementing NICHE is specified in the implementation framework and is the major focus on the Leadership Training Program. Oftentimes, leaders focus most of their time and energy on managing the behavioral aspects of managing change such as creating a sense of urgency, mobilizing stakeholders behind the change, and embedding new work practices into daily practice. Less attention is paid to demonstrating return on investment (ROI) generated by these projects or developing long-range business plans and funding. For the remainder of this chapter, we discuss strategies that nurse leaders can use to identify and garner financing to implement, grow, and sustain NICHE in their organizational settings.

Strategies to Finance Your NICHE Program

Healthcare organizations engaged with implementing NICHE should consider the following questions in an effort to foster ongoing program sustainability.

- How will your local NICHE effort be sustained beyond the period of initial funding?

- How will you measure the value NICHE provides to the organization and to the community? What is the ROI?

- How will your local NICHE program develop new funding sources or potentially generate a revenue stream?

Even as best practice becomes common practice, NICHE sites typically identify funding sources to cover the cost of NICHE membership and implementation of new clinical initiatives related to the care of older adults. Performance improvement initiatives are typically launched with internal resources from an organization's budget, which may cover needs such as staffing, travel, access to outside experts, and membership costs, as well as the costs related to improving care and evaluating outcomes.

During the period of the improvement initiative, it is key to produce clinical and financial outcomes and build a business case for the continuation of successful efforts.

There is a limited duration to budget lines or discretionary funds used in support of performance or quality improvement. During the period of the improvement initiative, it is key to produce clinical and financial outcomes and build a business case for the continuation of successful efforts. It is also critical to cultivate relationships with individuals and organizations that may be able to provide future funding for your work with NICHE. Fundraising is a skill nursing leaders must develop in order to implement capacity-building efforts such as NICHE.

The Role of Philanthropy

The role of philanthropy cannot be emphasized enough. Garnering outside support is a message to one's own community that there is valued work going on that is recognized externally. External philanthropy was essential to building the NICHE program as we know it today and without it, little would have happened related to true spread and scale. Some healthcare organizations are able to successfully garner external philanthropic funding in the form of grants to support NICHE or components of NICHE implementation. Philanthropic funding is considered "soft money" in that the monies are available for use over a defined period of time and are likely not renewable. New resources will need to be secured if the work is to continue and this can take the form of institutional self-funding, with NICHE becoming a line item in the budget. Using subscription fees such as charging for continuing education courses is another way to subsidize program expenses. The ability to identify and successfully acquire funding is of increasing value as nurses are positioned for greater impact and leadership within and beyond their organizations.

Identifying Needs and Matching With Funding Sources

Look at the types of funding you will need and look at the types of funding local foundations can offer. Know what types of funding your local foundations are more likely to approve as a grant. Foundation websites provide a wealth of information about the organization. Ask yourself if your work aligns with their mission, population, and geographical area, and if they have made similar types of grants to other organizations. If a local foundation funds training and has an interest in aging programs, ask for funds to train your GRN, offer staff training, and send a team to the NICHE conference. If the foundation focuses on research, ask for support to evaluate the outcomes related to your NICHE implementation.

Remember that you need a range of resources in order to be successful. Funding for NICHE can be used to support a GRN, educational programming, NICHE membership, travel to the annual NICHE conference, professional development for staff and your community-based clinical partners, and support for the evaluation of the impact of your efforts through development of a dashboard and the Geriatric Institutional Assessment Profile (GIAP) survey discussed in Chapter 5. Even small amounts of funds can garner the attention of leadership in your organization in support of your work.

The Role of Development in Securing Funding

Some hospitals and health systems have a development office that can assist in outreach for external funding. When a health system or setting has development staff, it is important to work with them, articulate identified needs, and share stories of the success or potential of your work so they can connect you with foundations and philanthropists that may be interested in supporting NICHE.

In institutions that lack professional development staff, there are a number of tools you may use to identify local and regional foundations that may be of support. One resource is the Foundation Center (www.foundationcenter.org), which includes the Foundation Directory Online. Another approach is to look at who funds other local efforts like yours. Always go to the foundation's website to see current funding priorities and requests for proposals (funding announcements), and look for instructions on applying for funding. If possible, it is best to speak with someone at the foundation and invite them to see what you are doing (or hope to do) related to the NICHE program.

Community Benefit

In order to maintain their tax-exempt status, nonprofit hospitals are required to provide benefits to the communities they serve. Nationwide, about 2,900 hospitals (60% of hospitals) are nonprofit (American Hospital Association, 2019), and community benefit dollars are estimated to be roughly 10% of the operating expenses of these nonprofit hospitals (Luthra, 2017). Community benefit dollars have been used to cover the cost of unreimbursed medical expenses, known as "free care," and research, and increasingly are used to benefit the community through initiatives addressing everything from health fairs and screenings to addressing social determinants of health such as food insecurity. Every not-for-profit hospital administers a community benefit program and an opportunity for you to secure funding (Young, Chou, Alexander, Lee, & Raver, 2013).

NICHE provides benefits to the community by helping older adults to avoid harm by reducing needless admissions and rehospitalizations and by proactively addressing the unique clinical needs of complex older adults. NICHE hospitals and health system–affiliated skilled nursing facilities should consider exploring whether they could apply for funding through community benefit. Opening your NICHE training to your community clinical partners is one way your work could be covered under community benefit.

According to the Catholic Health Association, community benefit dollars must address an identified community need and meet at least one of the following criteria:

- Improves access to healthcare services

- Enhances health of the community

- Advances medical or health knowledge

- Relieves or reduces the burden of government or other community efforts

For a guide to understanding community benefit, see the Catholic Health Association's *A Guide for Planning and Reporting Community Benefit* (2017).

ADDITIONAL EVIDENCE-BASED GERIATRIC NURSING RESOURCES

Institutions that are not yet ready to become members of the NICHE program, either because they currently lack the necessary internal support from leadership or have not yet garnered the requisite internal or external funding to implement NICHE, should still move forward and begin to improve care of older adults, even as they continue to cultivate buy-in and funding. There are a number of low or no-cost, high-quality geriatric nursing resources that can be used to improve the care of older adults.

- *The Handbook of Geriatric Assessment* (5th edition) by Terry Fulmer and Bruce Chernof. This textbook is a comprehensive resource on evidence-based assessment in the care of the older adult (Fulmer & Chernof, 2018).

- *Evidence-Based Geriatric Nursing Protocols for Best Practice* (5th edition) by Marie Boltz, Elizabeth Capezuti, Terry Fulmer, and DeAnne Zwicker. This text is for geriatric nurses in hospital, long-term, and community settings and delivers current guidelines, case studies, and evidence-based protocols (Boltz, Capezuti, Fulmer, & Zwicker, 2016).

- *Geriatric Models of Care* by Michael L. Malone, Elizabeth Capezuti, and Robert M. Palmer. This text reviews evidence-based models of care for the older adult population (Malone, Capezuti, & Palmer, 2015).

- Hartford Institute for Geriatric Nursing at New York University's Rory Meyers College of Nursing (www.hign.org). Established in 1996 through the generous support of the John A. Hartford Foundation, the Hartford Institute for Geriatric Nursing provides extensive evidence-based information, tools, and resources in support of geriatric nursing education, practice, policy, and research.

- ConsultGeri (consultgeri.org). This is the clinical website of the Hartford Institute for Geriatric Nursing; it offers evidence-based resources including clinical assessment tools and videos of evidence-based best practices in the care of older adults. Additionally, there are educational resources on common geriatric syndromes.

- *Try This Series* (consultgeri.org/tools/try-this-series). Developed by the Hartford Institute for Geriatric Nursing, these geriatric assessment tools with accompanying clinical actions if the assessment has positive findings are available for download. Some clinical sites opt to laminate these helpful tools for use at the bedside. The assessments are also available in a video format with demonstrations of the use of the assessment tools. There are assessments available for specialty practice and for dementia assessments. All resources in the *Try This Series* are offered for free for nonprofit educational use.

CHAPTER SUMMARY

The NICHE implementation framework was created to help leaders at member organizations identify clinical quality improvement priorities, establish clinical governance structures, and develop expertise in geriatric nursing practice. The framework consists of eight dimensions: guiding principles, organizational structures, leadership, staff competencies, interdisciplinary resources and processes, patient- and family-centered approaches, environment of care, and quality.

Following the framework, implementation occurs at four levels: early, progressive, senior-friendly, and exemplar. At the early level of implementation, the focus is on establishing leadership structures and clinical roles and setting clinical quality improvement priorities. At the progressive level, leaders establish a comprehensive geriatric acute care model and implement the GRN practice model on at least one nursing unit. At the senior-friendly level, the member organization is concerned with establishing family- and community-oriented programs to promote age-friendly care. At the exemplar level, leaders have institutionalized and sustained geriatric services throughout the organization and assumed a role of national leadership.

Sustaining a NICHE program requires consideration of cultural, financial, political, contextual, and timing factors related to implementation. It also requires identifying funding sources to match needs, which may involve working with development staff and establishing community benefits of the program.

REFERENCES

American Hospital Association. (2019). *Fast facts on U.S. hospitals 2019.* Retrieved from https://www.aha.org/statistics/fast-facts-us-hospitals

Boltz, M., Capezuti, E., Fulmer, T. T., & Zwicker, D. (Eds.). (2016). *Evidence-based geriatric nursing protocols for best practice.* New York, NY: Springer Publishing Company.

Boltz, M., Capezuti, E., Shuluk, J., Brouwer, J., Carolan, D., Conway, S., . . . & Galvin, J. (2013). Implementation of geriatric acute care best practices: Initial results of the NICHE SITE self-evaluation. *Nursing & Health Sciences, 15*(4), 518–524. doi:10.1111/nhs.12067

Buchanan, D. A., Fitzgerald, L., & Ketley, D. (Eds.). (2007). *The sustainability and spread of organizational change: Modernizing healthcare.* London and New York: Routledge.

Buchanan, D. A., Fitzgerald, L., Ketley, D., Gollop, R., Jones, J. L., Lamont, S. S., . . . & Whitby, E. (2005). No going back: A review of the literature on sustaining organizational change. *International Journal of Management Reviews, 7*(3), 189–205. doi:10.1111/j.1468-2370.2005.00111.x

Catholic Health Association. (2017). *A guide for planning and reporting community benefit.* Retrieved from https://www.chausa.org/store/products/product?id=3156

Fulmer, T., & Chernof, B. (2018). *Handbook of geriatric assessment* (5th ed.). Burlington, MA: Jones & Bartlett Learning.

Luthra, S. (2017). Nonprofit hospitals focused more on community needs under the ACA. That may change. *The Washington Post.* Retrieved from https://www.washingtonpost.com/national/health-science/nonprofit-hospitals-focused-more-on-community-needs-under-the-aca-that-may-change/2017/03/14/4214f3fe-080c-11e7-b77c-0047d15a24e0_story.html?noredirect=on&utm_term=.e1116faee66e

Malone, M. L., Capezuti, E., & Palmer, R. M. (2015). *Geriatric models of care.* New York, NY: Springer Publishing Company.

Young, G. J., Chou, C.-H., Alexander, J., Lee, S.-Y. D., & Raver, E. (2013). Provision of community benefits by tax-exempt U.S. hospitals. *New England Journal of Medicine, 368*(16), 1519–1527. doi:10.1056/NEJMsa1210239

Appendix 19.1

NICHE Implementation Framework

RECOGNITION STATUS	MEMBER		SENIOR FRIENDLY	EXEMPLAR
LEVEL OF IMPLEMENTATION	EARLY	PROGRESSIVE	SENIOR FRIENDLY	EXEMPLAR
DIMENSIONS		ATTRIBUTES		
Guiding Principles	• The institution has a NICHE mission statement that includes the older adult patient.	• The NICHE mission statement has been approved by the governing body of the facility.	• The facility website reflects NICHE membership.	• Previous requirements have been met.
Organizational Structures	• The NICHE Steering Committee includes representation from nursing management, quality management, clinical management, and staff education. • The NICHE Steering Committee has a 2-Year Action Plan that includes measuring specific quality outcomes.	• The NICHE Steering Committee includes GRN representation and representatives from the following disciplines at a minimum: medicine, rehabilitation therapies, pharmacy, and social work/case management. • The GRN model has been implemented on at least one unit. This includes GRN education and mentorship activity.	• The NICHE Steering Committee includes representatives from community-based programs (e.g., home health providers and palliative care). • The process of interdisciplinary, clinical decision making is implemented on GRN units (e.g., weekly rounds). • The GRN model has been implemented on more than one unit OR the ACE model has been implemented.	• Older adult stakeholders are represented on the NICHE Steering Committee. • The NICHE Steering Committee leads a system-level expansion of NICHE program(s) (e.g., geriatric service line). • The GRN model and GPCA training has been implemented on all units with > 40% older adults. • The GRN model has been extended to at least one specialty unit (e.g., orthopedic or neurosurgical).

(continued)

271

RECOGNITION STATUS	MEMBER		SENIOR FRIENDLY	EXEMPLAR
LEVEL OF IMPLEMENTATION	EARLY	PROGRESSIVE	SENIOR FRIENDLY	EXEMPLAR
DIMENSIONS		ATTRIBUTES		
Leadership	• A nurse who has completed GRN training, is certified in gerontology, is in the process of completing certification in gerontology, or is able to demonstrate geriatric expertise provides oversight for the GRN role. • The NICHE Coordinator is designated to lead Steering Committee functions, serve as the primary contact between NICHE at NYU and the facility, and disseminate NICHE materials and resources.	• The NICHE Coordinator and/or other members of the Steering Committee are represented on clinical practice committees or other bodies responsible for policy development within the facility. • GRNs are involved in leadership functions including quality improvement and GPCA training.	• The NICHE program has assumed a regional leadership role by hosting a state-level or network-wide conference OR by taking part in a state-wide quality initiative.	• The NICHE program has assumed a regional or national leadership role through one or more of the following: 1. Has become an official reviewer of NICHE resources 2. Has become a member of the NICHE Leadership Faculty 3. Is a NICHE Ambassador by speaking about NICHE at regional, national, or international conferences (this does not include the NICHE conference) 4. Has published examples of NICHE successes in an article, book chapter, or electronic communication 5. Has facilitated a NICHE Webinar Series
Geriatric Staff Competence	• At least one basic, geriatric-specific staff education program (e.g., NICHE interdisciplinary training modules) is provided in general orientation of nursing staff working on units serving older adults.	• Geriatric-specific staff education programs (e.g., the NICHE Introduction to Gerontology core curriculum course) are included in general orientation of all clinical and support staff working on units serving older adults.	• Geriatric nursing education (e.g., the NICHE Geriatric Resource Nurse core curriculum course) is provided to registered nurse (RN) staff on more than one unit. • Extended geriatric-specific staff education is provided to other disciplines (e.g., NICHE interdisciplinary training modules) on the NICHE expansion units.	• Participation in staff development programs that benefit the specific needs of older adults are integrated into the facility's clinical ladder or nurse advancement program. • The NICHE Coordinator and Managers evaluate the clinical needs of staff to meet the needs of older adult patients.

(continued)

RECOGNITION STATUS	MEMBER		SENIOR FRIENDLY	EXEMPLAR
LEVEL OF IMPLEMENTATION	EARLY	PROGRESSIVE	SENIOR FRIENDLY	EXEMPLAR
DIMENSIONS	ATTRIBUTES			
		• GRNs complete baseline GRN training and 6 hr/y of continuing education in gerontology content. • The NICHE Coordinator attended a regional geriatric conference or webinar in the past year.	• GPCA training is provided on all GRN units.	
Interdisciplinary Resources and Processes	• Information regarding NICHE is provided to other disciplines.	• Interdisciplinary evidence-based guidelines are implemented on medical, surgical, and medical–surgical units for at least two of the following: falls, restraints, pain, functional decline, skin care/pressure injuries, medications, sensory needs, transitional care, and palliative care. • Interdisciplinary care plans for older adults on NICHE units routinely address: falls, restraints, pain, functional decline, skin care/pressure injuries, infection, delirium, medications, sensory needs, transitional care, and palliative care.	• Interdisciplinary protocols are applied to critical care, ED, or other specialty units. • A method of maintaining geriatric-appropriate medication prescribing and/or utilization is implemented.	• Transitional care processes are implemented.
Patient- and Family-Centered Approaches		• One or more of the following is included in the organization's processes: 1. Education that addresses age-sensitive communication 2. Patient/family councils 3. Opportunities within the clinical unit for family to give feedback to staff and caregivers	• Transitional care including handoffs and discharge teaching is standardized and includes validation. • Policies address family involvement in care.	• Protocol implementation includes teaching materials for patients and families. • Specialty geriatric protocols include patient and family education and support tools.

(continued)

RECOGNITION STATUS	MEMBER		SENIOR FRIENDLY	EXEMPLAR
LEVEL OF IMPLEMENTATION	EARLY	PROGRESSIVE	SENIOR FRIENDLY	EXEMPLAR
DIMENSIONS			ATTRIBUTES	
Environment of Care		• A process to ensure accessibility to adaptive devices (e.g., meal aids, mobility devices) and/or sensory support (e.g., amplifiers, hearing aid batters) is implemented.	• The environment of care is an item on the Steering Committee agenda.	• The environment of care—functionality, safety, and comfort—is evaluated by the facility. • The physical environment on NICHE units reflects aging-sensitive principles, including basic safety provisions: nonglare flooring, adequate lighting, grab bars, access to adjustable high beds, call lights and controls, sensor alarms, and use of exit alarms.
Quality	• Two initial self-identified measures are identified as priorities with baseline data.	• Results of program evaluation and reports of follow-up activity are shared with staff, physicians, and other stakeholders. • At least one additional quality measure, beyond those identified in the original Action Plan, is added with both baseline and continuing data measurements.	• Quality measure activity is expanded and collected at least annually on two or more units.	• NICHE quality measures are evaluated annually post-implementation on at least half of units with functioning GRNs. This includes units where GRNs are engaged in personal quality improvement projects.

ACE, acute care of the elderly; ED, emergency department; GRN, geriatric resource nurse; NICHE, Nurses Improving Care for Healthsystem Elders; RN, registered nurse.

Moving to Age-Friendly Health Systems

20

Kedar S. Mate, Terry Fulmer, Amy Berman,
Leslie J. Pelton, and Mattia Gilmartin

John Beard and Alex Kalache have created the philosophy and language to help us
all think about an age-friendly world where older
people deserve and can demand an age-friendly city, community and
health system that are fully integrated across these sectors.
—Terry Fulmer, PhD, RN, FAAN, President of The John A. Hartford Foundation

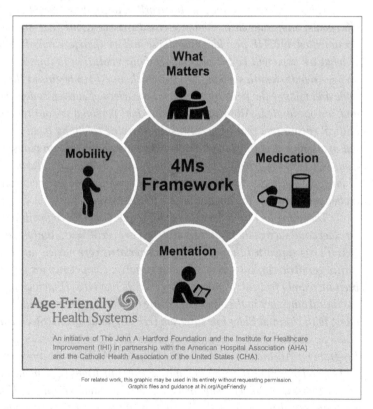

INTRODUCTION

Our NICHE journey has taught us a tremendous amount about the tenacity, will, and leadership required to spread and scale better care for older adults. As a result, NICHE has made many substantive contributions to improve care of older adults and prevent unnecessary harms and common geriatric errors among older adults (Fulmer et al., 2002; Mezey, Fulmer, & Fletcher, 2002). NICHE has also taught us many important lessons about what it takes to truly accelerate the pace of reliable implementation of best practice everywhere (Capezuti et al., 2013; Capezuti, Briccoli, & Boltz, 2013).

There can be no doubt that the work of improving care of older adults requires specific goals, alongside clear, evidence-based interventions that are measurable and clearly documented. NICHE provides all of these and we therefore refer to NICHE as the backbone of what we hope will be the next stage of our evolution to improved care for older adults: an age-friendly health system (AFHS). Such an AFHS begins at the older person's kitchen table and follows the person throughout a variety of care episodes that are often disjointed and uncoordinated. All of us have either had personal encounters or been told stories of clinical encounters that were confusing, directed solely by what the clinician decided and out of alignment with what other providers may have said previously. An AFHS, building from NICHE, age-friendly hospital efforts in Canada and Taiwan (Chiou & Chen, 2009; Huang, Larente, & Morais, 2011), and other foundational evidence-based geriatric care models, seeks to develop an alternative to these experiences.

The examples throughout this book provide clear and compelling evidence for better care for older adults across the healthcare system. For over 30 years, the John A. Hartford Foundation (JAHF) has supported the development of geriatric care models and training for present and future geriatric clinical specialists, and geriatric competence for generalists. This work has been incredibly fruitful, leading to care models like NICHE, which have seen improvements in clinical outcomes in the inpatient setting (Wald, Bandle, Richard, Min, & Capezuti, 2014), along with Hospital Elder Life Program (HELP) for delirium (SteelFisher, Martin, Dowal, & Inouye, 2011; Strijbos, Steunenberg, van der Mast, Inouye, & Schuurmans, 2013), the Program for All-Inclusive Care for the Elderly (PACE) in the ambulatory and home setting, and several programs that seek to improve care transitions (Coleman, 2014; Hirth, Baskins, & Dever-Bumba, 2009; Hirschman et al., 2017; Naylor et al., 2013). These models have been successful in research studies and in numerous pilot programs, demonstrating their robustness across a variety of clinical environments. Some, like NICHE, have been scaled to reach many hundreds of hospitals, affecting many tens of thousands of older adults. But the demographic shifts we face today in the United States and elsewhere demand an answer that can scale faster and more successfully than what we have managed in the past.

U.S. census data show that the population aged 65 and older is expected to nearly double over the next 40 years, from 43.1 million in 2012 to an estimated 83.7 million in 2050 (Ortman, Velkoff, & Hogan, 2014). This demographic shift is due to some remarkable societal and medical advances that have seen a steady increase in life expectancy. But the data on patient safety, overuse and lack of coordination of services, and inconsistent application of evidence-based practice suggest there is more to be achieved. As a result of our aging society, the demand for healthcare services is predicted to rise more than 200%, pushing our national investment in healthcare well beyond the $3 trillion mark where it currently stands (Ortman et al., 2014). Our current system design is producing suboptimal care at great expense.

> As a result of our aging society, the demand for healthcare services is predicted to rise more than 200%, pushing our national investment in healthcare well beyond the $3 trillion mark where it currently stands.

AFHS: WHAT IS IT, AND WHY IS IT IMPORTANT?

In the spring of 2016, JAHF began a partnership with the Institute for Healthcare Improvement (IHI) to create a national movement to retool our health systems to become "age-friendly." Now, just into our second year, our two organizations are pairing the JAHF aging expertise with IHI's national reputation and capacity to spread and scale care improvement (Fulmer & Berman, 2016; Fulmer, Mate, & Berman, 2018).

The project began with a vision of what an AFHS is. We believe such a system is one in which every day, every adult 65 and older:

- Gets the best care possible

- Experiences no healthcare-related harms

- Is satisfied with the healthcare they received

- Realizes optimal value

We recognize that this work will not be accomplished by any one health system, foundation, or organization. We will need the engagement and support of government, other foundations, our health systems, clinicians, social service agencies, community partners, and our older adults and their families.

Our goal is to try to reach 20% of hospitals and health systems (approximately 900 hospitals) by 2020 with a model of what it means to be age-friendly. Based on the diffusion of innovations theory from Everett Rogers and others, we recognize that this 20% threshold represents a tipping point (Moseley, 2004; Rogers, 2010). Beyond the 20% threshold, other health systems will take notice, the public interest and demand for age-friendly systems may grow, and policy makers, payers, and regulators are likely to begin creating a more optimal environment to allow

AFHSs to thrive naturally. In terms of business goals, we expect that by becoming age-friendly, the health systems will develop more sustainable business strategies regardless of whether they are in fee-for-service environments or in alternative payment models. The available evidence suggests that waste and redundancy can be reduced with a concerted effort to take better care of older people across the care continuum with concomitant improvements in communication and data sharing.

To help us define what it means to be age-friendly, JAHF and IHI convened a group of national geriatric experts along with leaders of several health systems, the American Hospital Association, and The Joint Commission at the IHI offices. Prior to the meeting, we reviewed 17 evidence-based geriatric care models to identify the primary discrete features of each care model. We found over 90 features, but after eliminating redundant and similar concepts, there were only 13 distinct features. We then asked the participants in the expert meeting to pick the most fundamental building blocks to optimal geriatric care and we arrived at what we now call the "4Ms." The 4Ms are the content focus of what it means to become an AFHS. The "4M" construct of what **m**atters most, **m**obility, **m**edications, and **m**entation is a simple way to "bundle" many of the most evidence-based and effective concepts in geriatric care.

The "4M" construct of what matters most, mobility, medications, and mentation is a simple way to "bundle" many of the most evidence-based and effective concepts in geriatric care.

"What matters" refers to inviting a dialogue with older adults to determine the focus of their care, while setting and reinforcing person-centered goals of care. We regard this concept as foundational to the AFHS, because the other three aspects of the 4Ms and associated care plans must follow on what matters to the older adult. "Mobility" reminds us of the importance of function to health and quality of life in older adults, and the potentially devastating consequences of falls. Even small gains in mobility can make the difference between living at home versus in a long-term care institution. Many falls that result in devastating injuries such as hip or knee fractures are preventable. Older adults with multi-morbidity often are prescribed multiple "medications" with overlapping side effects and potential for adverse events. Various strategies to reduce unnecessary polypharmacy and adverse medication effects is a cornerstone of good geriatric care. "Mentation" refers to the cognitive and affective disorders that are prevalent in older people across clinical settings. Specific attention is paid to depression, dementia, and delirium across care settings.

We know that these four elements are central to the health and well-being of older adults and also that they are interrelated. For example, if an older person has challenges with mobility, it is extremely important to understand any medications he or she is taking that might affect balance, gait, energy, or other factors that influence movement. Similarly, if an older adult has a change in mentation, for example showing signs of delirium or agitation, it may be that medication is causing the problem. Understanding what matters is critical to developing a treatment plan and a mobility strategy.

Most health systems are addressing these challenges already thanks, in part, to initiatives like NICHE. These systems have programs in place that focus on reducing falls, managing medications safely, and assessing cognition.

More recently, there has been some attention and focus on understanding and addressing patient preferences. Within care settings specific to older adults, this attention and focus has been informed by geriatric expertise. The challenge our systems face is that only a fraction of older adults can be cared for in such specialized care settings. In most cases, the care of older adults extends beyond these specialized care settings to places where geriatric expertise is limited. Our vision is a seamless approach to best practice for older adults where we can ensure reliable attention to the 4Ms for every older adult every day and in every point of clinical contact.

Implementation of the AFHS has begun with five health systems across the United States. These five systems, four large and one smaller, include Anne Arundel Medical Center, Ascension Health, Kaiser Permanente, Providence-St Joseph's Healthcare, and Trinity Health System. Scale-up will begin in 2018 in these initial five systems with planned national expansion beginning in 2019.

AFHS AND NICHE: HOW DO THEY WORK TOGETHER?

We believe that NICHE hospitals are in perfect position to initiate a cross-continuum interdisciplinary approach to age-friendly care. The annual NICHE conference, discussed in Chapter 4, is testimony to the strength of NICHE and the capacity of nursing leaders to make change in the quality of care for older adults in hospitals. JAHF, as previously noted, was the original funder of NICHE in 1992, and has given additional support over the course of the program's development. More recently, JAHF made a grant to the New York University (NYU) Rory Meyers College of Nursing to extend the nursing-led improvements of NICHE to long-term care settings (e.g., nursing homes and assisted living) and we look forward to those exciting results.

The AFHS and NICHE are different and complementary. NICHE, administered by NYU Rory Meyers College of Nursing, originated as a hospital-based, nursing-centered program and continues in most settings to be so, which has brought great strength to better care for older patients.

The AFHS was created to encompass a cross-continuum, system-wide, interdisciplinary approach that begins wherever the older adult is—in the physician office, in homecare, in rehabilitation care, or in inpatient settings.

The AFHS was created to encompass a cross-continuum, system-wide, interdisciplinary approach that begins wherever the older adult is—in the physician office, in homecare, in rehabilitation care, or in inpatient settings. We believe that NICHE serves, along with other major geriatric care programs, as a "backbone" to an AFHS. The active ingredients of the AFHS approach were derived from a thorough review of the core features of 17 geriatric care models, including NICHE.

Many of the features of the AFHS and NICHE are very similar (Table 20.1), which is why we see them as building blocks for one another. However, there are some notable distinctions between the two programs that are

TABLE 20.1 Similarities Between AFHS and NICHE		
	AFHS	**NICHE**
Mission	Improve care for older adults across the system of healthcare.	Improve care for older adults across the system of healthcare, leading with the inpatient care setting, and educate nurses in best practices and position them as leaders to implement evidence-based protocols for care of older adults.
Aims	Provide coordinated and consistent age-friendly care (as defined by the 4M construct) in every care setting encountered by an older adult.	Provide systematic approach to improving care to older adults using NICHE materials developed over 25 years through a membership model.
Dissemination	AFHS principles, scale-up plans, and resources will be available via the IHI website as they are developed. IHI has educational programs and conferences to help disseminate the care designs and best practices. IHI will always feature practical, usable, "how-to" resources that will be freely available to all participating systems and to a wider public audience as we seek to change national dialogue on what it means to have health systems that are age-friendly.	NICHE has a number of resources that can be obtained on a public website, and with paid membership, a rich array of materials on a secured website. NICHE has educational programs and conferences to help disseminate the care designs and best practices.
Initial funding	The John A. Hartford Foundation	The John A. Hartford Foundation
Measures	Uses existing measures and data systems.	Uses existing measures and data systems.
AFHS, age-friendly health system; IHI, Institute for Healthcare Improvement; NICHE, Nurses Improving Care for Healthsystem Elders.		

worth highlighting (Table 20.2). One obvious difference is that the AFHS model and approach are envisioned and shaped to go beyond the hospital admission to reach patients in their homes and community-based settings along with ambulatory care visits and postacute and long-term care. We recognize that NICHE is now moving beyond the inpatient care setting as well and this, we believe, will make the approaches even more complementary going forward.

Both programs bring important resources to support care improvement. NICHE has a 25-year history of convening care teams to consider ways to make change to their respective practice locations using the substantial resources of the program (Boxes 20.1–20.3). Both NICHE and IHI have educational programs and conferences to help disseminate the care designs and best practices.

TABLE 20.2 Unique Attributes of AFHS and NICHE

	AFHS	NICHE
Health system sponsorship	Health system-wide chief executive officer is engaged in the decision to pursue the system-wide transformation of becoming an AFHS.	Chief nursing officer and alignment at mid and unit level is needed to support NICHE. NICHE's nurse-driven model and practice interventions, along with the outcome measures, are specific to nursing practice.
Healthcare setting	The AFHS encompasses a cross-continuum, system-wide approach that begins wherever the older adult is—in the physician office, in homecare, in rehabilitation care, or in inpatient settings. The AFHS is envisioned and shaped to go beyond hospital admission.	Primary focus is the inpatient setting, though it has recently expanded into long-term care.
Value proposition	Provide reliable delivery of age-friendly care across healthcare settings—every older adult, every day, everywhere an older adult is part of the healthcare system. Provide safe and effective care for a rapidly growing population segment through the redirection of quality, safety, and care delivery resources to focus on delivery of proven, age-friendly practice.	NICHE develops the skills/competencies of the nursing workforce and galvanizes setting-specific change that can lead to system change. NICHE has a proven 25-year track record of galvanizing nurses.
Implementation team	Starts with an interdisciplinary approach and can be led by any discipline.	Starts with a nurse-led approach.
Outcome measures	Based on existing measures reported to Centers for Medicare & Medicaid Services and other regulatory and payor entities	Satisfaction and care improvement that are customized to the setting
Core of operations	IHI, Cambridge, MA, funded by JAHF for national movement	NYU Rory Meyers College of Nursing self-funded for hospital-based national movement and funded by JAHF for expansion into long-term care
Content framework	4Ms: what matters, mentation, mobility, and medications shaped into a prevention bundle, assessment checklist, and selected set of high-leverage (affecting multiple 4M elements) clinical interventions	Use of evidence-based assessment and evaluation tools including SPICES (skin problems, problems with eating/feeding, incontinence, cognition, evidence of falls, sleep disorders) and others to identify and address common geriatric syndromes

AFHS, age-friendly health system; IHI, Institute for Healthcare Improvement; JAHF, John A. Hartford Foundation; NICHE, Nurses Improving Care for Healthsystem Elders.

BOX 20.1 Cochairs

- Ann Hendrich, PhD, RN, FAAN, Senior Vice President and Chief Quality/Safety and Nursing Officer, Ascension Health

- Mary Tinetti, MD, Gladys Phillips Crofoot Professor of Medicine (Geriatrics) and Professor, Institution for Social and Policy Studies; Section Chief, Geriatrics

---

BOX 20.2 Advisory Group Members

- Don Berwick, MD, MPP, FRCP, President Emeritus and Senior Fellow, Institute for Healthcare Improvement, former Administrator of the Centers for Medicare and Medicaid Services

- Jay Bhatt, DO, Chief Medical Officer, President and CEO, Health Research and Educational Trust and American Hospital Association

- Alice Bonner, PhD, RN, Secretary, Executive Office of Elder Affairs, Commonwealth of Massachusetts

- Peg Bradke, MA, RN, Vice President, Post-Acute Care, UnityPoint Health—St. Luke's Hospital

- Jim Conway, MS, Adjunct Lecturer, Harvard School of Public Health, Senior Consultant, Safe and Reliable Healthcare

- Kate Goodrich, MD, Center for Clinical Standards and Quality, Director and Centers for Medicare and Medicaid Services Chief Medical Officer

- Maulik Joshi, PhD, Executive Vice President of Integrated Care Delivery and Chief Operating Officer, Anne Arundel Health System

- Doug Koekkoek, MD, Chief Executive, Providence Medical Group

- Lucian Leape, MD, Adjunct Professor of Health Policy, Harvard School of Public Health, retired

- Martha Leape, Writer, former Director of the Office of Career Services, Harvard College

- Bruce Leff, MD, Professor, Johns Hopkins Medicine, Director, The Center for Transformative Geriatric Research

- Eric Rackow, MD, President, Humana at Home; President Emeritus, NYU Hospital Center; Professor of Medicine, NYU School of Medicine

- Nirav Shah, MD, Senior Vice President and Chief Operating Officer for Clinical Operations, Kaiser Permanente

- Albert Siu, MD, Professor and System Chair, Geriatrics and Palliative Medicine, Mount Sinai Health System, Population Health Science and Policy, General Internal Medicine

- Steve Stein, MD, Chief Medical Officer, Trinity Health Continuing Care Group

---

BOX 20.3 The John A. Hartford Foundation and Institute for Healthcare Improvement Teams

- Terry Fulmer, PhD, RN, FAAN, President, The John A. Hartford Foundation

- Amy Berman, BSN, LHD, Senior Program Officer, The John A. Hartford Foundation

- Kedar Mate, MD, Chief Innovation and Education Officer, Institute for Healthcare Improvement

- Andrea Kabcenell, MPH, RN, Vice President, Institute for Healthcare Improvement

- Leslie Pelton, MPA, Director, Institute for Healthcare Improvement

- Richard Scoville, PhD, Improvement Advisor, Institute for Healthcare

- Karen Baldoza, MSW, Improvement Advisor, Institute for Healthcare

- Mara Laderman, MSPH, Senior Research Associate, Institute for Healthcare Improvement

- Catherine A. Mather, MA, Project Manager, Institute for Healthcare Improvement

- Betty Janey, MSW, Project Manager, Institute for Healthcare Improvement

- Kimberly Mitchell, Project Coordinator, Institute for Healthcare Improvement

---

NICHE is a nurse-driven model and the practice interventions, along with the outcome measures, are focused on nursing practice, which has led to great focus. The program develops much needed unit-level clinical leadership, which makes an enormous difference in the processes of leading change. The AFHS uses a theory of change that considers all settings of care and all professional disciplines with the patient/person at the center of care along with family caregivers.

The AFHS uses a theory of change that considers all settings of care and all professional disciplines with the patient/person at the center of care along with family caregivers.

All five of the aforementioned health systems that are implementing an AFHS have NICHE programs, along with other practice models (Acute Care for Elders [ACE] Transition Models, Program of All-Inclusive Care for the Elderly [PACE®] Model of Care, Hospital Elder Life Program [HELP], Better Outcomes for Older Adults Through Safe Transitions [BOOST], Geriatric Resources for Assessment and Care of Elders [GRACE] Team Care) embedded in their systems. That said, what we have found is that not all of a system's older adult population have the privilege of interacting with one or more of these programs and there are many disconnects as older adults transition from one care setting to another. The AFHS therefore focuses on a simpler set of principled actions, the "4Ms," with the idea of universalizing at least this set of core attributes of what it means to provide better care to older adults.

Finally, lack of coordination across the system leads to waste, harm, and lost value to patients and systems. Therefore, this fragmentation (and its attendant waste and harm) across the continuum represents the primary targets that the AFHS movement seeks to solve by guaranteeing a set of essential care principles to every older adult in the system at every point of contact with the system.

NICHE AS THE BACKBONE OF AN AFHS

In summary, we believe that NICHE serves, along with other major geriatric care programs, as a "backbone" to an AFHS in three important ways:

1. The active ingredients of the AFHS approach were derived from a thorough review of the core features of 17 geriatric care models, including NICHE.

2. Transformation of any healthcare system relies on a well-prepared workforce and leaders/managers committed to a strategic agenda to develop systems, structures, and strategies to achieve that transformation. NICHE engages nursing leadership and nurses in those elements of transformation in a profound way and as a fundamental step in the transformation of the full health system across disciplines.

3. The five health systems that are working with JAHF and IHI have NICHE programs, along with other practice models (ACE Units, Transitional Care Models, PACE, HELP, BOOST, and GRACE) embedded in their systems. The system experience unfortunately confirms that not all older adults have the privilege of interacting with one or more of these programs. This leads to disconnects as older adults transition from one care setting to another. The lack of coordination leads to waste, harm, and lost value to patients and systems. This fragmentation is the primary target for the AFHS initiative, which seeks to improve care for older adults by guaranteeing essential care principles (the 4Ms) to every older adult in the system.

The AFHS engages the full care team to achieve patient-centered care and builds on NICHE development of unit-level clinical leadership and the momentum of full frontline engagement.

CHAPTER SUMMARY

Through NICHE, health systems have learned and applied age-friendly practices that have contributed significantly to the health of older adults. AFHSs will build on this deep expertise to spread those elements that are most impactful and replicable system-wide.

The process and outcome of being a NICHE hospital has raised awareness among health system leaders about the needs of older adults. AFHSs will have leaders whose system strategic priorities align with AFHS outcomes. That focus and alignment will ensure that every day, irrespective of where older adults show up in the health system, they will receive excellent, age-friendly care that causes no harm, satisfies them, and ensures value for all involved.

REFERENCES

Capezuti, E., Boltz, M. P., Shuluk, J., Denysyk, L., Brouwer, J. P., Roberts, M.-C., . . . Secic, M. (2013). Utilization of a benchmarking database to inform NICHE implementation. *Research in Gerontological Nursing, 6*(3), 198–208. doi:10.3928/19404921-20130607-01

Capezuti, E. A., Briccoli, B., & Boltz, M. P. (2013). Nurses improving the care of healthsystem elders: Creating a sustainable business model to improve care of hospitalized older adults. *Journal of the American Geriatrics Society, 61*(8), 1387–1393. doi:10.1111/jgs.12324

Chiou, S.-T., & Chen, L.-K. (2009). Towards age-friendly hospitals and health services. *Archives of Gerontology and Geriatrics, 49*(Suppl. 2), S3–S6. doi:10.1016/S0167-4943(09)70004-4

Coleman, E. (2014). The Care Transitions Program: Health care services for improving quality and safety during care hand-offs. Retrieved from https://caretransitions.org

Fulmer, T., & Berman, A. (2016, November 3). Age-friendly health systems: How do we get there? [Blog Post]. Retrieved from http://healthaffairs.org/blog/2016/11/03/age-friendly-health-systems-how-do-we-get-there

Fulmer, T., Mate, K. S., & Berman, A. (2018). The age-friendly health system imperative. *Journal of the American Geriatrics Society, 66*(1), 22–24. doi:10.1111/jgs.15076

Fulmer, T., Mezey, M., Bottrell, M., Abraham, I., Sazant, J., Grossman, S., & Grisham, E. (2002). Nurses Improving Care for Healthsystem Elders (NICHE): Using outcomes and benchmarks for evidenced-based practice. *Geriatric Nursing, 23*(3), 121–127. doi:10.1067/mgn.2002.125423

Hirschman, K. B., Shaid, E., Bixby, M. B., Badolato, D. J., Barg, R., Byrnes, M. B., . . . Naylor, M. D. (2017). Transitional care in the patient-centered medical home: Lessons in adaptation. *Journal for Healthcare Quality, 39*(2), 67–77. doi:10.1097/01.JHQ.0000462685.78253.e8

Hirth, V., Baskins, J., & Dever-Bumba, M. (2009). Program of all-inclusive care (PACE): Past, present, and future. *Journal of the American Medical Directors Association, 10*(3), 155–160. doi:10.1016/j.jamda.2008.12.002

Huang, A. R., Larente, N., & Morais, J. A. (2011). Moving towards the age-friendly hospital: A paradigm shift for the hospital-based care of the elderly. *Canadian Geriatrics Journal, 14*(4), 100. doi:10.5770/cgj.v14i4.8

Moseley, S. F. (2004). Everett Rogers' diffusion of innovations theory: Its utility and value in public health. *Journal of Health Communication, 9*(Suppl. 1), 149–151. doi:10.1080/10810730490271601

Naylor, M. D., Bowles, K. H., McCauley, K. M., Maccoy, M. C., Maislin, G., Pauly, M. V., & Krakauer, R. (2013). High-value transitional care: Translation of research into practice. *Journal of Evaluation in Clinical Practice,19*(5),727–733.doi:10.1111/j.1365-2753.2011.01659.x

Ortman, J. M., Velkoff, V. A., & Hogan, H. (2014). *An aging nation: The older population in the United States* (Report Number P25-1140). Washington, DC: U.S. Census Bureau, Economics and Statistics Administration, US Department of Commerce. Retrieved from https://www.census.gov/library/publications/2014/demo/p25-1140.html

Rogers, E. M. (2010). *Diffusion of innovations* (5th Ed.). New York, NY: Simon & Schuster.

SteelFisher, G. K., Martin, L. A., Dowal, S. L., & Inouye, S. K. (2011). Sustaining clinical programs during difficult economic times: A case series from the Hospital Elder Life Program. *Journal of the American Geriatrics Society, 59*(10), 1873–1882. doi:10.1111/j.1532-5415.2011.03585.x

Strijbos, M. J., Steunenberg, B., van der Mast, R. C., Inouye, S. K., & Schuurmans, M. J. (2013). Design and methods of the Hospital Elder Life Program (HELP), a multi-component targeted intervention to prevent delirium in hospitalized older patients: Efficacy and cost-effectiveness in Dutch health care. *BMC Geriatrics, 13*(1), 78. doi:10.1186/1471-2318-13-78

Wald, H. L., Bandle, B., Richard, A. A., Min, S.-J., & Capezuti, E. (2014). A trial of electronic surveillance feedback for quality improvement at Nurses Improving Care for Healthsystem Elders (NICHE) hospitals. *American Journal of Infection Control, 42*(10 Suppl.), S250–S256. doi:10.1016/j.ajic.2014.04.018

Vignettes

We Improve Senior Health (WISH) Program

Denise L. Lyons

INTRODUCTION

Older adults occupy a majority of hospital beds and are at increased risk for hazards of hospitalization, which include adverse drug reactions, constipation, delirium, falls, functional decline, malnutrition, and pressure injuries. Because of these hazards of hospitalization, older adults have the potential for prolonged lengths of stay and higher hospital costs (Mattison, 2015; Wong, Ryan, & Liu, 2014). Delawareans over the age of 70 make up 13.5% of the total state population. This population is growing more rapidly than the other age groups in Delaware. It is projected that by 2030, 29% of the Delaware population will be over the age of 60 (Delaware Population Consortium, 2018; Substance Abuse and Mental Health Services Administration, 2012).

In 2000 at Christiana Care Health System, patients 65 and older accounted for 47% of all hospital admissions and 50% of hospitalized patient days. Senior leadership knew that this number would only be growing and that it was essential that all healthcare providers at the health system be prepared to care for the specialized needs of this vulnerable population. Unfortunately, most healthcare providers are ill prepared to care for this population due to the limited exposure to education in gerontology (Wendel, Durso, Cayea, Arbaje, & Tanner, 2010). Thus, there was an urgent need to provide basic geriatric knowledge and skills to the healthcare workforce caring for hospitalized older adults. Senior leadership also knew that Nurses Improving Care for Healthsystem Elders (NICHE) would provide the principles and tools to achieve systemic change within the health system in order to provide exemplary care to all hospitalized older adults.

HISTORY

The projected increase in the geriatric population prompted Christiana Care Health system to develop a strategic goal to create a system-wide awareness of the specialized needs of older adults through education of all staff including medical–dental staff, residents, and students. In order to meet this strategic goal, the We Improve Senior Health (WISH) program was developed in September 2001 (Lyons, Blum, Curtin, & Grimley, 2006). WISH was derived from the NICHE program. The WISH program is a collaborative effort among nurses, physicians, pharmacists, rehabilitative therapists, social workers, and other disciplines to improve the care that Christiana Care delivers to older adults in all settings. After 17 years, the senior leadership at Christiana Care Health System is still committed to this goal.

Christiana Care Health System is a not-for-profit large teaching health system based in Delaware with two campuses (1,071 beds), over 20 satellite offices, and a Visiting Nurse Association. Each campus has an acute care of the elderly (ACE) unit. The health system is the largest private employer in Delaware with more than 11,100 employees and among the top 10 in the Philadelphia region. Christiana Care Health System is recognized as a Magnet facility as well as a regional center for excellence in cardiology, cancer, and women's health services. The system is home to Delaware's only Level I trauma center, the only center of its kind between Philadelphia and Baltimore.

IMPLEMENTATION OF PROGRAM

WISH was designed to engage healthcare providers to cultivate a new way of thinking about caring for older adults (Lyons et al., 2006). The objectives of the program include:

- Provide organizational structure that will assist in the development of a senior-friendly healthcare organization.

- Focus on preventing and managing common geriatric syndromes such as delirium, depression, adverse drug reactions, pressure injuries, functional decline, falls, and bowel/bladder dysfunction.

- Ensure that staff is delivering care by utilizing the WISH principles (Appendix A) and evidence-based guidelines regarding constipation, continence, delirium, pressure injury prevention, sleep promotion, and fall prevention.

The key to implementing WISH was the development of the geriatric resource nurse (GRN) model. At Christiana Care Health System, the GRN model of care is referred to as the Senior Health Resource Team (SHRT). The SHRT comprises interprofessional healthcare professionals committed to improving geriatric care within the organization. Over 75% of SHRT members are nursing staff, which includes advanced practice nurses, registered nurses (RNs), licensed practical nurses, patient care technicians, and unit clerks. The other SHRT members are physicians, residents, pharmacists, social workers, rehabilitative therapists, respiratory therapists, nutritionists, and chaplains.

To become a SHRT member, they attend a live, in-person 16-hour educational course in specialized geriatric training. This course is based on the GRN modules from NICHE. Topics include:

- Normal aging changes
- Fall prevention
- Skin care
- Functional assessment
- Depression, dementia, and delirium
- Diversional activities
- Medication safety
- Continence
- Nutrition
- Constipation
- Sleep
- Pain
- Transitions of care

The 2 days of education include poems, videos, case studies, and a sensitivity experience. A Jeopardy!-like game is played at the end to review the information that was taught in the course. The participants receive a SHRT manual, a WISH pen, a WISH retractable badge holder, a SHRT certificate (Appendix B) and continuing education hours. The program is offered six times per year and is taught by interprofessional faculty, including geriatric advanced practice nurses, a geriatrician, a pharmacist, and a physical therapist. In spring 2018, we celebrated our 75th WISH training! Sixteen hours of education will not make anyone an expert so other geriatric educational opportunities are offered throughout the year. These offerings include 1-hour listen and learns, annual 8-hour retreats, and a geriatric review course for nurses. A WISH website (Appendix C) was also created and tips of the month are emailed to SHRT members.

The role of the SHRT (Appendix D) is to serve as unit-based resources to address the diverse problems of older adults on the patient care units (Lyons et al., 2006). In 2001, the SHRT team was piloted on four medical units. The pilot demonstrated positive outcomes in reduction in inappropriate medications, indwelling catheters, constipation, falls, pressure injuries, length of stay, and readmission rates. Currently, there are over 2,500 SHRT members on 12 general medical–surgical units, three emergency departments, five intensive care units, seven noncritical care–specialty units, two geriatric units, a rehabilitation unit, a psychiatric unit, and a medical observation unit. Some of the examples that have been worked on this past year include reduction in falls, pain interventions for older adults, preventing constipation, ensuring medication safety, reducing physician restraints, and reducing pressure injuries.

NICHE COORDINATOR ROLE

The NICHE coordinator (NC) is a master's-prepared nurse who is certified in gerontology as a clinical nurse specialist. The NC provides leadership and direction for all aspects of the WISH program including managing the cost center associated with the program. The coordinator incorporates best practice of the hospitalized older adult to promote positive patient outcomes. The coordinator serves as a role model for the SHRT. The role also includes working collaboratively with other disciplines to integrate innovative practices in the care of the older adult. The coordinator is also responsible for maintaining positive relationships with the NICHE team and NICHE community. The NC's other responsibilities include coordinating and teaching geriatric educational programs and providing clinical consultation. She is involved in many hospital projects that require geriatric expertise such as Senior Steer, system-wide fall prevention team, constipation team, and delirium team.

NICHE EXEMPLAR STATUS

In 2013, Christiana Care Health System was designated by NICHE as an exemplar site for the first time. Our health system was the first to receive exemplar status in the state of Delaware. This achievement was due to the implementation of the SHRT model and evidence-based protocols; implementation of system-wide aging-sensitive policies; and inclusion of input from patients and families in planning and implementation of initiatives. Since 2013, Christiana Care Health System has maintained exemplar status. The current state of the program is evaluated on an annual basis and future goals are set in order to maintain this prestigious status.

FUTURE PLANS

After being a NICHE site for 15 years, Christiana Care decided to administer the NICHE Acute Care Geriatric Institutional Assessment Profile (GIAP). In order for the health system to enhance the quality of care for older adult patients, it requires an understanding of the challenges and obstacles experienced by staff. These GIAP results will highlight where change or education is most needed in order to ensure quality care is being delivered to this vulnerable population. Based on the results, Christiana Care Health System had five areas of improvement regarding staffs' attitudes and perceptions toward the care of hospitalized older adults.

Knowledge

For total knowledge scores, the institution was in the "best possible score" range and considered statistically significant when compared with the other comparative groups. The institution also scored in the "best possible score" range in all six clinical areas with statistical difference between groups in four of the knowledge areas. These findings reveal that the institution has high knowledge scores in the six clinical areas for pressure ulcers, medications/sleep/pain, restraints and falls, functional decline and incontinence, dementia and delirium, and nutrition and hydration.

Attitudes

The institution scored in the "best possible score" range for total attitude regarding the care of the older adult and attitudes about evidence-based approaches in the six clinical areas of knowledge. The institution scored in the "neither good nor bad" score range for attitudes about restrictive approaches and these results were statistically significant compared with the all-hospital group. When compared with the other three groups, the institution respondents have more positive attitudes regarding the six clinical areas. An area that needs improvement is attitudes about restrictive approaches.

Professional Issues

The five factors that composed the professional issues section included disagreements among staff about older adult treatment, disagreements between staff/patient/family about older adult treatment, limited access to geriatric services, perceived vulnerability to legal actions, intensity of behavioral problems, and burden of behavioral problems. The perception scores for the institution were higher and statistically significant when compared with the comparison groups for disagreements among staff and between staff/patient/family about older adult treatment. The perception scores for the institution for burden of behavioral problems were higher than all three of the comparison groups and statistically significant for the peer hospitals by bed size and the all-hospital group.

The Geriatric Care Environment

The four factors that composed the total care environment scale included aging-sensitive care delivery, institutional values regarding older adults and staff, resource availability, and capacity for collaboration. The perception scores for the institution resided within the normal limits for three of the four areas. The perception scores for aging-sensitive care delivery were lower than the comparative groups and the difference was found to be statically significant. Therefore, aging-sensitive care delivery should be an area of focus. Since these scores were low and statically significant, they also lowered the score for the total geriatric care environment.

Based on the findings of the GIAP, a strategic plan (Appendix E) was developed to address the five areas of improvement.

SUMMARY

The NICHE program has provided organizational structure to Christiana Care in the development of a senior-friendly healthcare organization. The SHRT members are focused on preventing and managing common geriatric syndromes and are delivering evidence-based care by utilizing the WISH principles. As the "graying" of Delawareans continues to occur, the WISH program is preparing healthcare providers at Christiana Care Health System to care for the specialized needs of this vulnerable population.

REFERENCES

Delaware Population Consortium. (2018). Annual population projections. Retrieved from https://stateplanning.delaware.gov/demography/documents/dpc/DPC2018v1.pdf

Lyons, D. L., Blum, T., Curtin, P. M., & Grimley, S. M. (2006). Improving care of the older adult. *Medsurg Nursing, 15*(3), 176–177, 181.

Mattison, M. (2015). Hospital management of older adults. In J. Givens (Ed.), *UpToDate.* Retrieved from http://www.uptodate.com/contents/hospital-management-of-older-adults

Substance Abuse and Mental Health Services Administration. (2012). Delaware policy academy state profile. Retrieved from https://www.acl.gov/sites/default/files/programs/2016-11/Delaware%20Epi%20Profile%20Final.pdf

Wendel, V. I., Durso, S. C., Cayea, A. I., Arbaje, A. I., & Tanner, E. (2010). Implementing staff nurse geriatric education in the acute hospital setting. *Medsurg Nursing, 19*(5), 274–280.

Wong, K. S., Ryan, D. P., & Liu, B. A. (2014). A system-wide analysis using a senior-friendly hospital framework identifies current practices and opportunities for improvement in the care of hospitalized older adults. *Journal of the American Geriatrics Society, 62*(11), 2163–2170. doi:10.1111/jgs.13097

Appendix A

WISH Principles/Tools

Avoid complications associated with hazards of hospitalization for older adults such as:

- Adverse drug reactions
- Constipation
- Delirium
- Depression
- Falls
- Foley catheters
- Functional decline
- Malnutrition/dehydration
- Pressure ulcers
- Restraints

WISH Principles

- Ensure appropriate medication usage and avoid high risk medications such as benzodiazepines, hypnotics, or anticholinergic medication etc.
- Maintain functional status
  - Ambulate PT often
  - Obtain order for PT
  - Avoid bed rest orders
  - OOB to chair for meals
- Maintain nutrition and hydration
  - Feed patient
  - Encourage food/ fluids often (if clinically indicated)
  - Move bowels regularly
- Encourage family involvement
- Ensure usage of sensory aids (hearing aids/glasses/dentures)
- Minimize
  - FOLEY catheter use
  - Pressure ulcers
  - Restraint use

WISH Tools

- "All About Me" poster
- Constipation algorithm/protocol
- Continence CPG/FOLEY protocol
- Delirium algorithm/order set
- Diversional activity box
- Falls Prevention, Evaluation and Treatment guideline/post fall protocol
- Geriatric Depression Scale
- Mini Mental State exam
- AGS Beers Criteria®
- Skin Integrity guideline/protocol
- Sleep protocol
- WISH Team Assessment record

Appendix B

Senior Health Resource Team (SHRT) Certificate

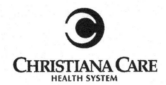

We Improve Senior Health (WISH) Program
Certificate of Achievement
Awarded to
Senior Health Resource Team Member

For successfully completing 16 hours of the New York University/Hartford Foundation NICHE curriculum.

_____   _____
President & CEO   Chief Nursing Officer

_____   _____
W.I.S.H. Program Coordinator   Section Chief, Geriatric Medicine

Appendix C

WISH Website

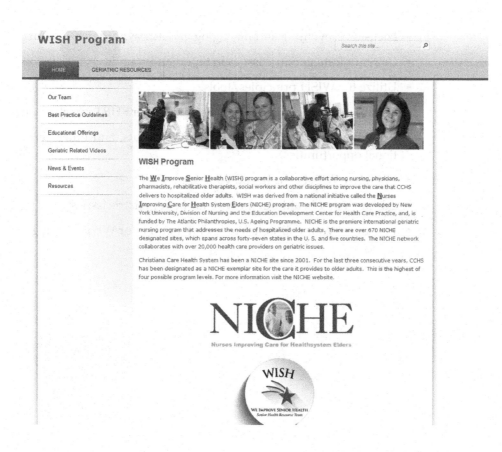

WISH Program

The **W**e **I**mprove **S**enior **H**ealth (WISH) program is a collaborative effort among nursing, physicians, pharmacists, rehabilitative therapists, social workers and other disciplines to improve the care that CCHS delivers to hospitalized older adults. WISH was derived from a national initiative called the **N**urses **I**mproving **C**are for **H**ealth System **E**lders (NICHE) program. The NICHE program was developed by New York University, Division of Nursing and the Education Development Center for Health Care Practice, and, is funded by The Atlantic Philanthropies, U.S. Ageing Programme. NICHE is the premiere international geriatric nursing program that addresses the needs of hospitalized older adults. There are over 670 NICHE designated sites, which spans across forty-seven states in the U. S. and five countries. The NICHE network collaborates with over 20,000 health care providers on geriatric issues.

Christiana Care Health System has been a NICHE site since 2001. For the last three consecutive years, CCHS has been designated as a NICHE exemplar site for the care it provides to older adults. This is the highest of four possible program levels. For more information visit the NICHE website.

Appendix D

Roles and Responsibilities of a Senior Health Resource Team (SHRT) Member

- Focus on preventing and managing geriatric syndromes on your patients.

- Communicate geriatric issues in report and rounds.

- Utilize the WISH principles/tools.

- Collaborate with your WISH Champion/other SHRT members on your unit.

- Attend WISH Listen 'N Learns, WISH retreats, and other geriatric educational opportunities.

- Complete WISH consults on your unit.

- Educate other healthcare providers about geriatric issues.

- Encourage your colleagues to attend the 16-hour WISH training.

Appendix E

GIAP Strategic Plan

	STRATEGY
Attitudes	• Work with unit-based educators to disseminate sleep protocol and mobility program
Professional Issues	• Place a portal announcement inviting all disciplines to attend WISH training • Attend a Hospitalist's monthly staff meeting to review WISH principles • Develop a one-page flyer for patients and their families to highlight WISH principles
	• Develop a clinical pathway for the care of patients with dementia
Geriatric Care Environment	• Work with IT to create an "All About Me" section in the electronic record
	• Meet with staff to highlight the importance of individualizing care regarding the specialized needs of the older population; discuss the importance of involving both the patient and family in making healthcare decisions; promote better communication between staff and patient/family; provide resources for patients and families and listen to staff, patients, and families

Finding My NICHE With NICHE

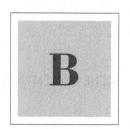

Carrie Hays McElroy

IN THE BEGINNING

The most exciting thing that can happen at work is being excited at work.

Sometimes the workday starts out just like any other day, and then, before you know it, your career dreams begin to start coming true. This was triggered for me on one particular day in 2010 when Dave Spivey, CEO of St. Mary Mercy Hospital Livonia, Michigan, walked in and said to me, "Would you be interested in heading up our Senior Services Programs?" No need for hesitation there, rather a response closer to "This is what my life has been leading to!" However, none of this, of course, is about my life—it is about our journey to improve the lives of older adults we serve.

The genesis of this conversation actually occurred a few weeks earlier. St. Mary Mercy Hospital is a 304-bed general hospital and a member of Trinity Health. Trinity Health, with headquarters located in Livonia, Michigan, is one of the largest multi-institutional Catholic healthcare delivery systems in the nation. It serves people and communities in 22 states from coast to coast with 93 hospitals, and 122 continuing care locations—including home care, hospice, PACE, and senior living facilities—that provide more than 97 million home health and hospice admissions. Senior Leadership from Trinity Health had challenged our Executive Leadership to consider the three things that our hospital should be known as being the best at doing. This led to discussions regarding our older adult population, our current energy with developing a senior emergency room (ER), and how we wanted to provide exemplary care for older adults in our community.

The essential component for successful implementation of programs for older adults is engagement and excitement by the Executive Leadership Team. As we explored what it would mean to be known as providing the best care for older adults, we quickly realized that obtaining NICHE designation would be a vital component of our strategy.

NICHE IMPLEMENTATION AT ST. MARY MERCY

The three *most* excited colleagues at St. Mary Mercy at that time were myself, Michelle Moccia, DNP, ANP-BC, CCRN, program director senior ER, and Sue Klotz, MS, BSN, RN-BC, clinical liaison and education coordinator; we embarked on the Leadership Training Program and developed our first NICHE action plan. At that time, Marie Boltz was the director at NICHE and she reviewed our action plan with us; I recall her giving us very positive feedback regarding the extensive plans the three of us developed. We were totally inspired by Marie and honored that she took such interest in our thoughts, hopes, and desires. The action plan covered all of the areas that we hoped to touch with regard to care of older adults over a span of 3 years. We included goals that encompassed the senior ER, Transition Coach Program, Patient Family Advisory Council, extensive RN geriatric education, comprehensive new hire orientation, delirium prevention program for surgical patients, and development of a Senior Wellness and Resource Center; the possibilities seemed endless. Our greatest challenge was realizing that we could not tackle everything at once. This was compounded when we attended our first NICHE conference in Las Vegas in April 2011. So much energy and similar souls in one place! So many great ideas that we took home with us. Every year since then we have all agreed that this is the best conference we attend.

With that realization of not being able to tackle everything at once, we took a step back and worked on determining our priorities; this was done by aligning our ideas and goals with those of the organization's strategic plan. Improving the patient experience and including the voice of the patient were things that the whole organization was looking into. One of our early accomplishments was the development of our Patient and Family Advisory Council, specifically focused on guiding our senior service programs. Our goal for this initiative included recruiting six to eight representatives for the Council, developing a charter, and commencing monthly Council meetings by the end of 2010. NICHE asked us to write an Organizational Strategy on the subject of Developing a Patient Family Advisory Council, which was published on the NICHE website. Between 2011 and 2015, we successfully implemented the senior ER, which continues to be spearheaded by Michelle Moccia. We expanded the ER attention on recognizing and preventing delirium to our pre-anesthesia and surgical areas. We provided education for over 1,000 new hires on care of older adults including a virtual aging and dementia experience, educated 208 RNs using the NICHE GRN curriculum, and supported achievement of the American Nurses Credentialing Center (ANCC) gerontological nurse certification for six RNs. We integrated aspects of older adult care into initiatives addressing venous thromboembolism (VTE) prevention and increased the rate of VTE risk assessments from 7.45% to 79%; appropriate mechanical prophylaxis increased 50% to 94% and appropriate pharmacological prophylaxis 54% to 79% within 15 months. We also sought grant funding for development of a volunteer patient companion program that was based on the Hospital Elder LIFE Program

(HELP), and developed the Senior Wellness and Resource Center. We presented on a number of our initiatives at NICHE conferences and achieved exemplar status in March 2015.

As we initiated NICHE, there was already a good deal of energy within the organization about the work underway to improve the care of our older adults and the Executive Leadership Team were kept abreast of the NICHE rollout on a regular basis. This helped to maintain engagement at that level, which also was a way to spread awareness of our initiatives across other departments. I feel it is important also to reference our steering committee. We pulled together a multidisciplinary group that included pharmacy, physicians, nurse leaders, patient experience, clinical documentation, human resources, and clinical informatics. Again, this group really helped to develop ongoing engagement and offered very valuable input into the work we were all doing.

The work at St. Mary Mercy Hospital continues, as part of a region of five Trinity Health hospitals which are all NICHE designated, with support and leadership from the Regional Director of Senior Services Joanne Grosh, MA, RN, Gero-BC; within the Trinity Health System there are 18 NICHE-designated hospitals.

EXPANDED NICHE INVOLVEMENT

On a more personal level, I have been honored to have been provided the opportunity to assist other healthcare organizations with their NICHE journey by serving as a Leadership Training Program (LTP) mentor. I started out as a mentor in 2011 with the acute care sites and have more recently transitioned to mentoring our recent long-term care (LTC) facilities. As NICHE began to expand into the LTC space, I also participated on a workgroup to review and begin the redesign of the GRN curriculum to be more inclusive of cross-continuum care settings.

In 2015, I was called to serve in a new role as VP clinical operations/chief nursing officer (CNO) for Trinity Health Programs of All-Inclusive Care for the Elderly (PACE), and a new Nirvana (defined as "an idyllic place") presented itself. Within Trinity Health we have 13 PACE organizations across eight states. PACE provides an environment that every gerontological nurse could hope for; I am currently working on the inclusion of PACE organizations into the NICHE community. PACE provides a truly person-centered, interdisciplinary approach to supporting frail elders in the community; this is an environment where all aspects of health and well-being are assessed, topics such as polypharmacy are taken very seriously, and social supports are available as considered appropriate by the team.

As I reflect on the summarized story above, I realize that NICHE is more than just a membership or status; it is a community of continuous learning. The opportunities are endless (even though you do not have to act on them all at once), the resources are extensive, and the support and encouragement are inspiring. I know that the work of improving care of older adults is what my life was meant for, and that is much to do. What is your life meant for?

MedStar Health: Accelerating and Sustaining NICHE Implementation Through Systemness

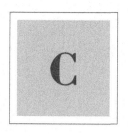

Karen Mack

THE ROLE OF AN ADVANCED PRACTICE NURSE AS A SYSTEM-LEVEL NICHE COORDINATOR

A targeted focus on improvement of care of older adults began at MedStar Health (MSH) in 2010 at MedStar Washington Hospital Center through the implementation of the NICHE program. NICHE implementation in the other nine MSH hospitals occurred in 2012 and 2013 when Maureen McCausland, DNSc, RN, FAAN, MSH, senior vice president and CNO, designated NICHE as a MedStar Nursing Signature Program for system-wide implementation. Dr. McCausland simultaneously created the role of the clinical practice program specialist (CPPS), which "supports a scholarly and rigorous approach to practice through the implementation of nationally recognized programs such as NICHE and the Iowa model of evidence based practice" (MedStar Health, 2017, para. 4). A CPPS role requirement is completion of a clinical nurse specialist educational program in a population focus included in the Advanced Practice Registered Nurse (APRN) Consensus Model (APRN Consensus Work Group & the National Council of State Boards of Nursing APRN Advisory Committee, 2008).

In September 2013, Karen Mack, MS, MBA, RN, APRN, CCNS, ACNPC, ACNP-BC, accepted the role as the first MSH CPPS. The role of CPPS in NICHE is to advance systemness, "a term that leaders use to define looking and acting more like a single integrated organization rather than a collection of independently functioning pieces" (McCausland, 2012, p. 307). Ms. Mack has presented the MSH systemness approach to NICHE implementation at NICHE annual conferences including abstracts on the following topics: (a) the MSH NICHE Program Gap Analysis; (b) the MSH NICHE Steering Committee (MSHNSC); and (c) the MSH NICHE Annual Report, which showcases the program business case (Mack, 2015, 2016; Mack & Mazard, 2017).

NICHE IMPLEMENTATION THROUGH SYSTEMNESS

In October 2013, the CPPS assumed monthly coordinating calls for the hospital NCs, which had been started in 2012 by Mary-Michael Brown, DNP, MSH, RN, vice president for Nursing Practice Innovation. The CPPS completed the NICHE

LTP in January 2014 during which she developed an action plan for system-level NICHE implementation. This initial action plan created a program leadership structure in which both hospital NCs and the CPPS shared complementary roles. As the program matured, the roles of nursing professional development specialists (NPDSs) and GRNs were integrated into the program leadership. The hospital NC's role is (a) implementation of a hospital action plan; (b) completion of the annual program evaluation; (c) facilitation of hospital NICHE leadership and steering committee meetings; (d) administration of the GIAP survey every 2 years; (e) oversight of education and development of GRNs, geriatric patient care associates (GPCAs), and other associates; and (f) development and completion of the MSHNSC annual goals (Boltz, Capezuti, Kim, Fairchild, & Secic, 2009). The CPPS role includes (a) facilitation of the MSHNSC meetings, (b) development of a timeline for execution of MSHNSC annual goals, (c) measurement and reporting of NICHE program outcomes in an annual report, (d) mentorship of new hospital NCs, (e) coordination of the MSH delegation to the NICHE annual conference, and (f) collaboration with the NICHE national program office to inform hospital NCs regarding requirements and program changes. NPDSs coordinate completion of NICHE education including (a) orientation; (b) NICHE courses, including live sessions; (c) age-specific competencies in simulation learning; and (d) ongoing geriatric education. GRNs provide direct care geriatric clinical expertise and participate in program design and implementation, both at the hospital and system level.

An initial tactic of the action plan was a *system-wide gap analysis* of each MSH hospital's achievement of the implementation criteria found in the NICHE Annual Program Evaluation (Capezuti et al., 2013; Mack, 2015). Assessment of each criterion determined gaps unique to individual hospitals as compared to those present at most MSH hospitals. This gap analysis was used to develop or modify individual hospital action plans and to refine the system-level action plan. A second tactic employed was creation of the system-level dashboard of Donabedian framework program measures that began in fiscal year (FY) 2014 (Donabedian, 1966). These measures, provided in Table C.1, are monitored for each MedStar Hospital and are featured in the MSH NICHE Annual Reports.

TABLE C.1 MedStar Hospital NICHE Implementation Donabedian Measures

STRUCTURE	PROCESS	OUTCOME
• Initial designation date • Annual membership date • NICHE implementation level • Most recent GIAP survey completion date	• NICHE action plan status • GRN model units • NICHE course completions • Registered nurses certified in gerontological nursing	• HCAHPS pain management satisfaction of older adults • GIAP results

GIAP, Geriatric Institutional Assessment Profile; GRN, geriatric resource nurse; HCAHPS, Hospital Consumer Assessment of Healthcare Providers and Systems; NICHE, Nurses Improving Care for Healthsystem Elders.

At the 2014 NICHE national conference, the Riverside Health System (RHS) presented the advantages of a system-level steering committee (Kennedy & Fletcher, 2014). This presentation was an impetus to move the MSH NICHE system-level implementation from monthly calls to a formally recognized system-level steering committee. On September 22, 2014, the MSHNSC convened and endorsed its charter. The MSHNSC charter notes its purposes, which are to (a) identify and advocate for evidence-based geriatric nursing care best practices; (b) identify and share NICHE programmatic best practices across the system; (c) optimize use of system resources through shared programming; (d) define and ensure timely reporting of MSH NICHE system program measures; and (e) develop tactics and actions for MSH's contribution to the NICHE national program (MedStar Health, 2014). The MSHNSC meets at the corporate office five times a year.

In FY 2017, the MSHNSC annual goal project was the creation and implementation of a GRN geriatric pain management education pilot. This project was led by the CPPS with support of the hospital NCs who identified a pilot unit, recruited a GRN project leader, mentored the GRN, and provided materials to support the program. The project focused on the GRN roles of peer consultant, educator, and quality and change agent. NPDSs and the CPPS developed the learning materials, which were then trialed by the GRNs. GRNs also completed a one-page implementation plan, publicized the project, distributed the learning materials, gathered process data, and evaluated the program. Remote meeting software, which allowed streaming of recorded meetings on demand, was used to deliver content to all 10 hospitals simultaneously. Data collection of process measures by the GRNs was devised in a simple one-page format. At the conclusion of the project, the hospital NCs awarded a certificate to each GRN project leader.

Other MSHNSC projects were (a) completion of *MedStar Alternative Medications for the Use of High-Risk Medications in Elders: A Guide for Clinicians*, in collaboration with the MSH Corporate pharmacists; (b) development and implementation of a standard orientation presentation about NICHE and elderspeak; and (c) development of GRN and NC role descriptions (Shah & Mack, 2017).

The MSHNSC accelerated NICHE implementation. Seven senior-friendly implementation hospitals and three exemplar hospitals made up the MSH NICHE program at the close of FY 2017. In comparison, the program included seven early implementations, two progressive implementations, and one senior-friendly hospital in September 2013. In a system-wide GIAP survey in 2016, 1,699 MSH associates completed the instrument. The GRN model has been implemented on 49 MSH units in 2017; this was an increase from 19 units in 2014. MSH nurses and other associates have completed 3,573 NICHE courses and 216 webinars during the period of FYs 2014 to 2017. In October 2017, 439 GRNs and 309 GPCAs were involved in the MSH NICHE program. The number of MSH nurses certified in gerontological nursing increased from one nurse in 2014 to 29 nurses in 2017.

SUMMARY

The future vision for the MSHNSC is to (a) strengthen the role of the GRN through an annual conference and quality improvement project; (b) provide visibility and recognition of the work of the hospital NCs; (c) implement additional NICHE clinical protocols; (d) determine and meet targets for NICHE course completions; and (d) achieve and sustain clinical outcome improvements. From an operational perspective, the goal is to increase the leadership role of the hospital NCs as MSHNSC committee chairs and project leaders.

REFERENCES

APRN Consensus Work Group & the National Council of State Boards of Nursing APRN Advisory Committee. (2008). Consensus model for APRN regulation: Licensure, accreditation, certification & education. Retrieved from https://www.ncsbn.org/Consensus_Model_for_APRN_Regulation_July_2008.pdf

Boltz, M., Capezuti, E., Kim, H., Fairchild, S., & Secic, M. (2009). Test—retest reliability of the Geriatric Institutional Assessment Profile. *Clinical Nursing Research, 18*(3), 242–252. doi:10.1177/1054773809338555

Capezuti, E., Boltz, M. P., Shuluk, J., Denysyk, L., Brouwer, J. P., Roberts, M. -C., . . . Secic, M. (2013). Utilization of a benchmarking database to inform NICHE implementation. *Research in Gerontological Nursing, 6*, 198–208. doi:10.3928/19404921-20130607-01

Donabedian, A. (1966). Evaluating the quality of medical care. *The Millbank Quarterly, 44*, 166–203.

Kennedy, T., & Fletcher, K. (2014). *Adapting Nurses Improving Care for Health System Elders (NICHE) as the nursing model of care for an integrated health care system.* Paper presented at the Nurses Improving Care for Healthsystem Elders Conference, San Diego, CA.

Mack, K. M. (2015). *Developing a gap analysis methodology to guide and improve NICHE implementation in a ten-hospital system.* Paper presented at the Nurses Improving Care for Healthsystem Elders Conference, Orlando, FL.

Mack, K. M. (2016). *Accelerating NICHE through systemness: The influence of a healthsystem steering committee on NICHE implementation.* Paper presented at the Nurses Improving Care for Healthsystem Elders Conference, Chicago, IL.

Mack, K., & Mazard, H. (2017). *NICHE 101: How to build a business case.* Paper presented at the Nurses Improving Care for Healthsystem Elders Conference, Austin, TX.

McCausland, M. P. (2012). Opportunities and strategies in contemporary health system executive leadership. *Nursing Administration Quarterly, 36*(4), 306–313. doi:10.1097/NAQ.0b013e3182669300

MedStar Health. (2014). *Medstar nurses improving care for HealthSystem Elders Steering Committee Charter.* Columbia, MD: Author.

MedStar Health. (2017). *NICHE hospital recognition levels.* Retrieved from https://www.medstarnursing.org/about-us/awards-recognition/niche-geriatric-care-designation

Shah, P., & Mack, K. (2017). *Alternative medications for the use of high-risk medications in elders: A guide for clinicians* [Reference guide]. Columbia, MD: MedStar Health.

NICHE Exemplar

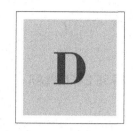

Kathleen Fletcher

INTRODUCTION

I have a long sustained history with NICHE at two different healthcare systems, one an academic institution and the other a community institution. While I was at the University of Virginia it was selected in 1997 as one of four dissemination sites for the NICHE model established by Dr. Terry Fulmer at Yale New Haven Hospital in 1989. I had been a geriatric nurse practitioner and educator since 1982 and the role of NC was a natural transition. The GIAP was conducted prior to implementation and indicated that though the staff completing the survey had positive attitudes about caring for the elderly, their knowledge base on how to care for the hospitalized elderly was limited. The GRN model was selected for implementation and it involved classroom time as well as bedside teaching rounds. We learned along the way that "one size did not fit all" and the model was implemented in different ways on medicine, intensive care, psychiatry, the emergency department, orthopedics, and in-home care. Several years later we established an ACE unit. The University of Virginia continues to sustain NICHE today, modifying and adapting the model to changing patient populations and staff needs and interests.

In 2013, I was recruited to RHS in Virginia to implement the NICHE model (GRN and an ACE unit). RHS had four hospitals, ten skilled nursing facilities, home care, and outpatient care including six PACE centers. This was my first opportunity to expand NICHE into LTC. It continues to survive today, but is now decentralized with individual facilities opting to select (or not) being a NICHE member. After 35 years as a geriatric nurse practitioner and educator and 20 years as a NICHE champion, I am now working part time as a research associate in the Riverside Center for Excellence in Aging and Lifelong Health. I have maintained a commitment to disseminating and generating knowledge and have published and presented extensively and exclusively in gerontological nursing. The following case study is intended to illustrate how NICHE can improve the care for older adults and their caregivers across the continuum of care.

CASE EXEMPLAR

EK is an 88-year-old frail female who currently lives in her own home and is being cared for by her youngest 52-year-old daughter who quit her job 10 years ago to be a full-time caregiver. EK married at age 16 (her husband passed away at age 62) and she had 10 children over a span of 19 years (and has now outlived two of them). Once all of her children were grown, she went to work for the first time at age 35 and worked full-time until she was 75 years of age. Social Security is currently her sole income.

EK's medical history includes hypertension, peripheral vascular disease, recurrent cellulitis with delirium, and the most debilitating, fibromyalgia, for which she has been treated by her primary care provider for more than 30 years with increasing doses of opioid analgesics. He has most recently begun to taper the medications with much resistance from EK; the daughter caregiver provides them to her mother as prescribed. EK has no direct access to these medications. EK has required multiple ER visits and hospitalizations over the past 10 years for pain control issues and falls, some with and some without injury. Her cognitive function is deteriorating and is complicated by the fact she is profoundly hard of hearing. She has a smoking history of half pack per day for 50 years and currently smokes less and only under supervision. She has no history of alcohol consumption. Her appetite has been diminished without any reported weight loss and largely consists of cream of wheat cereal with whole milk and heavily buttered and sugared white toast. She consumes about a liter of fluid per day primarily from coffee with heavy cream and sugar. She has a history of anxiety and takes alprazolam twice a day as scheduled. She gets no exercise except for the short walk assisted to the living room for meals and some socialization. She is a devout Catholic and is visited by the lay minister every Sunday.

EK is brought into the hospital by her daughter for a fall and pain control issues. Although she has an alarm device to call, EK frequently chooses not to use it, gets up unattended, and walks about six feet to the bathroom. This time she lost her balance in the bathroom and her left leg became lodged between the sink and the toilet. She complained of severe pain in the left leg and an inability to bear weight. She was seen in the ER and an x-ray revealed no evidence of fracture. She was given Dilaudid 4 mg IM for pain and subsequently admitted for pain control, delirium, and dehydration. Her current medications, all via oral route, include furosemide 40 mg once daily, potassium 20 mEq once daily, clopidogrel 75 mg once daily, pravastatin 40 mg once daily, alprazolam 0.5 mg twice daily, hydrocodone/acetaminophen 5/325 mg one tablet every 4 hours as needed for pain, and diphenhydramine 25 mg as needed nightly for sleep.

EK's course of hospitalization included fluid replacement as well as physical and occupational therapy consults for strength, gait and balance, and activities of daily living functioning. A dietary consult recommended increasing protein and fluid intake. Her delirium subsequently resolved and her physical therapist recommended short-term rehabilitation for fall prevention, gait and balance retraining, and general reconditioning. She failed to qualify for a short-term rehabilitation facility due to limitations in endurance and pain control and an LTC was selected.

EK's stay in LTC was complicated by the fact that she became more withdrawn and confused and was not always compliant with the therapeutic plan. Her caregiver daughter visited her daily with occasional visits from her other children who lived locally. Her daughter found her slumped in a chair and unresponsive. She was immediately transported by Emergency Medical Services (EMS) and was found in the emergency department to be dehydrated, overmedicated, and delirious and subsequently was readmitted. Her immediate problems were resolved, but pain control remained an issue and she was unable to participate in physical therapy and developed a stage 1 pressure injury. Her daughter refused LTC placement and elected to take her home with home health nursing and physical therapy. EK is increasingly frail and less mobile and independent than previously. She is tearful and has developed a fear of death and of being alone and uses her emergency whistle with increasing frequency at night. Her daughter, with guidance from the home care team, resolved the pressure injury. She is experiencing caregiver strain; she and her husband have not taken time away in over 5 years and she has neglected her own health issues. The home care nurse is recommending her to consider hospice care.

CASE STUDY DISCUSSION

Nurses (RNs and LPNs) have limited preparation in the care of the elderly and regardless of the practice area this is clearly evident. This becomes even more apparent during care transitions across settings. Without good role models and mentors working alongside of them in direct care, nurses and their patients/families are even more disadvantaged. The case study illustrates the impact of these areas of concern. How might the outcome be different if EK had been in a hospital and LTC facility where the nurses were well versed in the NICHE model and able to demonstrate knowledge and behaviors that reflect improved competencies to care for older adults and their families?

In the hospital, if EK were assigned to a GRN who worked closely with the interprofessional team, EK's outcomes likely would have been more positive. The team would have recognized that EK's previous and current medication regimen (i.e., opioids, benzodiazepines, and anticholinergics) and her previous deconditioning contributed to failure to meet the endurance level necessary to qualify for an inpatient rehabilitation facility. The team would have implemented a plan of care that proactively and more aggressively addressed the issues of pain control, delirium, and deconditioning. The team would also have recognized and better managed her long-standing pattern of inadequate protein and fluid intake and not just addressed this during the hospital stay. They could have educated EK and her daughter about how critical nutrition is to her health and well-being. Additionally, the team would have developed a transitional person-centered care plan focused on these concerns with the patient/family and communicated this to the LTC facility.

If the NICHE model had been implemented in the LTC facility, the nursing staff, in all likelihood, would have recognized and addressed EK's behaviors, including delirium, acting withdrawn, and noncompliance with the therapeutic plan. They would have recognized the impact of her previous and current medication use, her psychological needs, and her risk for pressure injury development. Finally, with improved communication between interprofessional staff in acute care, LTC, primary care, and home care settings, best practice in geriatric care could have been implemented and EK and her caregiver's long-term prognosis and quality of life would likely have been improved.

Outcomes of the NICHE model have demonstrated improvements in both the quality and costs of care, greater patient/family satisfaction, and strengthened interfacility communications. The challenge is that these outcomes have not been demonstrated consistently, there are limited incentives for staff nurses to participate in educational initiatives, and there is a serious lack in the number of advanced practice nurses with a geriatric specialty to serve as educators, mentors, or researchers. In terms of advanced practice nursing, we have yet to see what benefits there may be in the clinical setting from those educationally prepared and certified as adult-gerontology, acute or primary care, nurse practitioners.

Older adults have multiple, complex, interrelated issues. During institutionalization, older adults are more vulnerable to complications including functional decline and premature debility. Medication regimens are unnecessarily complex and overmedication or undermedication is too often seen. Families remain the primary caregivers and partnerships with healthcare providers are not well and consistently established. Geriatric interprofessional teams are the most desired approach, but teams are expensive and not always readily available particularly in LTC and in rural areas. Healthcare systems may be well intended to provide the highest quality of care to older patients and their families and to improve patient/family and nurse satisfaction, but less willing and able to prioritize it due to cost containment and competing priorities.

SUMMARY

The NICHE model has demonstrated positive outcomes and has expanded considerably since it was first established. But it "takes a village" to modify models of care to address the ever-changing needs and demographics. Partnerships with families need to be truly genuine and respectful ones that are tailored to their specific needs and relationships. Resources for healthcare providers and patients/families need to be available, accessible, and acceptable.

INOVA Fairfax Hospital NICHE

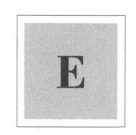

Deirdre M. Carolan Doerflinger

NICHE has positively impacted the culture of our institution, Inova Fairfax Hospital, and improved care of our older adult population. Inova Fairfax Hospital, in the late 1990s, was an 833-bed tertiary care, level 1 trauma center in the Washington, DC suburbs. Geriatrics had been a strength of this facility since the establishment of a geriatrics consult service, Geriatrics Team, pioneered in 1985 by Dr. Joanne G. Crantz, MD, FACP, medical director for geriatrics, and supported by Toni Ardabell, MSN, RN, director of medical surgical nursing. Ninety consultations were requested and completed in the first year; however, this service rapidly increased to 900 consultations per year by the late 1990s. Inpatients over the age of 65 hospitalized for various conditions who were having geriatrics issues due to their condition or hospitalization received a comprehensive geriatrics assessment and a personalized plan of care was designed and implemented to address their specific needs. These older adults had shorter length of stay, higher function and cognition at the time of discharge, lower readmission rates, and higher patient satisfaction than those not receiving geriatrics consultation.

The Geriatrics Team and the professional practice unit councils collaborated and identified deficits in care and a geriatrics issue on which to focus each year. These quality improvement projects were targeted to decrease negative events and improve the care of the older adult overall. The approach was interdisciplinary, and consequently, knowledge and practice deficits were identified in all disciplines. Nursing identified key elements of their practice self-identified as less than optimal and not evidence based. These priority areas for improvement were delirium identification and management, falls prevention, mobility, and appropriate design and furnishings. Simultaneously, a critical care colleague forwarded an article about a new program targeting increasing geriatrics focus and visibility in nursing specialty organizations. The article highlighted the NICHE program, still in its early stages. Much discussion, literature review, and administrative meetings ensued, and in March 2000, NICHE was selected as a model that we wanted to implement. The proposal for NICHE was funded by the Annual Inova Gala 2001. Our NICHE journey had begun!

A core group of multidisciplinary champions was recruited from invested disciplines, including nursing, pharmacy, nursing education, rehabilitation, and social work. Staff at all levels were included, from nursing assistants and unit secretaries, up to the director of nursing and the medical director of geriatrics. This diverse group organized and generated a plan that included data collection and analysis, needs assessment, implementation of geriatrics educational programs, and outcomes monitoring and evaluation data.

Falls were identified as a significant problem. Abundant data were already being collected. However, further analysis of event reports revealed that a large number of those falling were also delirious. Meetings with care team members to discuss this issue generated important aspects of this patient issue. The staff voiced concern regarding the lack of personnel for monitoring these patients, concern for the patients' safety, and minimization of their concerns by medical members of the care team as being problematic. Concurrently, the GIAP, conducted early in our journey, reflected distress on the part of the staff with patients who were confused and agitated. This population took more care hours due to their confusion, poor judgment and risk of falls, increased risk of inadvertent equipment removal, and lack of staff resources to stay in close proximity for safety. There was no standardized assessment of delirium or cognition in the documentation system, and retrospective review of the medical records of these patients demonstrated multiple diagnoses that reflected the presence of delirium.

The NICHE Steering Committee identified the unit with the highest number of confused older adults, a 65-bed general medicine unit. This particular unit was already committed to improving the care of the older adult population. The unit's unique strengths were a core experienced staff invested in improving the care of older adults, a supportive strong unit manager who was open to new approaches to improve the care on the unit, and the willingness to implement evidence-based practice. This unit nurse manager committed to this project and to the education of her staff on the issue of delirium due to its high delirium rate and high falls rate. Examination of risk and quality data demonstrated that, on this unit, the prevalence of delirium was over 50% and 80% of unit falls occurred in delirious older adults.

The action plan prioritized the identification of a delirium screening instrument. The medical reference librarians in the Jacob B. Zylman Health Sciences Library of Inova Fairfax Hospital provided expert assistance as the staff delved into the literature. A baseline delirium prevalence was collected on the pilot medical unit. Collaboratively, the team selected three tools to pilot, the Confusion Assessment Method (CAM), the Delirium Observation Scale (DOS), and the NEECHAM Confusion Scale (NEECHAM). All these instruments demonstrated strong validity and reliability. Each of the five team members used each instrument to assess 50 random inpatients on three different units. All usual care and usual assessments were done by the unit staff nurses. The units were medicine, general surgery, progressive coronary care, and the intermediate care unit. The NEECHAM was preferred as a guide for modification of care; however, the time to administer was longer than any other tool. The CAM was selected for use as it was a brief screen that was easy to remember and alternate versions were available, such as the CAM-ICU and the CAM-P.

After the tool was selected, implementation was started to facilitate tool adoption, process, and the development of a delirium order set. The work group included a pharmacist, critical care hospitalist, medical hospitalist, psychiatrist, neurologist, critical care clinical nurse specialist (CNS), and members of the NICHE Steering Committee. Regular (every shift) delirium screening using the CAM was approved and a delirium order set was created. Education via HealthStream was provided; this included NICHE educational materials regarding delirium, prevention, and treatment. This was supplemented with materials about the use of the CAM. All education was provided in multiple modalities, in addition to on-unit champion and CNS support, as each unit began including the CAM in its usual care. The education was completed by 96% of nursing staff on all units. Ongoing support was provided as issues were identified. Post implementation audits, by the NICHE Steering Committee, showed noncompletion or inaccuracies at 4 weeks of over 50%. Criteria were defined more succinctly and re-education was completed, increasing accuracy and compliance to over 80%. This has required continued re assessment and re-education due to arrival of new staff and other priorities.

This was our largest and most successful NICHE initiative. It was NICHE! The educational materials, the approach, and the nursing knowledge and confidence in their care of the older adult were all a result of NICHE. The results were most dramatic on the strongest NICHE unit. These gains have waxed and waned but have remained strong on this unit.

This unit used NICHE as the mechanism to improve care of our older adults and changed the culture of caring for them. They utilized the knowledge and skills from the NICHE program and implemented them using evidence-based practice. They correctly identified delirium as being the root cause of many of the nosocomial conditions experienced by their older adult population. Positive outcomes were seen in patient, clinical, and staff outcomes. Patient satisfaction and family satisfaction increased as nursing staff provided education for patients and families at high risk of delirium. Families enjoyed being actively involved in a positive and constructive manner. Educational materials were created by staff and given to family members, explaining the delirium and guiding family interventions. Open visitation had been on a case-by-case basis, but recognizing the importance of family presence in the prevention of delirium and increase in staff awareness in care of the delirious patient, families were more welcomed.

This NICHE unit effectively reduced rates of delirium by 33% and shortened the duration of delirium episodes by 0.4 days as a direct consequence of changing care. Accompanying these core improvements, the falls rate was reduced by 31% on the unit. Patients were out of bed for toileting, meals, and to maintain normal day/night cycles. Length of stay was shortened by a half day and readmissions were also reduced. Patients' medication regimens were reassessed more regularly. All of this resulted in improved nursing satisfaction and more interdisciplinary collaboration. During this entire process, sitter usage dropped as staff enlisted family and were more comfortable with managing the delirious patient. These significant improvements were accomplished in addition to maintaining a restraint-free care environment. The staff on this medical unit have remained committed to their older adult population. They freely share their knowledge and approaches to care of the older adult and teach students from all disciplines about older adults and evidence-based care.

The culture on this unit, specifically, and the facility have changed and best practice in the care of older adults is firmly embedded in all their care. There are competing priorities that challenge the staff to maintain these improvements. Change has slowly spread throughout other units as the positive results are highlighted and staff members transfer to different units. The CAM is now a component of all assessments on adults 60 years and older in the electronic medical record and in all areas of the facility. All units have access to the delirium order set. Ongoing education and focus on delirium is necessary on all units to maintain this significant practice improvement in the care of our older adults.

The Geriatric Resource Model: A Journey to Hardwiring Geriatric Excellence

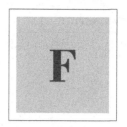

Dennise R. Lavrenz

It is an honor to contribute to celebrating 25 years of NICHE. My name is Dennise Lavrenz, MBA, BSN, RN, CENT, and I am currently the senior vice president of clinical and client services/chief clinical officer at the Milwaukee Center for Independence. I have worked as an executive clinical leader for over 30 years in a variety of healthcare settings including community and academic inpatient hospitals, outpatient clinics, and community programs. In this vignette, I am proud to share my experience on my special, career-changing relationship with NICHE. My inspirational journey began 18 years ago when I was introduced to NICHE, a geriatric "think tank" and best practice champion for our elderly patients, in 1999. The content of this vignette will focus on my role as the NICHE administrator, where I launched and sustained a successful NICHE program in a community hospital setting by hardwiring a GRN model into practice. I have served as a NICHE mentor and member of the NICHE annual conference planning committee, and also have been a speaker at the annual conferences and webinars. I have also collaborated as a NICHE grant facilitator for an elder caregiver project in partnership with the American Association of Retired Persons and *American Journal of Nursing* to improve transitions in care through a pilot to improve caregiver communication tools in acute care facilities.

In January 1999, while working as a nurse leader in a 400-bed community hospital in Wisconsin, I oversaw 153 adult medical–surgical, orthopedic, neurologic, and rehabilitation inpatient beds. After hearing about the NICHE program at a national nursing conference, our vice president of Inpatient Services requested that, as the director of the med/surg units, an aspiring med/surg clinical nurse specialist, and a surgical frontline RN, I attend the 1999 NICHE leadership training conference at New York University (NYU). This event, 18 years ago, would change my focus on caring for our elders for the rest of my career.

I recall sitting in a small conference room in the lower level at NYU with three colleagues and about 20 additional participants from several organizations throughout the country. We were provided several large binders of information and overwhelmed with ideas on how to raise the bar for geriatric care.

Following the conference, our team dug into the binders of best practice examples. We were overwhelmed and impressed with the content and structure. It did not take us long to decide to implement the geriatric resource model. I led the culture change as the administrative champion and the med/surg clinical nurse specialist would be our NC. Since I was responsible for all the med/surg beds, we began our journey to tackle all 153 beds on four nursing units.

We leveraged change theory concepts to ensure success. These included creating systems and structures necessary to hardwire excellence in the care of seniors into practice and to lead this change through a deliberate use of the stages of change by creating a shared need, shaping a vision, mobilizing commitment, implementing change, making change last, and monitoring outcomes.

Our first marching orders were to solicit support by presenting to our board and staff, sharing our vision top down and bottom up. We found that our desire to improve care for 54% of our population of elders resonated with so many similar initiatives around patient satisfaction, quality, safety, and finances. It seemed that NICHE was exactly what we needed to address common geriatric syndromes where we had been struggling to effectively impact outcomes and initiate best practice plans of care for many years. The idea of training our clinicians to proactively address the specific needs of our geriatric population by creating expertise on geriatric syndromes made practical sense for our system. NICHE was the answer we had been looking for.

We created a NICHE Steering Committee and developed a charter with specific, measurable, attainable, realistic, and time-sensitive goals. To aid us in our focus, we surveyed our nurses by using the GIAP to obtain baseline knowledge and attitude scores. Our strategy was to enlist those clinicians with knowledge and passion to train, role model, round, and essentially change a culture. The focus was on eliminating restraints, reducing falls, developing protocols, and implementing standards of clinical practice. Within the first 2 years we recruited 25 geriatric RNs to lead excellent care of our hospitalized elders; six of our RNs pursued national nursing certification as gerontological nurses during this timeframe. These GRNs on each of the med/surg units wore white lab coats with their name and "GERIATRIC RESOURCE NURSE" embroidered for all to see and ask about. As the GRNs rounded with our clinicians, our restraint and fall rates declined.

Our staff became excited about care for our elders. We promoted NICHE as a specialty like children's programs in which high-level skill was necessary for extraordinary outcomes. Through our NICHE steering team, we shared our story with anyone who would listen and invited ourselves to any meetings discussing elders. We learned early from our NICHE mentor, Mathy Mezey, to show up at everything. We hit the jackpot when we visited with our Foundation Board and realized that a board member's husband had Alzheimer's. For the next 11 years, our Foundation would support sending six to eight of our NICHE team to the annual NICHE conferences to advance our senior strategy. The level of elder expertise grew as we engaged more and more of our interdisciplinary team. Quoting our NICHE mentors, Terry Fulmer and Mathy Mezey, "Take no prisoners": find colleagues who have a passion for caring for your seniors and build your team.

Eleven years later, this organization created over 200 nurses and nursing assistants trained in geriatric best practice protocols. Eighteen would become nationally certified as gerontological nurses. As I reflect on how we hardwired

NICHE into our organization, it was by starting slowly with a core steering team, incrementally building on more advanced care strategies, and embedding best care into everything we did to the point that it was part of our culture. We created a culture that was laser focused on mentoring experts in care of our largest population of patients and some of our most vulnerable.

Thanks to NICHE, we are able to deliver on the value proposition of providing a plan of care for our seniors that is high quality, focused on wellness, delivering excellence in satisfaction, fiscally accountable with the right care in the right place at the right time, and leveraging measures to be proactive in our approach to prevent adverse geriatric syndromes. Our health system could effectively eliminate restraints, decrease preventable falls, improve our pressure ulcer rates, eliminate unnecessary catheters, develop a process to ensure appropriate medications, and address hospital-acquired delirium. We changed our facility to accommodate the unique needs of our elders through designing bathrooms that were within our senior's eye sight, ensuring effective lighting, installing heat lamps in the bathroom, creating color schemes that promoted healing and safety, purchasing glider rocking chairs and blanket warmers, and beginning to pay closer attention to font size and style and how we were engaging our elders in their plans of care. Our commitment was to address the uniqueness of our seniors by creating "All About Me" posters in each room to further understand the legacy of each individual and engage them in meaningful conversation, often leveraging pictures and reminiscence magazines. We worked with our team to be present by sitting down at the bedside and listening. We taught our nurses to be gentle with our frail elders and implemented benevolent touch to provide hand massages. We also used essential oils to support anxiety and to reduce urinary retention and nausea with great success. We engaged the ER and surgical intake units to hardwire geriatric-friendly environments and plans of care that would set our seniors up for success. Specifically, in our surgical patients we evaluated methods to prevent hospital-acquired delirium and promote early mobilization.

Since most of our population were located on the med/surg units, we created opportunities to make med/surg special. We encouraged nurses to become certified with the use of added reimbursement, a clinical ladder, and recognition. Those geriatric nurses who went above and beyond were rewarded with a trip to the annual NICHE conference. We also purchased white professional uniform coats embroidered with their name and GRN. Our steering team developed an annual celebration called the Academy of Medical–Surgical Nurses in which we awarded the Mathy Mezey Geriatric Excellence Award in Geriatric Leadership. Each awardee received a small Oscar-like statue with this engraved. Many of our RNs also utilized geriatric projects to advance within our clinical ladder.

We promoted our senior special care to our local newspaper and on our website and our CEO recognized our best practice as a key component and accomplishment within the hospital's strategic plan. We had overwhelming support from our Corporate and Foundation Boards. The Joint Commission applauded the performance improvement activities and benchmark outcomes that seniors were experiencing in our organization because of NICHE.

Several of my favorite NICHE conference moments included times when our GRNs dressed up for a panel presentation with gray wigs, having fun with NICHE and proudly presenting implementing pet therapy, activity aprons, and benevolent touch. Another special moment was yet another year when our GRNs presented compelling outcomes on the NICHE dashboard demonstrating improved outcomes to care while proudly wearing their GRN lab coats. The audience of 300 responded with a standing ovation. Tears ran down their faces with great joy for the acknowledgment of the pearls of wisdom that was just normal practice at our hospital.

I personally have not missed one NICHE conference since 1999. Reflecting on the growth of NICHE in my 18 years with the program, I recall the basement of NYU with 20 colleagues and fast forward to 2017 in Austin, Texas at the downtown Marriott, with over 800 colleagues present. I am proud of how NICHE has engaged the country. Regardless of the size of the conference, the spirit and passion remain the same: geriatric excellence!!!!

We have so many memories and colleagues from across the world with whom we have met and shared best practices through the Knowledge Center, discussion forum, and conferences. The NICHE family has created a strategy of not reinventing the wheel. Tools and best practice protocols are shared relentlessly for all to take and use. What started in 1999 as four nurse leaders meeting in a basement at NYU resulted in a culture change where senior population health measures were so embedded into daily work, it became how we practiced versus a special program for our elders. Thank you NICHE for changing my life as a nurse leader to mentor those I lead in geriatric excellence. You have made a difference in the lives of those we serve and those who serve.

Happy 25th anniversary NICHE!

Cedars Sinai Medical Center

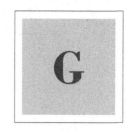

Flora B. Haus

Cedars Sinai Medical Center (CSMC) is an 886-bed teaching community hospital in Los Angeles, California. In July 2010, CSMC embarked on the journey to become NICHE designated. This coincided with a dual-track research study and performance improvement project on the rapid screening and early intervention of elder patients at risk of becoming frail. As we began designing the study and reviewed the NICHE resources, it was decided that Dr. Terry Fulmer's assessment tool SPICES was the gold standard, evidence-based instrument and would be used to meet the goal of rapid patient identification. SPICES not only had demonstrated validity and reliability, but also had the advantage of incorporating patient characteristics that were already collected during the admission process.

At the same time, we were on the verge of launching our electronic medical record based on the EPIC product. The system's functionality enabled extraction of discrete data and application of a decision support feature to create an alert for the treatment team regarding the patient's SPICES status. A major advantage was that the entire process could be accomplished without adding to the workflow of any member of the treatment team, most especially nursing. This was confirmed during the LTP, as we conducted a strengths, weaknesses, opportunities, and threats (SWOT) analysis. The ease of use of the SPICES tool and its lack of intrusiveness to the patient admission workflow for nursing became a critical advantage to both the research study and the process of becoming NICHE designated.

By April 2011, we were thrilled to achieve our NICHE designation. As we geared up to administer our GIAP, we pondered how best to advertise the survey and then capitalize on the robust resources as a NICHE facility. The realization that the GIAP was a 157-question survey was daunting. How were the staff supposed to complete this during their work shift? How long did it take? How could we sell it to them? Business management literature was replete with suggestions. Navigating the articles for advice on how to implement suggestions in our nursing environment was a little trickier. Experience had shown successful nurse participation frequently involved food; however, feeding 1,800 nurses was not even close to budget neutral. We did adopt and adapt various approaches. Here are some tips and how we found them successful:

- Communicate, communicate, communicate often and in various modalities (emails, posters, in person for unit practice and staff meetings).

- Get leadership on board through attending multiple nursing division leadership meetings and providing information on the benefits and details of the administration process.

- Make it fun! Encourage participation by putting units in competition with each other; those units receiving 100% participation were awarded bagel breakfasts.

- Explain the benefit to staff that each unit would determine which knowledge "gap" they could address first. This also afforded us the opportunity to share and dialogue the organizational clinical outcome goals related to decreasing hospital-acquired pressure ulcers (HAPUs), use of restraints, incidence of sleep deprivation–induced delirium, and catheter-associated urinary tract infections (CAUTIs). Staff were promised *no* cookie-cutter approaches. Each intervention to raise awareness would be tailored to the personality of the unit and its unique patient population issues.

- Hold managers accountable by sending daily alerts to apprise them of the percentage completion rates. The unit leadership was the linchpin in achieving high participation.

As the GIAP captures both knowledge and attitude scores, we decided to invite nurses beyond the typical inpatient units to participate. The intent was to utilize the GIAP to truly obtain an organizational measure. We therefore included all of the high-acuity critical care units, the emergency department, post anesthesia care, and ambulatory sites with high prevalence of geriatric populations.

The staff's voluntary participation of 84% ($n = 1,264$) exceeded not only the nursing leadership's expectations, but also the level of participation generally experienced with employee engagement surveys. Our excitement around staff participation, however, contrasted with our disappointment that we were below the mean in all four knowledge domains (physical restraints, incontinence, sleep disturbances, and pressure ulcers) in care of older adults. Organization-wide results were shared with nursing leaders, then divisional and department results were shared with applicable groups. Our promise to tailor instructional design to meet unit-identified clinical focus was kept and units chose performance improvement projects that were in alignment with the organization's clinical goals.

With over 1,264 nurses on 40 units responding, we next had to determine the best modality to provide the education they needed in the appropriate adult learner manner they wanted. The GRN course was ideal. This course was advertised to staff as an enhancement to one of the pillars of our mission, education. Advertisement of the NICHE learning site likewise used multiple approaches. Emails that were both informative and visually appealing were developed. A frequently asked questions (FAQ) sheet was provided to the leadership to share and encourage staff. A singular message regarding the value of cost-free access to the knowledge site and the earning of ANCC-approved continuing education units was met with overwhelming success. No restrictions on the number of nurses, or where they practiced, were placed on staff. Access was open to experienced staff as well as novice nurses. Our organization was on a parallel track to address the rapid identification of elders at risk for becoming frail and the access to NICHE resources fit into the overall approach.

Celebration and acknowledgment of completing the GRN course was accompanied by a certificate and GRN pin awarded at staff huddles or meetings held by the manager on behalf of the NC. Once GRN status was achieved, the nurses were encouraged and supported to seek ANCC certification in gerontological nursing with additional lectures, daily questions and answers (Q&A), and Certification Core Curriculum review courses. For many of the staff, the journey toward this certification was the second certification they were seeking. Their effort was matched not only by the public acknowledgment and praise, but also by a significant and well appreciated one-time financial bonus. Knowledge, acknowledgment, rewards, and support were the magic combination. Within 2 years we went from 20 to 512 GRNs; in the same period, we went from three gerontological certified RNs to 120. Both GRNs and certified nurses were present on both day and night shifts throughout the organization from inpatient to ambulatory; they represented clinical staff as well as educators and managers. It was clear our nursing staff was hungry for knowledge and thrived on self-motivated achievements.

The growth in the nursing staff's knowledge about the care of older adults was mirrored in the repeat GIAP of 2013. We went from below our peer mean in four domains to above the peer mean in all domains. We had lived the experience that using the GRN course could and would contribute and translate to increased knowledge scores. And once again, the staff surprised us with a 91% participation rate. The bagel breakfasts for 100% staff participation were provided to over 50% of the units and delivered by the NC.

Consumer Survey

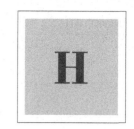

Melissa Botrell

(From May 1, 1995 *NICHE* report to the JAHF)

In 1995, to enhance the evaluation tools and support national implementation of NICHE, NICHE staff designed a consumer survey to capture family members' perceptions of the care their loved one received in a NICHE hospital.

While consumer surveys were being widely used in hospitals to assess patient satisfaction, at the time a literature review and contacts with consumer satisfaction survey developers identified no surveys specifically focused on the care of older patients. Available consumer surveys tended to ask general questions about the hospital food, the nursing care, preparation for discharge, and so on. We were interested in capturing the family perspectives on specific activities addressed in NICHE such as physical restraints, sleep management, skin care, pressure ulcer prevention, and pain management—creating data that would be useful for the facility, while tied directly to NICHE implementation.

To do so, the NICHE consumer survey was based on questions from the Institutional Assessment Profile (IAP, later GIAP) designed to assess the perceptions and knowledge of geriatric care of nurses (and others). By comparing family opinions of care with that of healthcare professionals using comparable questions, facilities could better understand how their activities improved the perceptions of care received by their patients. The consumer questionnaire was designed to be added directly to standard surveys already in use in the hospital or to be used as stand-alone measures. The intent was to allow hospitals to provide public service information about the quality of geriatric care or augment quality of care data with data from the consumer's perspective directly.

Questions most pertinent to areas likely to be valued by patients were abstracted from the IAP, rewritten using lay language (see the following Draft Consumer Survey) and assessed for health literacy reading level using available tools. Existing NICHE sites were approached about implementing the consumer survey in their current patient/consumer survey activities. All sites expressed support for the value of adding a consumer component to NICHE work, but most facilities were not able to use the questions due to a contracted standardized survey mechanism and the difficulty of changing that instrument. Baystate Medical Center committed to using the consumer survey questions, and other sites considered a more limited implementation, for instance with a subset of family members, or on a limited basis in certain units or settings. We were ahead of our time. Today, consumer surveys are routine and we are glad they are.

DRAFT

CAREGIVER CONSUMER QUESTIONS

1. **Do you provide care for a relative or close friend who is older than 65 and who is now in this hospital or was in this hospital/facility?**
(Question to be asked to close relatives, primary household caregivers, or other caregiver types)

   a. Yes   b. No   (If yes, go to #2. If no, **stop** here.)

2. **For your relative or friend, do you think the following treatments are used TOO LITTLE, APPROPRIATELY, or TOO OFTEN in this hospital?**

	Too Little	Appropriately	Too Often	Don't Know/ No Opinion
a. Physical restraints such as vests, mitts, or hands tied down	○	○	○	○
b. Sleeping medications or medications such as tranquilizers	○	○	○	○
c. Adult diapers	○	○	○	○
d. Pain medication	○	○	○	○
e. Tube feeding	○	○	○	○
f. Other:	○	○	○	○

3. **Thinking about this hospital, how satisfied are you about the extent to which:**

	Not Very Satisfied	Somewhat Satisfied	Very Satisfied	Don't Know	No Opinion
a. Hospital staff address issues specific to your relative	○	○	○	○	○
b. Your relative/friend got the care he/she needs (needed)	○	○	○	○	○
c. Staff are familiar with how aging affects patient's medical needs	○	○	○	○	○
d. Patients receive the information they need to make decisions about their care	○	○	○	○	○

(continued)

	Not Very Satisfied	Somewhat Satisfied	Very Satisfied	Don't Know	No Opinion
e. Families receive information and support they need to help elderly patients	○	○	○	○	○
f. What a patient's health was like before he/she came to the hospital	○	○	○	○	○
g. Medical care is coordinated when the patient moves from the hospital to home or the nursing home	○	○	○	○	○
h. Medical care is coordinated when a patient moves to different units or areas of the hospital	○	○	○	○	○
i. There are specialized services for the elderly	○	○	○	○	○
j. Elderly patients are included in decisions about their own medical care	○	○	○	○	○
k. Patients are protected from economic pressures to limit expensive treatments or the amount of time patients stay in the hospital	○	○	○	○	○

DEMOGRAPHIC INFORMATION

1. Age

2. Sex

3. Racial/ethnic background

4. Relationship to the patient in the hospital

5. Other information obtained in the hospital's forms

Hartford Institute for Geriatric Nursing Web Resources

Tara A. Cortes

For more than 20 years, the Hartford Institute for Geriatric Nursing (HIGN) at NYU Rory Meyers College of Nursing has been a global resource for health professionals delivering age-sensitive care to older adults. Included in its vision statement is that "Anyone involved in older adult care understands the unique needs of that population and has access to resources they need to decrease the incidence and mitigate the impact of chronic disease and social determinants of health." To address that vision, HIGN has developed hundreds of online, evidence-based resources including interactive modules, PDF information sheets, PowerPoints, webinars, a geriatric certification review course, and podcasts. Resources are available for nurses as well as physicians, nurse practitioners, and other members of the interprofessional team. The content addresses the care of older adults across the continuum, from the hospital to primary care, home care, and LTC. *Try This*® is one of the most frequently accessed resources. It includes an assessment series, a dementia series, and a quality improvement series. A new *Try This*® entitled "Virtual Patient Series" has been added.

The resources are located in the HIGN E-Learning Center, ConsultGeri. For many years, ConsultGeri was a separate website under the ConsultGeri.org name. In 2018, the decision was made to unite the two websites under hign.org. This unification of the two websites allows those accessing the resources to also gain knowledge from some of the gerontological research, policy initiatives, grant activity, and global outreach occurring at HIGN. During the 12 months before the two websites were consolidated, there were over 103,000 visitors to hign.org and consultgeri.org combined. They represent over 75% of the countries in the world. NICHE members and guests can access hign.org and all its resources directly from the NICHE website through the HIGN connect link. Conversely, visitors to the HIGN site can directly access the NICHE site through the NICHE connect link. In addition, there is a ConsultGeri app with algorithms to help nurses with geriatric issues including delirium, falls, and agitation. This app can be purchased through Apple's App Store.

Supplemental Material

Columbia University School of Nursing (Participant Letter)

Terry T. Fulmer, Ph.D., R. N., FAAN
Anna C. Maxwell Professor in Nursing Research
Associate Dean for Research
June 9, 1993

630 West 168th Street
New York, N.Y. 10032
(212) 305-4165
FAX (212) 305-6937

Dear Conference Participant:

We are delighted that you are able to attend this workshop. We are pleased to have with us a distinguished group of gerontological nursing experts who will present the nursing models developed in the recently completed *Hospital Outcomes Project for the Elderly* (HOPE), funded by the John A. Hartford Foundation of New York City.

Our goal today is twofold: (1) to continue the dissemination of knowledge gained in that important program, and (2) to describe a new initiative for which you can apply. The *Nurses Improving Care to the Hospitalized Elderly* (NICHE) project seeks to disseminate the nursing care models developed in the HOPE program to the broader hospital community. In this packet you will find a formal request for proposals to become part of the NICHE project, as well as:

- brief descriptions of each of the HOPE nursing care models

- a set of our nursing practice protocols on care for elderly patients with urinary incontinence, sleep disorders, pressure ulcers, and mechanical restraints. NICHE sites will implement one or more of these nursing practice protocols as an integral part of whichever model of care they adopt

- an Institutional Assessment Profile (IAP) that NICHE sites will use to survey nursing staff who care for elderly patients and develop a baseline measure of how well they are meeting their goals in delivering optimal care to elderly patients.

We believe that the NICHE project provides an outstanding opportunity for hospitals that seek to provide the very best of care to their elderly patients to take advantage of nursing models and tools that have demonstrated success in improving geriatric care and nursing satisfaction. If your hospital is interested in applying to participate, we urge you to complete a formal proposal.

Sincerely,
Terry Fulmer, RN, PhD, FAAN
Principal Investigator
Columbia University

School of Nursing
Mathy Mezey, RN, Ed.D, FAAN
Co-Investigator
New York University

School of Nursing
Rebecca Jackson
Project Director
Education Development Center, Inc.

Dissemination of the Hospital Outcomes Project for the Elderly

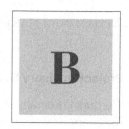

Request for Proposals

Columbia University School of Nursing
New York University School of Nursing
and
Education Development Center, Inc.

Principal Investigators

Terry Fulmer, RN, PhD, FAAN
Professor and Associate Dean for Research
Columbia University
School of Nursing

Mathy Mezey, RN, EdD, FAAN
Independence Foundation Professor of Nursing
Education
New York University
Division of Nursing

Project Staff

Kimberly Hamrick, MPH
Research Associate
Education Development Center, Inc.

Rebecca Jackson, BA
Project Director
Education Development Center, Inc.

Lydia O'Donnell, EdD
Associate Director of the Center for Health
and Human Development
Education Development Center, Inc.

Ann G. Pierce, RN, PhD
Assistant Professor
Columbia University
School of Nursing

Cheryl Vince-Whitman, EdM
Vice President
Education Development Center, Inc.

Margaret Wolf, RN, PhD
Professor
New York University
Division of Nursing

Project Advisory Board

Priscilla Ebersole, RN, PhD, FAAN
Professor Emerita
San Francisco State University

Mary Naylor, RN, PhD, FAAN
Associate Dean and Director of
Undergraduate Studies
Associate Professor
University of Pennsylvania
School of Nursing

Project Advisory Board (*Continued*)

Marquis Foreman, RN, PhD
Assistant Professor
The University of Illinois at Chicago

Denise Kresevic, RN, MSN
University Hospitals of Cleveland

Lorraine Mion, RN, PhD
Assistant Professor of Nursing
Yale University

Mary Walker, RN, PhD, FAAN
Associate Professor and Director
Division of Adult Nursing
University of Kentucky
College of Nursing

May Wykle, RN, PhD, FAAN
Florence Cellar Professor and Chair of
Gerontological Nursing Program
Case Western Reserve University
Francis Payne Bolton School of Nursing

The *Dissemination of the Hospital Outcomes Project for the Elderly* is funded by the John A. Hartford Foundation of New York City.

BACKGROUND

People 65 and over make up close to 45% of all hospital admissions nationally. While most elderly benefit from treatment provided in hospitals, a substantial number of elderly patients experience untoward events during and subsequent to hospitalization.

Unfortunately, little has been done to create models of geriatric nursing in hospitals. Very few hospitals have in place programs that specifically address the needs of elderly patients. There are few avenues for sharing "best practice" related to nursing management of common problems experienced by the hospitalized elderly. And nurses employed by hospitals by and large have had little exposure to the principles of geriatric nursing.

One of the few programs to specifically focus on care of the elderly in hospitals is the recently completed *Hospital Outcomes Project for the Elderly* (HOPE) of the John A. Hartford Foundation of New York City. Using nursing care models, the HOPE project was able to show both improved patient function as well as improved nurse attitudes and work satisfaction in caring for elderly patients.

THE PROJECT GOALS

The *Nurses Improving Care to the Hospitalized Elderly* (NICHE) project is an exciting opportunity to disseminate outcomes of the HOPE project to the broader hospital community. We invite you to compete to be one of four hospital sites that will be chosen to implement the NICHE project. The goals of the project are to assist hospitals to:

1. Implement and analyze institutional assessment of the needs of elderly patients.

2. Select and implement a nursing care model for care of elderly patients.

3. Implement one or more practice protocols on areas of nursing care for elderly patients with urinary incontinence, sleep disorders, pressure ulcers, and mechanical restraints.

4. Develop a database from which to monitor progress in achieving the hospital's goals for care of elderly patients.

Over a 6-month period, participating hospitals will receive technical assistance from project staff at Columbia and New York University, the Education Development Center, and members of the project Advisory Board. Each participating hospital will receive:

1. An Institutional Assessment Profile of the care currently provided to their elderly patients.

2. Technical assistance in identifying and selecting a nursing model of care and practice protocol(s) appropriate to the hospital's care of elderly patients.

3. Two days of on-site consultation and follow-up telephone consultation by experts who have implemented the selected nursing model and practice protocol(s).

4. Consultation on development of a database to monitor ongoing care of elderly patients.

We believe that the NICHE project provides an important impetus to institutions that are enthusiastic about improving their programs of care for geriatric patients. Hospitals interested in participating should complete the attached materials and return them by **June 30, 1993** to:

Terry Fulmer, RN, PhD, FAAN
NICHE Project
Columbia University School of Nursing
630 West 168th Street
New York, NY 10032

Phone no. 212-305-4165
Fax no. 212-305-6937

APPLICATION

Please limit the body of the application to no more than 10 double spaced pages.

We are delighted with your interest in the HOPE Dissemination Program, NICHE. It signals an important and vital step toward improving the care of hospitalized geriatric patients. **Please complete the following questions:**

PART A

1. Hospital: _____

   Address: _____

   _____

   _____

2. Name and Title of Person Responsible for Application:
   (Please attach resume or curriculum vitae.)

   _____

   Address: _____

   _____

   _____

   Telephone number: _____

   Facsimile (fax) number: _____

3. Name of Chief Executive Officer: _____

   Address: _____

   _____

   _____

   Telephone number: _____

   Fax number: _____

4. Name of Nurse Executive Officer: _____
   (Please attach resume or curriculum vitae.)

   Address: _____

   _____

   _____

Telephone number: _____

Fax number: _____

5. Please name a nursing coordinator who will be responsible for the oversight of the project. The person named should have some familiarity with survey research, marketing, or evaluation, including knowledge of response rates and data management.

Name and title of coordinator: _____
(Please attach resume or curriculum vitae.)

Address: _____

_____

_____

Telephone number: _____

Fax number: _____

PART B

1. Describe your hospital. Please include the size, patient population/mix, description of staff (RN, LPN, NA, mix), facilities, affiliations, accreditation, and mission statement.

2. Describe the nursing model or models for nursing practice currently used by the hospital.

3. Describe the hospital commitment to geriatric care, including a statement of current and future goals. Provide evidence that nurse managers are prepared to support this project.

4. Describe how this project will relate to existing programs already in place.

5. Describe the incentive plan that the hospital will provide to encourage participation in an on-site program related to the improvement of geriatric nursing care (clinical support, time to fill out instruments, clerical support as necessary, and coverage when there are educational sessions).

6. Articulate self-identified priorities that you would like to address (i.e., continuity of care).

7. What are the products and/or outcomes you hope to achieve by participating in this project?

8. How will you evaluate your progress in geriatric care in the future?

Dissemination of the Hospital Outcomes Project for the Elderly

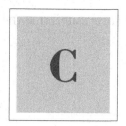

Models of Nursing Care for the Hospitalized Elderly

Columbia University School of Nursing
New York University School of Nursing
and
Education Development Center, Inc.

THE HOPE PROJECT

MODELS OF NURSING CARE FOR THE HOSPITALIZED ELDERLY

While most elderly patients benefit from treatment provided in hospitals, a substantial number of those patients experience untoward events during and subsequent to hospitalization. One of the few programs to specifically focus on care of the elderly in hospitals is the recently completed *Hospital Outcomes Project for the Elderly* (HOPE), funded by the John A Hartford Foundation of New York City. This project yielded five models of nursing care that acute care hospitals can implement to improve geriatric health.

Unit-Based Geriatric Care

In a model developed at Yale-New Haven Hospital, a unit-based, nurse-centered Geriatric Care Program (GCP) integrated geriatric resource nurses (GRNs), gerontological nurse specialists (GNSs), primary nurses, and a geriatrician on the geriatric care team (GCT). The program was based on the beliefs that: (1) primary nurses know the most about the day-to-day patterns and problems of the elderly who come to their units; (2) primary nurses, by serving as GRNs, are more likely to integrate new behaviors into practice because of the unit-based visibility and regular feedback available; and (3) a GRN program can recognize expertise and later might be reflected in a clinical ladder program for primary nurses. To support the learning needs of the GRNs, a monthly geriatric nursing interest group conference was established for teaching purposes and the exchange of ideas.

From the outset, the overall project was divided into two parallel programs: the GCP, concerned with the clinical intervention; and the GCP Evaluation

Project, which evaluated the efficacy of the project. Four target conditions, referred to as "geriatric vital signs," were selected to serve as markers of general functional decline in the hospitalized elderly: delirium, decline in physical functioning, incontinence, and pressure ulcers. The overall hypothesis of the study was that through improved recognition, prevention, and effective remedial therapy, the target conditions would be reduced in the intervention group as compared to the nonintervention group. High-level, mid-level, and control interventions were implemented on both medical and surgical services. The high-level units received the full intervention model (GRNs, geriatric nurse specialists, and physician-based GCT). The mid-level units received only the nursing component (GRNs and GNSs) but not the physician-based GCT. Standard care was provided on the control units.

Acute Care of the Elderly Medical–Surgical Nursing Unit

This model was developed at University Hospitals of Cleveland in conjunction with the Frances Payne Bolton School of Nursing at Case Western Reserve University. A 29-bed medical–surgical specialty unit was renovated and dedicated as an Acute Care of the Elderly (ACE) unit to prevent functional decline in this targeted group of patients. The unit was designed with special attention to the physical environment, collaborative team building, and development of nurse-initiated clinical protocols of care. Clinicians worked with designers to adapt the environment to enhance patient function. Soft colors, which have a calming effect, were used for patients' rooms. Geometrical hallway carpeting helped patients pace their activity. An activity room for congregate meals, visiting, and art and music therapy was decorated in vivid colors. Levers replaced door knobs for easy access. Patients' rooms contained recliner sand low beds with automatic lights. Collaborative team building began with interdisciplinary in services and workshops. Nurses developed clinical protocols as appropriate. And, unlike previous models using geriatric experts as consultants, in this model the geriatric medical director and clinical nurse specialist held dual roles.

Improving Nurses' Accuracy and Speed in Detecting and Managing Delirium

This model, developed at the University of Chicago hospitals, provides for consultation and education by a doctorate-level GNS to improve nurses' accuracy and speed in detecting and managing delirium in hospitalized elderly patients. Specifically, nurses were taught:

(1) the use and interpretation of simple bedside tests for assessing cognition; (2) the clinical features that distinguish delirium, dementia, and depression; (3) when and how to communicate patients' symptoms to physicians; (4) common causes of delirium in this patient population; (5) independent, interdependent, and dependent strategies for preventing and managing delirium; and (6) how to

document findings in the medical record. Nurses received direct instruction on all study units and on every shift. The instruction was repeated once for reinforcement. Preprinted assessment forms and a large poster that summarized all instrumental components of the approach were placed in a prominent position in each nursing station. In addition, the model provides for consultation from the GNS. While the GNS model has been used in a few other hospitals to provide geriatric support to nurses, no prior program has measured the effect of the GNS model in alleviating one discrete clinical problem.

Comprehensive Discharge Planning for the Elderly

The Discharge Planning Model currently being implemented at the University of Pennsylvania has two major objectives: (1) to use a comprehensive discharge planning protocol developed specifically for the hospitalized elderly and implemented by GNSs and (2) to evaluate the effectiveness of this model as compared to the hospital's general discharge planning procedures. Preliminary findings from the first 3 years of implementation of this model indicate that this clinical intervention has lengthened the time between rehospitalizations for subjects in the experimental group.

This intervention targets elders at high risk for poor postdischarge outcomes. The intervention includes direct care by a clinical nurse specialist from the time of admission, and availability of this nurse through the postdischarge period (4 weeks postdischarge). The assumption is made that GNSs have advanced knowledge and skill in caring for high-risk elderly and their caregivers. The GNSs, therefore, provide care under a general protocol and adapt this protocol to the specific needs of the elderly. GNSs see patients soon after admission and at least every 48 hours during the course of the patient's hospital stay. The GNS is accessible to patients and family members by telephone 7 days a week and works with the unit staff in helping to customize care to the needs of individual patients. By coordinating care of multiple healthcare providers involved in discharge planning, the GNS becomes the one consistent person to whom patients and families can turn to during and soon after hospitalization. This model thus fosters continuity of care. Emphasis is placed on documentation, notably written discharge summaries provided by the GNS to patients, caregivers, primary physicians, and other health team members.

Managed Care

The overall objectives of the Managed Care Model are to: (1) provide outcome-oriented patient care; (2) use appropriate resources based on specific case type; (3) promote the integration and coordination of clinical services; (4) monitor the use of patient care resources; (5) support collaborative practice and continuity of care; and (6) enhance patient and provider satisfaction.

Within the Managed Care Model, selected staff nurses are upgraded to the role of case manager. Case managers serve as coordinators and facilitators of resources to the patients. Each case manager is responsible for their patients from the time of admission to the time of discharge from the unit. It is crucial that case managers be clinically expert and able to project patient needs for the entire course of the patient's hospital stay. An integral aspect of the case management model is standards of care called multidisciplinary action plans (MAPS). The MAP is a time-lined plan of care designed to guide all healthcare practitioners toward the achievement of the highest possible quality and cost-effective care.

In addition, case managers serve as role models and informal educators for other staff members (although this is not a formal job responsibility). This role modeling has a "trickledown" effect, ultimately leading to an upgrade in the quality of care delivered by the entire nursing staff. The case manager is also the link to the physician in the development and ongoing evaluation of the MAP. Thus, the case manager's role is pivotal to the full integration of the MAP on any nursing unit.

NICHE: Draft Text for Newsletter 1993

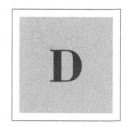

FINDING OUR NICHE AT "INSTITUTION NAME"

Patients age 65 and older make up about half of our admissions and about two-thirds of our hospital days. Caring for older adults is a major community responsibility of "Institution Name." We strive to provide the best possible care to older adults, and to achieve the highest possible patient satisfaction.

How prepared are we for this challenge? What are our strengths, and what are our weaknesses? How can we build on these strengths to improve our care? How can we empower our nursing staff in caring for older adults and their families?

In the next month or so, "Institution Name" will be conducting a survey on geriatric care among its nursing staff—part of NICHE (Nurses Improving Care to Hospitalized Elderly), a national initiative to assist healthcare organizations in meeting the needs of acutely ill elderly. The survey, the Geriatric Institutional Assessment Profile, assesses nurses' (a) attitudes toward caring for the elderly; (b) knowledge of guidelines for care of the elderly; (c) knowledge of common geriatric syndromes; and (d) perceptions of barriers to best nursing practice for elderly patients.

The findings will be critical in our efforts to provide quality care to our older patients and their families. In addition, by linking our results to a national database, we will be able to assess how we compare to their healthcare providers. Where do we do better, and where don't we? What can we learn from other NICHE hospitals, and what can we teach them?

The survey will be another step in our CQI efforts. It will also help us plan for the future—an important task considering the changing demographics of this community and the local area.

We encourage all nursing staff to participate in this survey. We want to hear your voice!

We need your help in finding our NICHE at "Institution Name"!

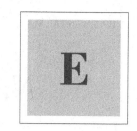

NICHE

Institutional Assessment Profile

This institution is about to embark on the *Nurses Improving Care to the Hospitalized Elderly* (NICHE) program. NICHE is a multidisciplinary worksite-based program that addresses the care of the hospitalized elderly. This Institutional Assessment Profile identifies the particular issues and concerns regarding the care of elderly patients at this institution.

In answering these questions, consider only the care provided to elderly patients (those aged 65 or older).

DO NOT PUT YOUR NAME ON THIS QUESTIONNAIRE. This will ensure that your responses remain anonymous. The questionnaires will be analyzed by Education Development Center, Inc. Results will be provided to the program faculty for distribution at this institution.

It is important that we receive this information from you as soon as possible. It will help us to update and strengthen clinical policies and practices and thereby improve the quality of care we provide to elderly patients and their families.

PLEASE COMPLETE THIS PROFILE AND RETURN IT TO THE NICHE PROGRAM COORDINATOR.

INSTRUCTIONS

- Please use a blue pen, a black pen, or a number 2 pencil.
- Make heavy marks that fill the ovals.
- Make no stray marks on the survey portion of the form.
- Do not fold this form.

Nurses Improving Care to the Hospitalized Elderly

INSTITUTIONAL ASSESSMENT PROFILE

1. **Please check your profession:**

   Nurse

Nursing Assistant	BSN
AD	**MSN**
LPN	Clinical Specialist
RN	

   Staff/Attending Physician

   House Officer

   Social Worker

   Physical Therapist

   Occupational Therapist

   Other, specify _____

2. **How many years of experience do you have in this profession?** _____

3. **How many years have you been working at this institution?** _____

4. **Which of the following best describes the unit where you currently spend the majority of your time?** *(Check one.)*

General medical	ER
General surgical	Rotating
Medica V surgical	Non critical care specialty unit (e.g., on colony, AIDS)
MICU	Geriatric unit
SICU	
CCU	

5. **For the elderly patients you care for, do you think the following treatments are used:**

	Too Little		Appropriately		Too Often
a. mechanical restraints (e.g., posey vests, geri-chairs)	1	2	3	4	5
b. sleeping medications or chemical restraints (i.e., tranquilizers)	1	2	3	4	5
c. incontinence pads	1	2	3	4	5
d. adult diapers	1	2	3	4	5
e. urinary catheters	1	2	3	4	5
f. pressure mattresses	1	2	3	4	5
g. adaptive devices (e.g., foam wedges, bed alarms)	1	2	3	4	5
h. pain medication	1	2	3	4	5
i. tube feeding	1	2	3	4	5

6. **How often do disagreements among staff (disciplines) arise over the use of these treatments?**

	Almost Never		Sometimes		Almost Always
a. mechanical restraints (e.g., posey vests, geri-chairs)	1	2	3	4	5
b. sleeping medications or chemical restraints (i.e., tranquilizers)	1	2	3	4	5
c. incontinence pads	1	2	3	4	5
d. adult diapers	1	2	3	4	5
e. urinary catheters	1	2	3	4	5
f. pressure mattresses	1	2	3	4	5
g. adaptive devices, (e.g., foam wedges, bed alarms)	1	2	3	4	5
h. pain medication	1	2	3	4	5
i. tube feeding	1	2	3	4	5
j. pressure ulcer treatment (e.g., turning bedridden patients)	1	2	3	4	5

7. **How often do disagreements between staff and patients and/or their families arise over the use of these treatments?**

	Almost Never		Sometimes		Almost Always
a. mechanical restraints (e.g., posey vests, geri-chairs)	1	2	3	4	5
b. sleeping medications or chemical restraints (i.e., tranquilizers)	1	2	3	4	5
c. incontinence pads	1	2	3	4	5
d. adult diapers	1	2	3	4	5
e. urinary catheters	1	2	3	4	5
f. pressure mattresses	1	2	3	4	5
g. adaptive devices, (e.g., foam wedges, bed alarms)	1	2	3	4	5
h. pain medication	1	2	3	4	5
i. tube feeding	1	2	3	4	5
j. pressure ulcer treatment (e.g., turning bedridden patients)	1	2	3	4	5

8. **At your institution, how satisfied are you about the extent to which**

	Not very Satisfied		Somewhat Satisfied		Very Satisfied
a. staff individualize care for the geriatric patient	1	2	3	4	5
b. geriatric patients get the care they need	1	2	3	4	5
c. issues about geriatric patient care are discussed by the staff	1	2	3	4	5
d. staff are familiar with how aging affects response to treatment	1	2	3	4	5
e. aging is considered a factor in planning and evaluation	1	2	3	4	5
f. patients receive the information they need to make decisions about their care	1	2	3	4	5
g. families receive the information and support they need to help elderly patients	1	2	3	4	5
h. staff obtain information about elderly patients' prehospital baseline	1	2	3	4	5
i. there is adequate continuity of care across settings	1	2	3	4	5
j. there is adequate continuity of care between units	1	2	3	4	5

9. **The following are obstacles to making good decisions about the care provided to elderly patients. To what extent does each interfere with care at your institution?**

	Does Not Interfere	Somewhat Interferes			Greatly Interferes
a. lack of knowledge about care of the elderly	1	2	3	4	5
b. lack of or inadequate written geriatric policies and procedures	1	2	3	4	5
c. differences of opinion among staff (disciplines) regarding common geriatric problems	1	2	3	4	5
d. lack of specialized services for the elderly (e.g., oral care, podiatry)	1	2	3	4	5
e. lack of special equipment (e.g., raised toilet seats, special mattresses)	1	2	3	4	5
f. exclusion of nurses from geriatric care decisions	1	2	3	4	5
g. economic pressures to limit expensive treatment or length of stay	1	2	3	4	5
h. staff shortages/time constraints	1	2	3	4	5
i. communication difficulties with geriatric patients and their families	1	2	3	4	5
j. exclusion of the elderly from care decisions	1	2	3	4	5
k. confusion over who is the appropriate decision maker	1	2	3	4	5

10. **How many geriatric nurse specialists or geriatric nurse practitioners does your institution have on staff?**

0	1	2	3	4	5+	Don't know

11. **How often do you use their consultative services?**

Daily	Weekly	Monthly	Less Than Monthly	Hardly Ever	Not Available
1	2	3	4	5	6

12. **How often do you use these other geriatric support services?**

	Daily	Weekly	Monthly	Less Than Monthly	Hardly Ever	Not Available
a. geriatric nurse specialist or geriatric nurse practitioner	1	2	3	4	5	6
b. geriatrician	1	2	3	4	5	6
c. geriatric social worker	1	2	3	4	5	6
d. geriatric psychologist/psychiatrist	1	2	3	4	5	6
e. geriatric rounds and in services	1	2	3	4	5	6
f. geriatric texts and journals	1	2	3	4	5	6
g. regional/national geriatric conference/workshops	1	2	3	4	5	6

13. **How would you rate the Job your institution has done educating the staff about the care of the elderly?**

Poor		Adequate		Excellent
1	2	3	4	5

14. **How knowledgeable do you consider yourself to be about basic principles and issues surrounding the care of the elderly?**

Not Very Knowledgeable		Somewhat Knowledgeable		Very Knowledgeable
1	2	3	4	5

15. **How vulnerable do you feel to legal liability arising from:**

	Not At All Vulnerable		Somewhat Vulnerable		Very Vulnerable
a. the development of pressure ulcers in hospitalized patients	1	2	3	4	5
b. patient falls	1	2	3	4	5
c. charges of unlawful restraint	1	2	3	4	5
d. injuries from use of restraints	1	2	3	4	5
e. nosocomial infection from catheter use	1	2	3	4	5
f. injuries resulting from use of sedating medication	1	2	3	4	5

16. **Within the last 12 months, approximately what proportion of the patients in your care have been 65 years of age and older?**

Almost None	Less Than Half	Half	More Than Half	Almost All
1	2	3	4	5

17. Approximately what proportion of the elderly patients in your care:

	Almost None	Less Than Half	Half	More Than Half	Almost All
a. come from nursing homes	1	2	3	4	5
b. have families or loved ones who participate in their care	1	2	3	4	5
c. are discharged to a nursing home	1	2	3	4	5
d. are discharged home alone	1	2	3	4	5
e. are discharged home with home healthcare or a caregiver	1	2	3	4	5
f. have a continuing care plan	1	2	3	4	5
g. are Black/African American	1	2	3	4	5
h. are Hispanic/Latino	1	2	3	4	5
i. are Asian	1	2	3	4	5
j. are White	1	2	3	4	5
k. do not speak English	1	2	3	4	5
l. are not insured	1	2	3	4	5

18. Approximately what proportion of your shift is spent caring for elderly patients in your unit?

Almost None	Less Than Half	Half	More Than Half	Almost All
1	2	3	4	5

19. Some elderly patients can exhibit behaviors that are upsetting. How often are the elderly patients in your care:

	Never	Sometimes (1–4×/wk)	Often (5+×/wk)
a. demanding	1	2	3
b. argumentative	1	2	3
c. uncooperative	1	2	3
d. seeking reassurance	1	2	3
e. up during the night	1	2	3
f. wandering during the day	1	2	3
g. confused/agitated	1	2	3

20. How much does it bother you when the elderly patients in your care:

	Does Not Disturb Me	Disturbs Me Somewhat	Disturbs Me Very Much
a. are demanding	1	2	3
b. are argumentative	1	2	3
c. are uncooperative	1	2	3
d. seek reassurance	1	2	3
e. are up during the night	1	2	3
f. wander during the day	1	2	3
g. are confused/agitated	1	2	3

21. Overall, how much difficulty would you say you are experiencing caring for the elderly patients on your unit?

No Difficulty		Some Difficulty		Great Difficulty
1	2	3	4	5

22. How rewarding is your work with elderly patients?

Not Rewarding		Somewhat Rewarding		Very Rewarding
1	2	3	4	5

23. How burdensome do you find your work with elderly patients?

Not Burdensome		Somewhat Burdensome		Very Burdensome
1	2	3	4	5

24. To what extent do you disagree or agree with these statements about your hospital:

	Strongly Disagree				Strongly Agree
a. Clinicians and administrators work together to solve geriatric patient problems	1	2	3	4	5
b. It is acceptable to disagree with your supervisor regarding geriatric patient care	1	2	3	4	5
c. Input from staff is sought in determining policies and guidelines about geriatric care	1	2	3	4	5
d. Geriatric patients are always treated with respect	1	2	3	4	5
e. Appropriate staff is involved with decisions about geriatric practice	1	2	3	4	5
f. Personal growth is encouraged	1	2	3	4	5
g. The rights of elderly patients are protected	1	2	3	4	5

Indicate the degree to which you disagree or agree with the following statements:

	Strongly Disagree				Strongly Agree
25. Most pressure ulcers are preventable.	1	2	3	4	5
26. Pressure ulcers occur in about half of the hospitalized elderly.	1	2	3	4	5
27. It is almost always possible to prevent skin breakdown.	1	2	3	4	5
28. Heels are one of the most susceptible regions to break down in a bedridden patient.	1	2	3	4	5
29. Pressure ulcers can lead to osteomyelitis.	1	2	3	4	5
30. Regular massage over bony prominences reduces skin breakdown.	1	2	3	4	5
31. Time spent preventing pressure ulcers is valued at this institution.	1	2	3	4	5
32. I don't have time to perform daily skin assessment on my elderly patients.	1	2	3	4	5
33. Adequate nutrition is the most essential element in preventing skin breakdown.	1	2	3	4	5
34. Changes in sleep patterns are a normal part of aging.	1	2	3	4	5
35. Sleep problems in hospitalized patients contribute to poor hospital outcomes.	1	2	3	4	5
36. Sedatives prevent hallucinations and agitation in elderly patients with sleep disorders.	1	2	3	4	5
37. Most sleeping problems in hospitalized elderly patients require the use of sedatives.	1	2	3	4	5
38. Sleep disturbances should always be aggressively treated.	1	2	3	4	5
39. We do a good job identifying and preventing sleep disorders.	1	2	3	4	5
40. Time spent preventing sleep problems is valued at this institution.	1	2	3	4	5
41. I don't have the time to help prevent sleep problems without relying on sedatives.	1	2	3	4	5
42. Prevalence of incontinence in hospitalized elderly patients is about 20%.	1	2	3	4	5

	Strongly Disagree				Strongly Agree
43. Problems with urinary continence are a normal part of aging.	1	2	3	4	5
44. Kegel exercises are good for all types of incontinence problems.	1	2	3	4	5
45. Constipation can lead to urinary incontinence.	1	2	3	4	5
46. Time spent managing urinary incontinence without the use of catheters or diapers is valued at this institution.	1	2	3	4	5
47. I try to avoid using indwelling catheters for elderly patients even if this means they are occasionally well.	1	2	3	4	5
48. We use diapers at night for most of our incontinent elderly patients.	1	2	3	4	5
49. Indwelling urinary catheters are appropriate in the management of incontinence as long as they are discontinued after 10 days.	1	2	3	4	5
50. Reducing the use of indwelling catheters creates significant demands on staff time.	1	2	3	4	5
51. Indwelling catheters are the single leading cause of septicemia in hospitalized elderly.	1	2	3	4	5
52. Confused elderly patients are safer when restrained in bed or a chair.	1	2	3	4	5
53. Nerve injuries can result from the use of restraints.	1	2	3	4	5
54. Using restraints often contributes to patient confusion.	1	2	3	4	5
55. I check my restrained patients at least every hour.	1	2	3	4	5
56. When the use of mechanical restraints goes down, the use of sedating drugs goes up.	1	2	3	4	5
57. At this institution, all reasonable alternatives are tried before restraining elderly patients.	1	2	3	4	5

	Strongly Disagree				*Strongly Agree*
58. Clinicians need better guidelines to help determine what care is appropriate for the elderly	1	2	3	4	5
59. Many elderly patients prefer to let their caregiver make the decision about what treatment is best	1	2	3	4	5
60. My opinion about the proper care of geriatric patients is valued by my colleagues.	1	2	3	4	5

61. **What is your age?** _____

62. **What is your gender?**

Male _____ Female _____

63. **What is your religion?**

Protestant

Jewish

Catholic

None

Other/specify _____

64. **How do you describe yourself?**

Black/African American

White

Hispanic/Latino

Asian

Other/specify_____

65. **How many years of school have you completed?** _____
(High school = 12, 2-year college = 14, MD = 20)

66. **What are the most pressing issues you currently face in caring for the elderly?**

_____

_____

_____

_____

_____

_____

_____

_____

_____

67. **Do you have any other comments or reactions to particular issues raised by this questionnaire?**

_____

_____

_____

_____

_____

_____

_____

_____

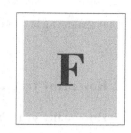

NICHE

Geriatric Institutional Assessment Profile

Instructions:
- You may use a blue or black pen or a pencil to fill in the ovals
- Make marks that fill the ovals   Like this: ●   Not Like this ⊘   or this ⊗
- Do not make stray marks outside of the ovals
- Do not fold this form

1. In what position do you spend the majority of your time?

○ Nursing Assistant/Aid
○ Staff Nurse
○ Head Nurse/Nurse Manager
○ Clinical Specialist/Nurse Practitioner
○ Nursing Faculty
○ Patient Educator

○ Staff Educator
○ Administrator
○ Staff/Attending MD
○ House Officer/Resident/ Fellow
○ Other (specify)

○ Pharmacist
○ Social Worker
○ Occupational Therapist
○ Physical Therapist
○ Respiratory Therapist
○ Lab Technician
○ Dietician

2. *For Nurses,* please fill in highest nursing degree. *(Select One)*

○ Nurse Assistant
○ LPN/LVN

If RN: highest degree/licensure
○ Diploma   ○ Masters
○ AD   ○ Doctorate
○ BSN

○ Not Applicable

3. Please fill in your highest non-nursing degree. *(Nurses and Non nurses)*

○ BS, BA
○ MS, MA
○ PhD, EdD, SciD

○ Other professional degree (MD, JD, etc.)
○ Not applicable

4. How many years of experience do you have in this profession?

5. How many years have you been working at this institution?

6. Unit where you spend the most time:

○ General Medical
○ General Surgical
○ General Medical/Surgical
○ ER
○ ICU-critical care
○ CCU-coronary care
○ Noncritical care specialty unit (e.g., step down, oncology, AIDS)

○ Geriatric Unit
○ OB/GYN
○ Long-Term Care Unit/ Hospice
○ Ambulatory Care Unit
○ Rehabilitation
○ Home care
○ Psychiatric Unit
○ Rotating
○ Other (specify)

7. For the elderly patients you care for, do you think the following treatments are used:

	Too Little	Appropriately			Too Often
a. mechanical restraints (e.g., posey vests, geri-chairs)	○	○	○	○	○
b. sleeping medications or chemical restraints (i.e., tranquilizers)	○	○	○	○	○
c. incontinence pads	○	○	○	○	○
d. adult diapers	○	○	○	○	○
e. urinary catheters	○	○	○	○	○
f. pressure mattresses	○	○	○	○	○
g. adaptive devices (e.g., foam wedges, bed alarms)	○	○	○	○	○
h. pain medication	○	○	○	○	○
i. tube feeding	○	○	○	○	○
j. pressure ulcer treatment (e.g., foam wedges, bed alarms) . .	○	○	○	○	○

8. How often do disagreements among staff (between disciplines) arise over the use of these treatments?

	Almost Never		Sometimes		Almost Always
a. mechanical restraints (e.g., posey vests, geri-chairs) . .	○	○	○	○	○
b. sleeping medications or chemical restraints (i.e., tranquilizers)	○	○	○	○	○
c. incontinence pads	○	○	○	○	○
d. adult diapers	○	○	○	○	○
e. urinary catheters	○	○	○	○	○
f. pressure mattresses	○	○	○	○	○
g. adaptive devices, (e.g., foam wedges, bed alarms)	○	○	○	○	○
h. pain medication	○	○	○	○	○
i. tube feeding	○	○	○	○	○
j. pressure ulcer treatment (e.g., turning bedridden patients)	○	○	○	○	○

9. How often do disagreements between staff and patients and/or their families arise over the use of these treatments?

	Almost Never		Sometimes		Almost Always
a. mechanical restraints (e.g., posey vests, geri-chairs) . .	○	○	○	○	○
b. sleeping medications or chemical restraints (i.e., tranquilizers)	○	○	○	○	○
c. incontinence pads	○	○	○	○	○
d. adult diapers	○	○	○	○	○
e. urinary catheters	○	○	○	○	○
f. pressure mattresses	○	○	○	○	○
g. adaptive devices, (e.g., foam wedges, bed alarms)	○	○	○	○	○
h. pain medication	○	○	○	○	○
i. tube feeding	○	○	○	○	○
j. pressure ulcer treatment (e.g., turning bedridden patients)	○	○	○	○	○

10. At your institution, how satisfied are you about the extent to which:

	Not Very Satisfied		Somewhat Satisfied		Very Satisfied
a. staff individualize care	○	○	○	○	○
b. geriatric patients get the care they need	○	○	○	○	○
c. staff address issues about geriatric patients	○	○	○	○	○
d. staff are familiar with how aging affects response to treatment	○	○	○	○	○
e. aging is considered a factor in planning and evaluation	○	○	○	○	○
f. patients receive the information they need to make decisions about their care	○	○	○	○	○
g. families receive information and support they need to help elderly patients	○	○	○	○	○
h. staff obtain information about elderly patients' prehospital baseline	○	○	○	○	○
i. there is adequate continuity of care across settings	○	○	○	○	○
j. there is adequate continuity of care across hospital units	○	○	○	○	○

11. The following are obstacles to making good decisions about the care provided to elderly patients. To what extent does each interfere with care at your institution?

	Does Not Interfere		Somewhat Interferes		Greatly Interferes
a. lack of knowledge about care of the elderly	○	○	○	○	○
b. lack of or inadequate written geriatric policies and procedures	○	○	○	○	○
c. differences of opinion among staff (between disciplines) regarding common geriatric problems . . .	○	○	○	○	○
d. lack of specialized services for the elderly (e.g., oral care, podiatry)	○	○	○	○	○
e. lack of special equipment (e.g., raised toilet seats, special mattresses)	○	○	○	○	○
f. exclusion of nurses from geriatric care decisions	○	○	○	○	○
g. economic pressures to limit treatment or high length of stay	○	○	○	○	○

h. staff shortages/time constraints .... ○ ○ ○ ○ ○

i. communication difficulties with geriatric
patients and their families .... ○ ○ ○ ○ ○

j. exclusion of the elderly from care decisions .. ○ ○ ○ ○ ○

k. confusion over who is the appropriate decision
maker .... ○ ○ ○ ○ ○

12. How many geriatric nurse specialists or geriatric practitioners does your institution have on staff?

0	1	2	3	4	5 +
○	○	○	○	○	○

13. How often do you use their consultative services?

Daily	Weekly	Monthly	Less Than Monthly	Hardly Ever	Not available
○	○	○	○	○	○

14. How often do you use these other geriatric services?	Daily	Weekly	Monthly	Less Than Monthly	Hardly Ever	Not Available
a. geriatric nurse specialist or geriatric nurse practitioner	○	○	○	○	○	○
b. geriatrician	○	○	○	○	○	○
c. geriatric social worker	○	○	○	○	○	○
d. geriatric psychologist/ psychiatrist	○	○	○	○	○	○
e. geriatric rounds and in services ..	○	○	○	○	○	○
f. geriatric texts and journals	○	○	○	○	○	○
g. regional/national geriatric conferences, workshops	○	○	○	○	○	○

15. How would you rate the job your institution has done educating the staff about the care of the elderly?

Poor		Adequate		Excellent
○	○	○	○	○

16. How knowledgeable do you consider yourself to be about basic principles and issues surrounding the care of the elderly?

Not Very Knowledgeable		Somewhat Knowledgeable		Very Knowledgeable
○	○	○	○	○

---

17. How vulnerable do you feel to legal liability arising from:

	Not At All Vulnerable		Somewhat Vulnerable		Very Vulnerable
a. the development of pressure ulcers in hospitalized patients	○	○	○	○	○
b. patient falls	○	○	○	○	○
c. charges of unlawful restraint	○	○	○	○	○
d. injuries from use of restraints	○	○	○	○	○
e. nosocomial infection from catheter use	○	○	○	○	○
f. injuries resulting from use of sedating medication	○	○	○	○	○

---

18. Within the last 12 months, approximately what proportion of the patients in your care have been 65 years of age and older?

Almost None	Less Than Half	Half	More Than Half	Almost All
○	○	○	○	○

---

19. Approximately what proportion of the elderly patients in your care:

	Almost None	Less Than Half	Half	More Than Half	Almost All
a. come from nursing homes	○	○	○	○	○
b. have families or loved ones who participate in their care	○	○	○	○	○
c. are discharged to a nursing home	○	○	○	○	○
d. are discharged home alone	○	○	○	○	○
e. are discharged home with home health care or a paid caregiver	○	○	○	○	○
f. have a continuing care plan	○	○	○	○	○
g. are Black/African American	○	○	○	○	○
h. are Hispanic/Latino	○	○	○	○	○
i. are Asian	○	○	○	○	○
j. are Caucasian	○	○	○	○	○
k. are other ethnicity	○	○	○	○	○
l. are not insured	○	○	○	○	○

20. Approximately what proportion of your shift is spent caring for elderly patients in your unit?

Almost None	Less Than Half	Half	More Than Half	Almost All
⚬	⚬	⚬	⚬	⚬

21. Some elderly patients can exhibit behaviors that are upsetting. How often are the elderly patients in your care:

	Never	Sometimes (1–4×/wk)	Often (5+×/wk)
a. demanding	⚬	⚬	⚬
b. argumentative	⚬	⚬	⚬
c. uncooperative	⚬	⚬	⚬
d. seeking reassurance	⚬	⚬	⚬
e. up during the night	⚬	⚬	⚬
f. wandering during the day	⚬	⚬	⚬
g. confused/agitated	⚬	⚬	⚬

22. How much does it bother you when the elderly patients in your care:

	Does Not Disturb Me	Disturbs Me Somewhat	Disturbs Me Very Much
a. are demanding	⚬	⚬	⚬
b. are argumentative	⚬	⚬	⚬
c. are uncooperative	⚬	⚬	⚬
d. seek reassurance	⚬	⚬	⚬
e. are up during the night	⚬	⚬	⚬
f. wander during the day	⚬	⚬	⚬
g. are confused/agitated	⚬	⚬	⚬

23. Overall, how much difficulty would you say you experience caring for the elderly patients on your unit?

No Difficulty		Some Difficulty		Great Difficulty
⚬	⚬	⚬	⚬	⚬

24. How rewarding is your work with elderly patients?

Not Rewarding		Somewhat Rewarding		Very Rewarding
⚬	⚬	⚬	⚬	⚬

25. How burdensome do you find your work with elderly patients?

Not Burdensome		Somewhat Burdensome		Very Burdensome
○	○	○	○	○

26. To what extent do you disagree or agree with these statements about your hospital:

	Strongly Disagree ←——————→ Strongly Agree				
a. Clinicians and administrators work together to solve geriatric patient problems	○	○	○	○	○
b. It is acceptable to disagree with your supervisor regarding geriatric patient care	○	○	○	○	○
c. Input from staff is sought in determining policies and guidelines about geriatric care	○	○	○	○	○
d. Geriatric patients are always treated with respect	○	○	○	○	○
e. Appropriate staff are involved with decisions about geriatric practice	○	○	○	○	○
f. Personal growth is encouraged	○	○	○	○	○
g. The rights of the elderly patients are protected	○	○	○	○	○

Indicate the degree to which you disagree or agree with the following statements:

	Strongly Disagree ←——————→ Strongly Agree				
27. Most pressure ulcers are preventable	○	○	○	○	○
28. Pressure ulcers occur in about half of the hospitalized elderly	○	○	○	○	○
29. It is almost always possible to prevent skin breakdown	○	○	○	○	○
30. Heels are one of the most susceptible regions to skin breakdown in a bedridden patient ...	○	○	○	○	○
31. Pressure ulcers can lead to osteomyelitis	○	○	○	○	○
32. Regular massage over bony prominences reduces skin breakdown	○	○	○	○	○
33. Time spent preventing pressure ulcers is valued at this institution	○	○	○	○	○
34. I don't have time to perform daily skin assessments on my elderly patients	○	○	○	○	○

	Strongly Disagree	⟷			Strongly Agree
35. Adequate nutrition is the most essential element in preventing skin breakdown	○	○	○	○	○
36. Changes in sleep patterns are a normal part of aging	○	○	○	○	○
37. Sleep problems in hospitalized patients contribute to poor hospital outcomes	○	○	○	○	○
38. Sedatives prevent hallucinations and agitation in elderly patients with sleep disorders	○	○	○	○	○
39. Most sleeping problems in hospitalized elderly patients require the use of sedatives	○	○	○	○	○
40. Sleep disturbances should always be aggressively treated	○	○	○	○	○
41. We do a good job identifying and preventing sleep disorders	○	○	○	○	○
42. Time spent preventing sleep problems is valued at this institution	○	○	○	○	○
43. I don't have the time to help prevent sleep problems without relying on sedatives	○	○	○	○	○
44. Prevalence of incontinence in hospitalized elderly patients is about 20%	○	○	○	○	○
45. Problems with urinary continence are a normal part of aging	○	○	○	○	○
46. Kegel exercises are good for all types of incontinence problems	○	○	○	○	○
47. Constipation can lead to urinary incontinence	○	○	○	○	○
48. Time spent managing urinary incontinence without the use of catheters or diapers, is valued at this institution	○	○	○	○	○
49. I try to avoid using indwelling catheters for elderly patients even if this means they are occasionally wet	○	○	○	○	○
50. We use diapers at night for most of our incontinent elderly patients	○	○	○	○	○
51. Indwelling urinary catheters are appropriate in the management of incontinence as long as they are discontinued after 10 days	○	○	○	○	○

	Strongly Disagree	←——————————→			Strongly Agree
52. Reducing the use of indwelling catheters creates significant demands on staff time	○	○	○	○	○
53. Indwelling catheters are the single leading cause of septicemia in hospitalized elderly . .	○	○	○	○	○
54. Confused elderly patients are safer when they are restrained in bed or a chair	○	○	○	○	○
55. Nerve injuries can result from the use of restraints	○	○	○	○	○
56. Using restraints often contributes to patient confusion	○	○	○	○	○
57. I check my restrained patients at least every hour	○	○	○	○	○
58. When the use of mechanical restraints goes down the use of sedating drugs goes up	○	○	○	○	○
59. At this institution, all reasonable alternatives are tried before restraining elderly patients . .	○	○	○	○	○
60. Clinicians need better guidelines to help determine what care is appropriate for the elderly	○	○	○	○	○
61. Many elderly patients prefer to let their caregiver make the decision about what treatment is best	○	○	○	○	○
62. My opinion about proper care of geriatric patients is valued by my colleagues	○	○	○	○	○

63. What is your age? ☐☐

64. Are you?   ○ Male   ○ Female

65. What is your religion?   ○ Protestant   ○ Catholic   ○ Jewish   ○ None
○ Other (specify) ☐☐☐☐☐☐☐☐☐☐☐☐☐☐☐☐☐☐☐☐

66. How do you describe yourself?   ○ Black/African American   ○ Hispanic/Latino   ○ Caucasian
○ Other (specify) ☐☐☐☐☐☐☐☐☐☐☐☐☐☐

67. How many years of school have you completed?
(High school = 12, 2-year college = 14, MD = 20)

---

68. What are the most pressing issues you currently face in caring for the elderly?

---

69. Do you have any other comments or reactions to a particular issue raised by this questionnaire?

NICHE

Nursing Standard of Practice Protocols

Columbia University School of Nursing
New York University School of Nursing and
Education Development Center, Inc.

NURSING STANDARD OF PRACTICE PROTOCOL: SLEEP DISTURBANCES IN ELDERLY PATIENTS

I. **Background**
  A. Sleep disturbances are abnormal difficulties in initiating and maintaining sleep.
  B. Sleep disturbances are associated with poorer outcomes of hospitalization. Adequate, uninterrupted sleep is essential to good outcomes.
  C. Older people do not normally have sleep disturbances.
  D. Most sleep disturbances of elderly persons have a diagnosable cause and are amenable to treatment.

II. **Assessment Parameters**
  A. Conduct a thorough, individualized sleep assessment of all patients' subjective evaluation of sleep, that is, verbal comments by the individual of:
    • not sleeping well
    • not feeling rested
    • being tired
    • being awakened earlier than usual
    • having interrupted sleep
  B. Observe and document daytime behavior and/or performance. Note whether the individual is:
    • irritable
    • restless
    • lethargic
    • listless
    • apathetic
  In addition, note:
    • difficulty concentrating
    • an increased reaction time
    • a greater sensitivity to pain
    • diminished daytime alertness

C. For individuals with sleep disturbance, identify and document:
1. Usual sleep/wake patterns (e.g., usual times for retiring and rising, time required for falling asleep, daytime physical and social activity)
2. Bedtime routines/rituals (e.g., snacks, beverages, personal hygiene, baths, prayer)
3. Diet and drug use (e.g., stimulants such as coffee or tobacco before bedtime, prescribed and over-the-counter medications, sleep aids, diuretics, laxatives)
4. Environmental factors (e.g., noise, light, temperature, ventilation)
5. Illness factors (e.g., pain, depression, worry, discomfort, anxiety, respiratory disturbances)

III. **Care Strategies**
A. Develop an *individualized* sleep protocol. Strategies for promoting sleep include:
1. Maintain normal sleep pattern (e.g., arrange medications and therapies to minimize sleep interruptions)
2. Encourage daytime activity (e.g., discourage daytime naps)
3. Support bedtime routines/rituals (e.g., enable bedtime reading, listening to music, or quiet television)
4. Promote comfort (e.g., make sure the bed is comfortable, including pillows as requested, wrinkle-free linen, and loose bedcovering)
5. Promote relaxation (e.g., provide warm milk or soup, offer a backrub)
6. Avoid/minimize stimulation before bedtime (e.g., no caffeinated drinks after dinner and reduce fluid intake prior to sleeping; individuals should also refrain from smoking)
7. Avoid/minimize drugs that negatively influence sleep (see Ebersole and Hess [1990] for a list of drugs that adversely affect sleep patterns)
8. Create a restful environment (e.g., turn off lights as desired, reduce or eliminate noise, minimize disruptions for therapy or monitoring)
B. Pharmacological treatment, prescription and administration of a sedative/hypnotic, should be implemented to correspond with patient practices at home, that is, low dosage. Pharmacologic treatment should be considered an intervention of last resort for individuals who have not been using sedatives or hypnotics at home.

IV. **Evaluation of Expected Outcomes**
A. Patient
1. Patients will report that they are sleeping well or feeling rested.
2. Patients will demonstrate an increased ability to concentrate and a reduction in behaviors indicative of sleep deprivation (e.g., restlessness).
B. Health care provider
1. Assessment of sleep disturbances will be more accurate.
C. Institution
1. Prevalence and incidence of sleep disorders will decrease.
2. Use of sedatives for patients with sleep disturbances will decrease.

V. **Follow-Up to Monitor Condition**
A. Continue to track incidence and prevalence of sleep disturbances.
B. Educate caregivers to continue assessment process.

REFERENCES

Bachman, D. L. (1992). Sleep disorders with aging: Evaluation and treatment. *Geriatrics, 47*(9), 53–61.

Ebersole, P., & Hess, P. (1990). *Toward healthy aging: Human needs and nursing response* (pp. 185–191). St. Louis, MO: Mosby.

Gillin, J. C., & Byerley, W. F. (1990). The diagnosis and management of insomnia. *New England Journal of Medicine, 322*(4), 230–248. doi:10.1056/NEJM199001253220406

National Institutes of Health. (1990, March 26–28). Treatment of sleep disorders of older people. *NIH Consensus Development Conference Statement, 8*(3), 1–22.

Wooten, V. (1992). Sleep disorders in geriatric patients. *Clinics in Geriatric Medicine, 8*(2), 427–439.

NURSING STANDARD OF PRACTICE PROTOCOL: URINARY INCONTINENCE IN ELDERLY PATIENTS

I. **Background**
A. Urinary incontinence is the involuntary loss of urine sufficient to be a problem to the patient (Agency for Health Care Policy Research, 1992).
B. Older people are not normally incontinent.
C. The loss of control associated with urinary incontinence and the use of catheters is personally devastating to the patient.
D. The majority of incontinent episodes in the hospital are reversible and preventable with nursing interventions. Urinary incontinence that is mild or controlled at home can be made worse by hospitalization (e.g., changes brought on by medication and difficulty getting to the bathroom).
E. Indwelling catheters predispose elderly persons to urinary tract infections—the most common cause of septicemia in older adults—and to fistula formation, both of which prolong hospital stay and increase mortality.

II. **Assessment Parameters**
A. Document the pattern of voiding of all patients prior to and during hospitalization to determine the presence or absence of incontinence. Note/ask for at 2-hour intervals:
- whether the patient is wet or dry
- whether the patient voided
- what volume of urine was voided
- any other comments (e.g., whether there was pain during urination)
B. Document the presence or absence of an indwelling urinary catheter.

C. Identify risk factors for incontinence developing during the hospital stay. (Etiology and contributing factors are described below.)

D. For patients who are incontinent:

1. Determine whether the problem is established (i.e., existed prior to hospitalization), transient and reversible (i.e., resulting from factors associated with hospitalization or treatment decisions), or both.

2. Identify and document the etiology of the problem.

   a. *Urge incontinence* is involuntary urine loss that occurs with a strong and abrupt desire to void. It is usually associated with the following conditions:
      - stroke
      - Parkinson's disease
      - Alzheimer's disease
      - cystitis
      - bladder stone
      - multiple sclerosis

   b. *Stress incontinence* is involuntary urine loss that occurs with increased abdominal pressure such as sneezing, coughing, or high-impact exercise. It is associated with:
      - pelvic floor muscle laxity
      - sphincter incompetence (rare)

   c. *Overflow incontinence* is involuntary urine loss that occurs with overdistention of the bladder, resulting in overflow or dribbling. Contributing factors include:
      - prostate enlargement
      - fecal impaction
      - tumor
      - atonia

   d. *Functional incontinence* is involuntary, unpredictable urine loss or the inability to reach the toilet on time due to environmental or host barriers. Contributing factors include:
      - disorientation
      - confusion
      - functional limitations (personal and environmental)
      - gait and balance impairment

   e. *Iatrogenic incontinence* results from treatments controlled by health care providers and is reversible. Contributing factors include (DIAPERS mnemonic):
      - delirium
      - infection
      - atrophic vaginitis or urethritis·
      - pharmaceutical considerations
      - excessive urine production
      - restricted mobility
      - stool impaction

III. **Care Strategies**
   A. General principles that apply to preventing and treating *all forms of incontinence*:
      1. Identify and continue successful prehospital management strategies for patients with established incontinence.
      2. Provide a regular toileting schedule: assisted toileting every 2 hours with some exceptions for nighttime shifts (as this may disrupt normal sleep patterns). Or develop a personalized toileting regimen using the data from the patient's incontinence assessment.
      3. Modify the environment to facilitate continence. Examples include: appropriate toilet location, good lighting, prompt response to calls for assistance, clothing with Velcro closures, and raised toilet seats with safety bars.
      4. Monitor fluid intake and maintain appropriate hydration schedule. During the daytime, maintain fluid intake to 1 to 2 L. Ask patients to refrain from alcohol and caffeine use as well as to restrict fluids prior to bedtime.
      5. Avoid medications that contribute to incontinence.
      6. Avoid use of indwelling catheters whenever possible.
      7. Provide patients with usual undergarments in expectation of continence. Be positive.
      8. Treat constipation to regularize bowel function.
      9. Use absorbent pads as needed to improve perineal hygiene if other measures fail.
   B. Additional strategies for patients with *storage problems*:
      1. Teach Kegel exercises. Help patients identify the proper muscle and exercise the muscle appropriately.
      2. Encourage bladder retraining.
      3. Prescribe habit training.
      4. Try prompted voiding.
      5. For women, add estrogen to therapeutic regimen if not contraindicated (for treatment of atrophic vaginitis).
   C. For patients with *release problems* not amenable to other interventions, provide clean, intermittent catheterization.

IV. **Evaluation of Expected Outcomes**
   A. Patient
      1. Patients will have fewer or no incontinent episodes.
      2. Patients will have fewer episodes of urinary tract infections and septicemia.
   B. Provider
      1. Assessment of incontinence will be more accurate.
      2. Evening chart will include documentation of voiding pattern.

C. Institutional
1. Hospital will require the adoption of assessment and documentation procedures.
2. Hospital will have available the Agency for Health Care Policy and Research *Guidelines* for urinary incontinence.

V. **Follow-Up to Monitor the Condition**
A. Assure follow-up through adequate discharge planning and appropriate community referral, that is, monitor patients after discharge, determine whether they are still incontinent, and plan accordingly.
B. Adopt a facility-wide effort to incorporate continuous quality improvement criteria into the clinical thinking of every practitioner.

REFERENCES

Agency for Health Care Policy Research. (1992). *Urinary Incontinence in Adults: Clinical Practice Guidelines* (Publication No. 92-0038). Rockville, MD: U. S. Department of Health and Human Services.

Resnick, N. M., Yalla, S. V., & Laureno, E. (1989). The pathophysiology of urinary incontinence among institutionalized elderly persons. *New England Journal of Medicine, 320*(1), 1–7. doi:10.1056/NEJM198901053200101

Rousseau, P., & Fuentevilla-Clifton, A. (1992). Urinary incontinence in the aged. Part 2: Management strategies. *Geriatrics, 47*(6), 37–40.

Thomas, A. M., & Morse, J. M. (1991). Managing urinary incontinence with self-care practices. *Journal of Gerontological Nursing, 17*(6), 9–14.

NURSING STANDARD OF PRACTICE PROTOCOL: USE OF MECHANICAL RESTRAINTS WITH ELDERLY PATIENTS

I. **Background**
A. Physical restraint is the use of any manual method or physical/mechanical device that the patient cannot remove, that restricts the patient's physical activity or normal access to his/her body, and that
- is not a usual and customary part of a medical, diagnostic, or treatment procedure indicated by the patient's medical condition and/or symptoms
- does not serve to promote the patient's independent functioning
B. The standard of care for hospitalized elderly patients is nonuse of mechanical restraints except under exceptional circumstances, after all reasonable alternatives have been tried.

    C. Risk factors for use of mechanical restraints in the acute care setting include:
- fall risk
- tubes or IVs that need stability
- severe cognitive and/or physical impairments
- diagnosis or presence of a psychiatric condition
- surgery

    D. Morbidity and mortality risks associated with mechanical restraint use include:
- nerve injury
- new-onset pressure ulcers
- pneumonia
- incontinence
- increased confusion
- inappropriate drug use
- strangulation/asphyxiation

    E. Appropriate alternatives exist to the use of mechanical restraints.

II. Assessment Parameters

    A. Request information about the use of mechanical restraints from prehospital settings.

    B. On admission, identify as at risk for restraint use any elderly patient who is agitated, at risk of falling, or disrupting therapy.

    C. Use 1:1 observation and/or behavior monitor logs to identify and document specific risks. For example, for fall risk, assess impaired cognition, poor balance, impaired gait, orthostatic hypotension, impaired vision and hearing, and the use of sedatives and/or hypnotics.

III. Care Strategies

    A. Prevention
1. Develop a nursing plan tailored to the patient's presenting problem(s) and specific risk factors.
2. Consider several alternative interventions. See attached appendices for suggested alternatives to restraints.
3. Refer to occupational and physical therapy for self-care deficits or mobility impairment; use adaptive equipment as appropriate.
4. Document use and effect of alternatives to restraints.

    B. Treatment
1. Use restraints only after exhausting all reasonable alternatives.
2. When using restraints:
   - choose the least restrictive device
   - reassess the patient's response at least every hour
   - remove restraints every 2 hours
   - renew orders q24 hours, after reassessment

3. Modify the care plan to compensate for restrictions imposed by restraint use:
   - change position frequently and provide skin care
   - provide adequate range of motion
   - assist with ADLs, such as eating and toileting
4. Continue to address underlying condition(s) that prompted restraint use (e.g., gait impairment). Refer to geriatric nurse specialist, occupational or physical therapy, and so forth as appropriate.

IV. **Evaluation of Expected Outcomes**
   A. Patient
      1. Mechanical restraints will be used only under well-documented exceptional circumstances, after all reasonable alternatives have been tried.
   B. Health care provider
      1. Providers will use a range of interventions other than restraints in the management of patient care problems.
   C. Institution
      1. Incidence and prevalence of physical restraint use will decrease.
      2. Use of chemical restraints will not increase.
      3. The number of serious injuries related to falls, agitated behavior, and other presenting problems for use of restraints will not increase.
      4. Referrals to occupational and physical therapy will increase, as will availability of adaptive equipment.
      5. Staff will receive ongoing education on the prevention of restraints.

V. **Follow-Up to Monitor Condition**
   A. Document incidence of restraint use on an ongoing basis.
   B. Educate caregivers to continue assessment and prevention.
   C. Identify patient characteristics and care problems that continue to be refractory and involve consultants (geriatric nurse specialist, etc.) in devising an expanded range of alternative approaches.

REFERENCES

Evans, L. K., Strumpf, N. E., & Williams, C. C. (1992). Limiting use of physical restraints: A prerequisite for independent functioning. In E. Calkins, A. Ford, & P. Katz (Eds.), *The practice of geriatrics*, (2nd ed.). Philadelphia, PA: Saunders.

Mion, L. C., & Frengley, J. D. (1993). Physical restraints in the hospital setting. In J. V. Braun & S. Lipson, (Eds.), *Toward a restraint free environment*. Baltimore, MD: Baltimore Health Professions Press.

National Nursing Home Restraint Minimization Program. (1991). *Retrain, don't restrain* (Field Test Version: Reference Curriculum). New York, NY: Jewish Home for the Aged.

Stillwell, E. M. (1991). Special issue: Nurses' use of restraints. *Journal of Gerontological Nursing, 17*(2), 3–30. doi:10.3928/0098-9134-19910201-03

Strumpf, N., Wagner, J., Evans, L., & Patterson, J. (1992). *Reducing restraints. individualized approaches to behavior.* Huntington Valley, PA: The Whitman Group.

NURSING STANDARD OF PRACTICE PROTOCOL: PRESSURE ULCERS IN ELDERLY PATIENTS

I. **Background**
   A. Eleven percent to 28% of hospitalized elderly have pressure ulcers.
   B. Complications of pressure ulcers include:
      - pain and discomfort
      - cellulitus
      - osteomyelitis
      - sepsis
      - increased hospital stays
      - increased mortality
   C. Risk factors for pressure sores include:
      - pressure, shearing forces, and friction
      - poor nutrition
      - immobility
      - skin moisture
      - incontinence
      - altered level of consciousness
   D. With aggressive care most pressure ulcers can be prevented.
   E. Prevention of pressure ulcers saves patient discomfort and prevents the need for intensive rehabilitation.

II. **Assessment Parameters**
   A. Request information about skin care regimen from prehospital setting on all patients.
   B. On admission, identify as *at risk for pressure ulcers* any elderly patient who has *either* impaired nutrition *or* whose ability to move is impaired by disease condition or treatment.
   C. Assess all at-risk patients using a standardized risk assessment instrument. For example, the Braden scale, which takes roughly 10 minutes to administer.
   D. Document risk factors, skin assessment, and plan for prevention and treatment, including a schedule for administering the risk assessment instrument and treatments.

III. **Care Strategies**

A. Prevent skin breakdown.

1. Educate patients and caregivers.

   a. Implement education programs for patients, families, and caregivers as to:
      - etiology of and risk factors for pressure ulcers
      - risk assessment tools and their application
      - skin assessment
      - selection and/or use of support surfaces
      - individualized program of skin care
      - positioning to reduce risk of tissue breakdown
      - accurate documentation

   b. Assign responsibility for pressure ulcer prevention.

   c. Develop, implement, and evaluate programs using principles of adult learning. Present audience-appropriate level of information.

   d. Develop clearly defined quality assurance standards and mechanisms.

2. Maintain and improve skin integrity.

   a. Use a standardized skin assessment instrument (and/or body chart) to check skin daily; document results.

   b. Keep skin clean and dry. Avoid hot water and strong soap. Keep irritating agents such as urine and wound drainage off skin.

   c. Use humidifiers and moisturizers to keep skin moist. Keep patient well hydrated (eight glasses of noncaffeine fluid per day unless there is a fluid restriction).

   d. Do not massage skin over bony prominences because it can lead to deep tissue trauma.

   e. Provide adequate calories, protein, vitamin C, and zinc.

   f. Keep patient active. Ambulate where possible, teach aerobic exercises, or administer passive exercise.

   g. Document treatments and outcomes.

3. Avoid pressure, friction, and shearing of skin.

   a. Move or change the position of patients on bed rest every 2 hours.

   b. Keep legs apart with pillows or foam wedges when the patient lies on his/her side. Avoid direct pressure on the trochanter.

   c. Lift heels off the bed with pillows or other devices (not donuts).

   d. Use pressure-reducing mattresses and chair cushions for patients unable to change position without assistance.

   e. Lower the head of the bed as much as possible and limit the amount of time the head of the bed is elevated.

   f. Document treatments and their outcomes.

B. Treat all skin breakdown immediately.
1. Inspect skin lesion daily and document location, 11t size (cm), stage (1–4), odor, skin surrounding lesion, drainage.
2. Treat pressure ulcer according to lesion stage (Agency for Health Care Policy and Research, 1992)
3. Educate patient, family, and caregivers on assessment, prevention, and treatment.

IV. **Evaluation of Expected Outcomes**
A. Patients
1. Skin integrity will be maintained.
2. Patients will leave the hospital with no pressure ulcers.
3. Patients (and/or caregivers) will be knowledgeable about prevention and assessment of pressure ulcers.
4. Preexisting pressure ulcers will be improved or stabilized.
B. Health care provider
1. Documentation of prevention, treatment, and outcomes will be improved.
C. Institution
1. Incidence and prevalence of pressure ulcers will decrease.

V. **Follow-Up to Monitor Condition**
A. Educate caregivers to continue assessment process.
B. Show evidence of transfer of information to discharge setting.
C. Continue to track incidence and prevalence of pressure ulcers among patients admitted.

REFERENCES

Agency for Health Care Policy and Research. (1992). *Pressure ulcers in adults: Prediction and prevention. Clinical practice guidelines, Number 3* (Publication No. 92-0047). Rockville·, MD: U.S. Department of Health and Human Services.

Allman, R. M. (1989). Pressure ulcers among the elderly. *New England Journal of Medicine, 320*(13), 850–853. doi:10.1056/NEJM198903303201307

Bergstrom, N., Braden, B. J., Laguzza, A., & Holman, Z. (1987). The Braden scale for predicting pressure sore risk. *Nursing Research, 36*(4), 205–210.

Meehan, M. (1990). Multisite pressure ulcer prevalence survey. *Decubitus, 3*(4), 14–17.

Letter From Tracie Kientz

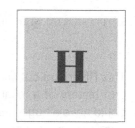

Tracie Nolan Kientz
3544 Dutchman Rd.
Charlottesville, VA. 22901

Terry Fulmer
Columbia University School of Nursing
630 West 168th St.
New York, NY. 10032
June 30, 1994

Dear Terry,

It's been in my mind to write you for a while. I think now is a good time because it is truly NICHE EVE here for me at UVA. Kathy Fletcher and I will begin rounds in the CCU early in July. Two of my coworkers had the opportunity to meet Kathy at a physical assessment class given at the School of Nursing this past week. They both said they now see why I've been so excited to work with Kathy. They found her a wonderful teacher and could tell how much she cares about the elderly. I'm excited that they feel this way and think it can only help the whole process we are about to begin.

I had a difficult spring but have bounced back nicely. I had a cervical laminectomy April 5. Talk about a threat to one's functional capacity! But what good lessons I learned as a nurse—especially one that wants to help our elderly patients. I'm doing very well, with complete relief of my symptoms.

When I got back to work after my surgery I felt a little overwhelmed by all of the geriatric issues I saw in our patients. There really are many issues once your assessment skills expand beyond the immediate concerns of blood pressure and oxygenation. It seems I see the issues more clearly than before and I'm learning all the time.

I am feeling more and more support toward improving the care of our geriatric patients. One of our nursing attendants told me she was glad someone was bringing this information into the unit. This same person figured out how to clear up a skin problem in one of our long-term patients. She received written praise for this.

We had an elderly patient from a nursing home this week. The RN caring for her was concerned about the patient's mental status and anxiety level. This RN called the nursing home from which the elderly woman came and discovered she was on Ativan TID. The RN obtained an order for the Ativan and the patient was able to relax and have a good visit with her family. This same woman died the next night.

Another RN I work with did a wonderful pre-op assessment of an elderly woman going for coronary bypass.

This RN found out information about the patient's history of urinary incontinence, difficulty ambulating, and history of a fecal impaction on a previous hospitalization. As you know, any one of these issues could have a huge impact on the woman's post-op course. We wrote the information in the chart for her post-op nurses. I told my coworkers what a great job they did and how much they helped these two elderly patients.

It was such a wonderful experience to be able to spend time with you back in March. There are times and people in one's career that turn out to be real pointers for the future. I will never forget how you bent down to speak to that elderly patient we visited, or how you spoke to and praised the nurse that was caring for that patient. That's the essence of all this for me, right there, in that moment.

It's the magic part of leadership in nursing that we both get to share. Thanks for bringing me in and I hope our paths cross again.

Sincerely,

Tracie Nolan Kientz

Finding Your NICHE ...

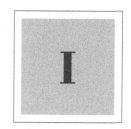

Sample Work Plan

1. Phase I Promotional Activities
   a. Article for staff newsletter
   b. Sample briefing to managers and other key staff
   c. Idea: general posting during week of the nurse

2. Conducting the GIAP
   a. Getting prepared to do the GIAP memo from NYU
   b. Conference call with NYU to discuss sample, distribution, and return

3. Phase II Promotional Activities for the GIAP
   a. Memo to nursing staff—2 weeks before distribution (sample included)
   b. Alert posting—10 days before distribution
   c. Dates and channels (distribution and return) posting—3 days before distribution
   d. Reminder return date and channel posting—5 days after distribution

   Guidelines re: 1 and 2
   - repeat key message(s)
   - common/recognizable format
   - consistency across messages
   - contact person(s)

4. Distribution Channels
   a. Institution order proper number of questionnaires from NYU
   b. NYU to mail proper number of questionnaires to site
   c. In-house distribution per suggestions made during preparation conference call

5. Return Channels
   a. In-house return per suggestions during preparation conference call
   b. Site will pick up after grace period at date TBA
   c. Site will mail completed surveys or data disk to NYU per conference call decisions

6. Help Desk—suggested for staff concerned about completing the GIAP
   a. Site will make arrangements

7. Cover Letter for Survey
   a. Site to draft (see enclosed sample)

8. Dissemination
   a. Presentations (ideas for which to make)
      i. Nursing management group
      ii. Staff development days
      iii. Follow-up for nurses unable to attend staff development days
      iv. Administrative executive committee
      v. Medical executive committee
      vi. Board
   b. Publications (Suggestions)
      i. Institutional reports or flyers
      ii. Mailings to patients or other interested parties

SAMPLE TIME TABLE
V.1—APRIL 23, 1997

Start Date	End Date	Suggested Time Period	Activities
23 April	4 May	2 weeks	Develop work plan Design phase 1 and 2 promotional activities
5 May	18 May	2 weeks	Implement phase 1 promotional activities
19 May	25 May	1 week	Implement phase 2 promotional activities
26 May	6 June	3 weeks	Distribution of surveys with 6/6 return deadline Access to "help desk"
7 June	15 June	1 week	Grace period for survey returns Continued "help desk" access
16 June	6 July	3 weeks	Collection of surveys at institution Shipping of surveys to NYU Data entry
7 July	30 August	6–7 weeks	Statistical analysis, tabulation, and graphics by NYU Outline dissemination activities
1 September			Dissemination activities at site

GRN Rounds

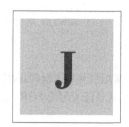

High-Risk Patient	SPICES Assessment	SPICES Plan
GRN of the Day: _____ _____ _____ **GOAL:** Improve quality of life of patient as well as their function; Decrease admission to SNF. Date/Time: _____ Patient Name: _____ MRN: _____ DOA: _____ CC: _____ Dx: _____ **Is this patient at high risk for delirium:** Age > 75 years: _____ Dementia: _____ Surgery < 48 hours: _____ Multiple chronic comorbidities (>10): _____ Hx of delirium: _____ **Living situation:** Home? SNF? ALF? _____ With who? _____ **Prior level of function:** Eating: Walking: Dressing: Bathing: Toileting: Transfer: Mood: Memory: High-risk meds Transition of care/Plan for discharge: _____	**Sleep Problems:** RLS? Y/N Insomnia? Y/N Sleep Apnea? Y/N C-pap? _____ Sleep aids? _____ Routine @ home? Hours of sleep? _____ Nocturia? _____ Sleeping pattern at home _____ Patient's sleep/behavior last night? _____ Poor sleep due to? Pain, agitation, noise, _____ --- **Sensory Aids:** Visual/hearing impairment? **Y/N** ☐ eyeglasses ☐ hearing aids ☐ **pocket talker** Sensory aids used as outpatient? Y/N _____ --- **Pain:** ☐ Chronic pain? _____ ☐ Current pain? _____ ☐ Relieving/worsening factors? _____ PAIN Med _____ DOSE _____ Frequency? _____ Time Last given _____ --- **Problems with eating:** Weight loss? Y/N 3 months _____ 6 months? _____ Albumin: _____ Prealbumin: _____ Dentures? Y/N Diet? _____ Dietitian Consult? Y/N Date: _____ Swallowing issues? Or refusal of meds/food? Y/N --- **Polypharmacy/High-Risk Meds (given while in ED/Unit):** **MEDICATIONS:** More than 5 meds? High-risk medications (e.g., Benadryl, Benzodiazepines, anticholinergic, psychotropic)? _____ Last Administered? _____ **Administration issues?** _____ --- **Incontinence/Constipation:** Foley? Y/N Indication? _____ Removal Date _____ Straight cath? Y/N # of times tried: _____ Condom cath? _____ Toilet rounds done? Y/N Anticholinergic Meds: _____ Last BM _____ Laxatives/Stool Softeners: Y/N --- Confusion: ☐ Dementia ☐ Depression ☐ Delirium High-risk meds used? _____ CAM? _____ --- **Evidence of Falls:** Past 6 months? Y/N PT Consult? Y/N _____ Fall precaution in place? Restraints? _____ Alternatives used? _____ Ambulate 3× _____ OOB with meals _____ --- **Skin:** Braden Score: _____ Wound: _____ Skin Issues/PU:	1. Sleep --- 2. Sensory Aids --- 3. Pain --- 4. Nutrition --- 5. Polypharmacy --- 6. Incontinence Urine/BM and Constipation --- 7. Confusion --- 8. Falls/Function and activity --- 9. Skin

Source: Created by Tmeris, Geriatric CNS/NP-C last updated 10/12/15

KAISER PERMANENTE WOODLAND HILLS—5 SOUTH NKE + (*NURSE KNOWLEDGE EXCHANGE*)/ ACUTE CARE FOR ELDERS (ACE) REPORT FORM

SITUATION Pertinent HX affecting current TX and POC	RM/BED _____ PT NAME _____ AGE/SEX_____ TEAM _____ ADMIT/OBS _____ Isolation(s)_____ CODE: Full/DNR/Modified _____ DX _____ C/O _____ Surgical Date _____ ADV Directive: NO/HC/Paper Chart/Requested from _____ **Evidence of Falls** □ History of Falls w/in last 6 months? □ During this admission? _____ SCHMID Score _____ **Fall Risk w/INJURY: A B C D S** _____ **Current Braden Score** _____ **Precaution: F/Asp/Skin/Sz/Orthos**	
BACKGROUND **Previous shift's issues and concerns** **S** (Summary) PER, orders **M** (eMAR) **I** (I & O) IV, credits, (NGT) **L** (Labs) results, pending **E** (Education/Plan)	□ NKDA Allergies _____ IV/HL ACCESS _____ **Central Lines/PICC** _____ **Insertion Date**_____ **ACCU √ AC and HS/Q4H/Q6H** _____ **Abnormal Labs** _____ **Procedures** □ **Specimens?** _____ □ **MRSA Swab/Screen?** _____	**PAIN** □ Chronic pain? _____ □ Current pain? _____ □ Relieving/worsening factors? _____ **PAIN Med** _____ **Frequency?** _____
ASSESSMENT Abnormal/Changes/V/S I&Os/Mobility/Activity Nutrition/Hydration Elimination **MEDICATION TIMES**	**NEURO**: A and O x _____ Neuro √ Q _____ Deficits _____ **CONFUSION/AGITATION**: ISSUES:_____ Baseline mental status: □ Alert □ Confused □ Lethargic □ Any acute changes? _____ **CAM** □ Negative □ Positive, MD notified? Date_____ Behavior? _____ □ **Fluctuating? Yes/No? Time of Day** ____Restraint Use? Type? _____ Indication? _____Alternatives used? _____ □ Sitter? _____ - **RESP**: □ **Room Air** □ O_2 **via** _____ @ _____L SpO$_2$ _____% □ **On home O_2** _____ □ **HHN Q** _____ **Lung sounds** _____ □ **Cough** _____	
07/19 - 08/20	**CARDIAC**: _____ □ Daily wt. _____ □ Pacemaker_____ □ Edema _____ V/S _____	
09/21 - 10/22 - 11/23 - 12/00 - 13/01	**GI**: BRP/BSC/INC **Last BM** _____ NGT/GT/_____ Diet _____ **NUTRITION: Diet** _____ **Issues:** _____ □ Dentures? _____ □ Swallowing? _____ □ Assist w/meals, set-up/feeding _____ **GU**: BRP/BSC/Urinal/INC/**Toileting Issues?** _____ □ **FOLEY?** (*insertion date*) _____ Indication? _____ □ Straight Cath? _____ Reason? _____ □ Dialysis Access _____ Dialysis Schedule _____	

14/02 ------------------------ 15/03 ------------------------ 16/04 ------------------------ 17/05 ------------------------ 18/06 ------------------------	**SKIN:** □ **INTACT** □ Bruise/Ecchymosis_____ □ Wound(s) _____ □ Pressure Ulcer(s)_____ □ Incision(s) _____ □ Drain(s)_____ □ Dressing(s) _____ □ Other_____ Mattress? Type? _____ **ACTIVITY/MOBILITY/FUNCTION: SCORE _____ PLOF_____** **CLOF_____ ADLs: _____** _____ □ **Ambulatory?** □**Assistive Device? @ home vs. current** _____ □ **Other** _____	
RECOMMENDATION Plan for next shift Discharge POC/education Update Care Boards Teaching	**CONSULTS:** □ PT/OT/SPEECH □ MSW □ CDRP □ Nutrition □ Pharmacy (Coumadin) □ WOCT RN □ **Geri Rounds** □ Geriatrician/CGNS □ Geri-Clinic □ Other _____ **TRANSITION: Current Living Situation?** _____ **Lives with?** _____ **DISCHARGE PLANS?** _____ Core Measures: □ Stroke □ AMI □ CHF □ SCIP □ CAP □ VTE	**SAFETY √/H.E.A.L.** (High-alert med, Equipment, Alarms, Lines)

Source: Created by Anne Loewenthal MSN, RN-BC, CNL 8/29/16, updated.

Fulmer SPICES

An Overall Assessment Tool for Older Adults

By: Terry Fulmer, PhD, RN, FAAN
The John A. Hartford Foundation

WHY: Normal aging brings about inevitable and irreversible changes. These normal aging changes are partially responsible for the increased risk of developing health-related conditions within the older adult population. Prevalent issues experienced by older adults include: sleep disorders, problems with eating or feeding, incontinence, confusion, evidence of falls, and skin breakdown. Familiarity with these commonly occurring issues helps the nurse prevent unnecessary iatrogenesis and promote optimal function of the aging individual. Flagging conditions for further assessment allows the nurse to implement preventative and therapeutic interventions (Fulmer, 1991, 2007).

BEST TOOL: Fulmer SPICES is an efficient and effective instrument for obtaining the information necessary to prevent health alterations in the older adult patient (Fulmer, 1991, 2001). SPICES is an acronym for the common syndromes of the elderly requiring nursing intervention:

S is for Sleep Disorders

P is for Problems with Eating or Feeding

I is for Incontinence

C is for Confusion

E is for Evidence of Falls

S is for Skin Breakdown

TARGET POPULATION: The problems assessed through SPICES occur commonly among the entire older adult population. Therefore, the instrument may be used for both healthy and frail older adults.

Fulmer, T. (2019, updated). *Try This:*® Issue 1: Fulmer SPICES: An overall assessment tool for older adults. *Try This:*® Series: Best practice in nursing care to older adults. Hartford Institute for Geriatric Nursing, NYU Rory Meyers College of Nursing. Retrieved from https://consultgeri.org/try-this/general-assessment/issue-1

VALIDITY AND RELIABILITY: The instrument has been used extensively to assess older adults in the hospital setting, to prevent and detect the most common complications. Full psychometric testing has not been done; however, validation has been conducted (Aronow, Borenstein, Haus, Braunstein, & Bolton, 2014; Fulmer, 2007; Mitty, 2010). Used in the acute care setting within 24 hours of admission, SPICES has been shown to be valid and predictive of adverse events, as well as significantly correlated with age and other validated assessments for vulnerability, comorbidities, and depression (Aronow et al., 2014).

STRENGTHS AND LIMITATIONS: The SPICES acronym is easily remembered and may be used to recall the common problems of the elderly population in all clinical settings. It provides a simple system for flagging areas in need of further assessment and provides a basis for standardizing quality of care around certain parameters. SPICES is an alert system and refers to only the most frequently occurring health issues of older adults. Through this initial screen, more complete assessments are triggered. It should not be used as a replacement for a complete nursing assessment.

MORE ON THE TOPIC:

Best practice information on care of older adults: https://consultgeri.org

Aronow, H. U., Borenstein, J., Haus, F., Braunstein, G. D., & Bolton, L. B. (2014). Validating SPICES as a screening tool for frailty risks among hospitalized older adults. *Nursing Research and Practice, 2014*, 1–5. doi:10.1155/2014/846759

Fulmer, T. (1991). Grow your own experts in hospital elder care. *Geriatric Nursing, 12*, 64–66.

Fulmer, T. (2001). The geriatric resource nurse: A model of caring for older patients. *American Journal of Nursing, 102*, 62.

Fulmer, T. (2007). How to try this: Fulmer SPICES. *American Journal of Nursing, 107*(10), 40–48; quiz 48–49. doi:10.1097/01.NAJ.0000292197.76076.e1

Mitty, E. (2010). Iatrogenesis, frailty, and geriatric syndromes. *Geriatric Nursing, 31*(5), 368–374. doi:10.1016/j.gerinurse.2010.08.004

FULMER SPICES: AN OVERALL ASSESSMENT TOOL FOR OLDER ADULTS

Patient Name: Date:

SPICES	EVIDENCE	
	Yes	No
Sleep Disorders		
Problems with Eating or Feeding		
Incontinence		
Confusion		
Evidence of Falls		
Skin Breakdown		

Source: Adapted from Fulmer, T. (1991). The geriatric nurse specialist role: A new model. *Nursing Management, 22*(3), 91–93.
© Copyright Lippincott Williams & Wilkins, http://lww.com. The Hartford Institute for Geriatric Nursing recognizes Meredith Wallace Kazer, PhD, APRN, A/GNP-BC as one of the original authors of this issue.

Index

Printed in the United States
By Bookmasters